"*Resources are needed if audit is to be successful and worthwhile. The critical resource is an attitude of mind*".

The application of audit to resource allocation and clinical practice has emerged as a fundamental principle in sophisticated medical systems over recent years. The implementation of audit procedures is now an important and necessary part of the clinician's responsibilities. Used effectively, audit can result in wide-ranging benefits for both patients and practitioners, by ensuring the best use of limited resources and continuously evaluating and improving the quality of care. However, the setting up of an efficient and productive audit facility requires careful planning and may encounter resistance.

This book provides a detailed account of audit processes and discusses the application of audit in a variety of medical settings. It describes the factors which should be considered in order to choose the best audit system, gives guidance on the successful implementation of such systems and discusses the advantages which can be obtained from effective audit. Attention is drawn to the place of audit in continuing medical education, in research and in modulating the purchaser–provider relationship in health care. The book contains contributions from clinicians and managers who describe their own experience of medical audit, in the UK as well as in Europe and the United States.

This is both a thoughtful review and a practical guide to successful medical audit and includes advice on the collection and utilisation of information for effective resource management and improved patient care. It gives clear guidance and helpful advice for the clinician and manager on how to create and maintain an effective system for the measurement of medical performance, whether in hospital or in the community.

MEDICAL AUDIT

MEDICAL AUDIT:

Rationale and Practicalities

Edited by
SIMON P. FROSTICK, PHILIP J. RADFORD AND
W. ANGUS WALLACE

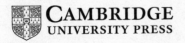
CAMBRIDGE
UNIVERSITY PRESS

Published by the Press Syndicate of the University of Cambridge
The Pitt Building, Trumpington Street, Cambridge CB2 1RP
40 West 20th Street, New York, NY 10011–4211, USA
10 Stamford Road, Oakleigh, Melbourne 3166, Australia

© Cambridge University Press 1993

First published 1993

Printed in Great Britain at the University Press, Cambridge

A catalogue record for this book is available from the British Library

Library of Congress cataloguing in publication data available

ISBN 0 521 44604 X paperback

Contents

List of contributors

James Barrie
British Orthopaedic Association Research Fellow in Orthopaedic Surgery, Department of Orthopaedic Surgery, Clinical Sciences Building, Hope Hospital, Salford, Manchester M6 8HD, UK

Maurice W. Beaver
Managing Director, Information and Computing and Senior Lecturer in Public Health Medicine, University of Nottingham, Nottingham Health Authority, Forest House, Berkeley Avenue, Nottingham NG3 5AF, UK

Julian F. Bion
College and Association of Anaesthetists' Senior Lecturer in Intensive Care Medicine, Birmingham University and Director of Intensive Care, Queen Elizabeth Hospital, Birmingham, University Department of Anaesthesia and Intensive Care, North 5A, Queen Elizabeth Hospital, Birmingham B15 2TH, UK

Ian R. Bowns
Director of Public Health, Department of Public Health Medicine, Barnsley Health Authority, Hillder House, Gawber Road, Barnsley S75 2PY, UK

Jonathan Boyce
Associate Director, Health Studies, The Audit Commission, 1 Vincent Square, London SW1P 2PN, UK

Audrey Bradford
Information Manager, University Hospital, Queen's Medical Centre, Nottingham NG7 2UH, UK

George Brown
15, Barrack Crescent, Attenborough, Nottingham, UK

Christopher J. K. Bulstrode
Clinical Reader in Trauma and Orthopaedic Surgery, University of Oxford, Nuffield Department of Orthopaedic Surgery, Nuffield Orthopaedic Centre, Headington, Oxford OX3 7LD, UK

Andrew Carr
Senior Registrar in Orthopaedic Surgery, Nuffield Orthopaedic Centre, Headington, Oxford OX3 7LD, UK

H. Brendan Devlin
Chairman, Clinical Audit and Quality Assurance Committee, The Royal College of Surgeons of England, 35–43, Lincoln's Inn Fields, London WC2A 3PN, UK

Michael J. Dinsmore
Commercial Manager, University Hospital, Queen's Medical Centre, Nottingham NG7 2UH, UK

Robert B. Duthie
Nuffield Professor of Orthopaedic Surgery, University of Oxford, Nuffield Department of Orthopaedic Surgery, Nuffield Orthopaedic Centre, Headington, Oxford OX3 7LD, UK

Trevor J. Dyson
Director of Business and Strategy, Department of Information and Computing Services, Nottingham Health Authority, Forest House, Berkeley Avenue, Nottingham NG3 5AF, UK

Simon P. Frostick
Senior Lecturer, Department of Orthopaedic and Accident Surgery, University Hospital, Nottingham NG7 2UH, UK

C. S. B. Galasko
Professor of Orthopaedic Surgery, University of Manchester, Department of Orthopaedic Surgery, Clinical Sciences Building, Salford, Manchester M6 8HD, UK

Helen K. Gordon
Consultant Obstetrician and Gynaecologist, Bellshill and Hairmyres Hospitals, Bellshill Maternity Hospital, Bellshill, Lanarkshire, ML4 JN, UK

Robert Gumpert
Consultant General Surgeon, Department of Surgery, Royal Sussex County Hospital, Eastern Road, Brighton, Sussex BN2 5BE, UK

Philip C. Holland
Consultant Paediatrician, Department of Paediatrics, Clarendon Wing, The General Infirmary at Leeds, Leeds LS2 9NS, UK

Robert B. Keller
Executive Director, The Maine Medical Assessment Foundation, PO Box 4682, Augusta, Maine, 04330, USA

Michael B. Lagaay
Consultant Surgeon, Red Cross Hospital, 600 Sportlane, 2566 MJ The Hague, Holland

Duncan A. MacPherson
Senior Medical Officer, Department of Health, Richmond House, 79, Whitehall, London SW1A 2NS, UK

David R. Marsh
Senior Lecturer in Orthopaedic Surgery, University of Manchester, Department of Orthopaedic Surgery, Clinical Sciences Building, Hope Hospital, Salford, Manchester M6 8HD, UK

Naren B. Patel
Consultant Obstetrician and Gynaecologist and Honorary Senior Lecturer, University of Dundee, Department of Obstetrics and Gynaecology, Ninewells Hospital and Medical School, Dundee DD1 9DY, UK

Malcolm Pendlebury
Regional Advisor in Dental Vocational Training, c/o 15, Barrack Crescent, Attenborough, Nottingham, UK

Harry W. Purser
Director of Planning and Contracting, Directorate of Planning and Contracting, Bloomsbury & Islington Health Authority, 100 Hampstead Road, London NW1 2LJ, UK

Paul Pynsent
Nuffield Department of Orthopaedic Surgery, Nuffield Orthopaedic Centre, Headington, Oxford OX3 7LD, UK

Philip J. Radford
Senior Registrar, Department of Orthopaedic and Accident Surgery, University Hospital, Nottingham NG7 2UH, UK

M. D. Rawlins
Wolfson Unit of Clinical Pharmacology, Department of Pharmacological Sciences, The University, Newcastle upon tyne, NE1 7RU, UK

James D. Read
Director, National Health Service Centre for Coding and Classification, Wood Gate, Loughborough, Leicestershire LE11 2TG, UK

David W. Riddington

Clinical Research Fellow, University Department of Anaesthetics and Intensive Care, University of Birmingham, Queen Elizabeth Hospital, Birmingham B15 2TH, UK

Jonathan Secker-Walker

Consultant Anaesthetist and Senior Lecturer in Audit Studies, Department of Medical Audit, University College and Middlesex School of Medicine, 25 Grafton Way, London WC1E 6DB, UK

Charles D. Shaw

Director, Bristol Clinical Audit Unit, University of Bristol, Department of Epidemiology and Community Health Medicine, Canynge Hall, Whiteladies Road, Bristol BS8 2PR, UK

J. M. Smith

Wolfson Unit of Clinical Pharmacology, Department of Pharmacological Sciences, The University, Newcastle upon Tyne, NE1 7RU, UK

Karl-Göran Thorngren

Professor of Orthopaedics, University of Lund, Department of Orthopaedics, Lund University Hospital, S - 22185 Lund, Sweden

W. Angus Wallace

Professor of Orthopaedic and Accident Surgery, Department of Orthopaedic and Accident Surgery, University Hospital, Nottingham NG7 2UH, UK

Manfred J. W. Wildner

Orthopaedic Resident, Freiburg University Hospital, Orthopadische Abteilung Der Universitatskliniken, Hugstetter Str. 55, D-7800 Freiburg, Germany

John Wing

Director of the Research Unit, The Royal College of Psychiatrists, 17 Belgrave Square, London SW1X 8PG, UK

David W. Yates

Professor of Emergency Medicine, University of Manchester, Department of Accident and Emergency Medicine, Hope Hospital, Salford, Manchester M6 8HD, UK

Foreword

I am pleased to have the opportunity of writing the foreword to this book. Improving the quality of patient care is a vital part of the NHS reforms and the improvement of the medical element of that care is central. Medical audit as we know it now has been practised for well over a decade, some would arguably say for centuries, but this book is a timely and helpful addition to the subject.

Medical and patient centred clinical audit have the potential to lead to the delivery of consistently higher standards of care than hitherto. The practice of medical audit should lead to improved outcomes.

There is a systematic specialty account of the current state of progress in the subject. Other chapters deal with experience from abroad. The important issue of information and medical audit is covered from several angles and the organisational aspects which will be increasingly important are also included. In short, there is something in this book for everybody involved in delivering health care.

Professor Kenneth Calman
Chief Medical Officer of Health
Department of Health

Foreword

By the breadth of their intention, the Editors of this book set themselves an ambitious task. Their declared purpose was to establish the philosophy of audit in medical practice; to examine the sort of information needed by the different groups interested in audit; to describe how audit is currently practised in certain specialties; and to suggest a coherent pattern for audit and make recommendations for the acquisition and storage of large volumes of information. To this end, they recruited a wide panel of experts who have contributed to their theme. The end result is both timely and impressive and one which should provide a useful source of reference for clinicians, health economists, systems analysts and managers.

Each of these has a legitimate interest in and involvement with audit. The first step in the classical 'audit cycle' is that of observation and documentation. This helps to define a range of practice in whatever is being observed and hence to allow identification of substandard practice. Explicit recommendations for changes in process and practice are then made, so that performance is improved. After a period of time, this is followed by re-examination to ensure that standards set have been achieved and progress maintained.

The common bond uniting the four groups described above is the capacity of audit to enhance the quality of medical practice. Clinicians are also very conscious of the educational potential of audit and would argue that confidentiality of audit meetings is essential if failures are to be examined with frankness and examples of substandard practice corrected.

One of the most challenging aspects of audit is the development of appropriate outcome measures against which performance can be assessed, and it is here that both health economists and systems analysts can have useful roles to play. Finally, the NHS and Community Care Act (1990) put quality very firmly on the agenda for the reformed health service and increasingly we can expect to see quality specifications built into contracts between purchasers and providers. Managers, therefore, will need to have access to anonymised results of audit carried out in their hospitals and to be satisfied that these, in turn, compare well with national standards.

Audit becomes very much 'a state of mind' for those who participate in it. The process of measurement itself often seems to improve performance and the continual search for improvements in procedure and outcome adds to the culture of the organisation. Furthermore, the generation of best practice guidelines can be a natural sequel to the audit of a particular clinical problem.

I believe that during the last few years the medical profession has done much to embrace audit as part of its regular responsibilities. Much, however, remains to be done – not least the challenge of how to help those clinicians who have been identified by audit as performing less well than their colleagues. I have no doubt that this book will provide a useful contribution to the continuing debate and congratulate the editors for this.

Sir Terence English
Past President
The Royal College of Surgeons of England

1

Introduction

SIMON P. FROSTICK, PHILIP J. RADFORD AND
W. ANGUS WALLACE

The audit of medical practice is neither a new concept nor a new activity.
All medical practitioners have examined the effects of their treatment and
have assessed outcome for centuries. The major advances in medical
practice, particularly during the twentieth century, would not have
occurred without observing and assessing the effects of treatment regimes.
The main effect of the changes indicated in the HM Government White
Paper 'Working for Patients' and subsequently the National Health
Service and Community Care Act (1990) and the directives from the
various Royal Colleges has been to emphasise the need for audit activity
and to introduce a more formal basis to audit. Audit has also been linked
to the need for the cost-effective use of resources.

The purposes of this book are firstly to describe the philosophy of audit
in medical practice; secondly to establish the types of information required
by the different groups interested in audit; thirdly to outline the ways in
which audit activity is being undertaken in various specialties; and fourthly
to suggest a coherent pattern for audit and make recommendations for the
acquisition and storage of large volumes of information.

Definitions

The general public concept of audit is the annual review of the 'books' of
a business. This is a retrospective analysis of the debit and credit of a
business. This analysis, however, has the prospective effect of allowing a
financial plan to be formulated for the next year. This is a positive feedback
loop. The profits and deficits of one year will have a direct effect on the
developments of the next year, and in turn on the profits and deficits of the
following year.

Audit in medical practice should be viewed in a similar fashion, as a

1

positive feedback loop. The specific methodology is irrelevant, but unless change follows review, then audit of medical practice will have no effect whatsoever and is a waste of time.

There is a great deal of confusion at present over the definitions that are used in relation to the audit of medical activity. The various authors in this book use the following definitions for medical and clinical audit:

1. Medical audit is defined as the review of the clinical care of patients provided by the medical staff only.
2. Clinical audit is the review of the activity of all aspects of the clinical care of patients by medical and paramedical staff.

A third definition is required, as the above two ignore the effects of resources on the review process. It is the view of the editors that it is impossible to separate clinical practice from resource management and so audit by the medical profession must take into account the effects of resource changes on their clinical practice. A third definition of audit is therefore suggested, called 'patient care audit', and this is defined as the review of all activity within the health service that has a direct effect on patient care. Many clinicians object to, and are frightened by, the resource management aspects of modern day health care. However, any change in clinical practice will have effects on resources and any change in resources will have an effect on clinical practice, and so the two cannot be regarded as separate entities. It is still possible to review clinical treatment separately from resource management in order to improve the day-to-day care of patients, but it must be continually borne in mind that clinicians are expected to provide an efficient and cost-effective service.

Audit versus clinical research

There is a great deal of controversy at present as to what constitutes audit and what constitutes clinical research. We would suggest that clinical research is undertaken when a prospective *controlled* clinical trial is instituted. Clinical trials should, like all forms of scientific research, be based upon an hypothesis and will be subject to statistical analysis. Audit of clinical care is the assessment of the quality of care provided for an individual or group of patients. The audit is undertaken retrospectively (on, hopefully, prospectively acquired patient data) and will examine the usual form of treatment that a particular clinician provides. In order for this to be meaningful it will be necessary for there to be a standard against which to compare; for example, comparing the length of stay following a hernia repair between two general surgical units or the rate of dislocation after total hip replacement. The value of audit data improves if the collection is systematic and the data are validated.

There will always be a grey area where clinical research and audit do and should overlap but in terms of the day-to-day review of patients the two must not be confused.

A basic concept

A recurring theme throughout this book will be the concept of *structure–process–output (outcome)*. The term '*structure*' refers to the provision of staff hospital facilities, equipment, etc; '*process*' refers to the activity of providing medical care for patients; '*output (outcome)*' refers to the effect of the process on the community as a whole and on individual patients. The closing part of the loop is that measuring outcome must result in a change in process, and this will also have an effect on structure.

Outcome

An intrinsic part of audit in medical practice is the ability to measure outcome. This is a very thorny question and will be covered in many chapters in this book. If we consider outcome as scientists requiring objective, even quantitative, measurement of our activity, then it becomes extremely difficult to define outcome measures. In the area of orthopaedic surgery, the only obvious remotely objective outcome measures are death rates, revision rates for major joint replacement surgery and possibly the rate of non-union of fractures. If we wish to measure outcomes such as the rate of deep venous thrombosis or the rate of wound infection, for example, we have major problems. The problems are one of definition and another of accurately diagnosing these conditions. Measures of outcome in these areas, therefore, become significantly subjective. Further, if we consider patient satisfaction and quality of care then the outcome measures become wholly subjective. However, we cannot entirely base our measurement of outcome on scientific methodology. We are expected to maintain an acceptable standard of medical care which requires us to achieve an 'excellent' or 'good' result with the minimum of complications for each individual patient. We must therefore accept a degree of subjectivity in assessing outcome and accept that we cannot apply statistical methods with any degree of accuracy in order to compare one unit's outcome with another.

Guidelines

Two important statements are made in the White Paper '*Working for Patients*'. Both statements appear in the introduction in the White Paper and are called 'key changes'. The first key change is defined as 'to make the Health Service more responsive to the needs of patients, as much power and responsibility as possible will be delegated to the local level'. The second definition of importance to this book is the seventh key change, 'to ensure that all concerned with delivering services to the patient make the best use of the resources available to them, quality of service and value for money will be rigorously audited'. The guidelines in the White Paper for medical audit are fairly clear cut. These guidelines, together with the recommendations from the various Royal Colleges and the King's Fund should be used as the basis for the clinical and medical aspects of audit. However, the guidelines are certainly not rigorous, and it is up to the individual specialties, and also to some extent the local audit committees, to define how audit will be undertaken. It would seem that the central bodies have purposely allowed the local medical audit committees to define the medical audit activity and have not imposed rigorous requirements. The development of audit is an evolutionary process. Structured audit has no experts at present and it is the role of the interested clinician to define the guidelines for the day-to-day running of medical audit. It is not the intention of this book to impose our view as to how audit should be undertaken, but to provide the essential information that is required so that individual units can decide how best to undertake this activity.

The unenthusiastic clinician

Only a small number of clinicians are real enthusiasts for clinical audit. The majority of consultants see audit simply as another activity, which will only have the effect of taking them away from their clinical activities. Further, some clinicians at senior and junior level will be frightened at the prospect of having their clinical activity examined by another clinician. The answer to the first problem is for the enthusiasts to demonstrate that the review of clinical activity can actually make the provision of services more efficient and more effective for the patients. In order to ensure that fear of criticism or embarrassment is eliminated it is essential that confidentiality is maintained but that defects of practice become apparent to the individual concerned so that they can effect change.

2

Audit: historical and future perspectives

ROBERT B. DUTHIE

Historical aspects

'*Audit* can be defined as a hearing; especially a judicial hearing of complaints or a judicial examination or an official examination of accounts with verification by reference to witnesses and vouchers, or a judgement upon any matter, a critical evaluation. An *auditor* is one who learns by aural instruction, one who listens judicially and tries cases as in the Audience Court of 1640. However, *quality Assurance* is the quality of a person or of a character, deposition, nature, capacity and ability of skills and things; an attribute property which specifically features the degree or grade of excellence possessed by a thing. *Assurance* is a promise making a thing certain, with the intention of insuring and securing the value of things' (from *The Shorter Oxford English Dictionary on Historical Principles*, 1980).

Historically, audit has been carried out for many centuries, beginning with the development of national statistics of births and deaths in the Domesday Book of 1066, the Parish Registers of 1597, the Population Act of 1840 and the first National Population Census in 1801. To improve upon earlier attempts required the development of statistics as a science, beginning with the formation of the Statistical Society of London in 1833. This history has been recently reviewed extensively by Pollock and Evans.[1] These authors also give credit to Joseph Lister for introducing the concept of clinical audit by his analysis of the therapeutic effects of phenol in compound fractures in his paper published in the *British Medical Journal* in 1867. Burdett[2] presented a paper in 1882 to the Statistical Society, in which he analysed the results of the Listerian system from over 60 hospitals throughout the country and compared their results of amputation for injury and disease with those in the several surgical meccas of the world.

5

Ernest Hey Groves[3] gave a paper to the BMA pointing out how most surgical papers, because of poor statistics, were very inadequate by only representing the 'best and not the average results'. He proposed a national organisation to collect records in an uniform way and approached 15 large hospitals to discover operating mortalities for certain acceptable operations. This resulted in very little interest and certainly no support for such an epoch making concept. Joseph Bell,[4] the prototype of Conan Doyle's Sherlock Holmes, another brilliant thinker and teacher of general surgery in Edinburgh began, in 1887, to analyse and publish statistical results on the treatment of injuries and tuberculosis in children.

Surgeons then became more aware of the importance of mortality and morbidity conferences as part of their teaching and learning programmes. Sir James Learmonth[5] of Edinburgh began, in 1946, a monthly conference in which each surgical firm in turn presented their careful analysis of not only deaths and complications, but also of outcome. Thus began the breakdown of the rigidity and the autocracy of the surgical firm system by exposing its results to a general discussion by colleagues. This was the beginning of peer review. It is of interest that 43 years later the Royal College of Surgeons of England[6] issued guidelines on clinical audit and surgical practice. The college has defined audit as a 'systematic appraisal of the implementation and outcome of any process in the context of prescribed targets and standards. Clinical audit is a process by which medical staff collectively review, evaluate and improve their practice.' The college pointed out that deaths and complications traditionally have been considered, but the quality of life after surgery and the degree of patient satisfaction should also be assessed as far as possible.

The Royal Colleges of Surgeons and of Anaesthetists have sponsored the *National and Confidential Enquiry into Perioperative Deaths* (NCEPOD) in order to improve standards of surgical practice.[7] As a result of this they have set up a hospital recognition committee, which will now be responsible for arranging a routine quinquennial inspection. From January 1990 the committee will initiate a routine scrutiny of hospital records and audit records to ensure optimum standards of surgical care.

The Government has become very interested and concerned about medical audit and issued a Department of Health circular in January 1991[8] with a definition of medical audit as being:

The systematic, critical analysis of the quality of medical care, including the procedures used for diagnosis and treatment, the use of resources and the resulting outcomes in quality of life for the patient.

This has been built into the new reorganisation of the National Health Service, where responsibility has been given to the deans and directors of postgraduate medical education in the various regions. Equally important are the funds now specifically allocated to the regions for the development of medical audit.

Ralph Johnson,[9] in a paper on 'the purpose and conduct of medical audit – an educational perspective', defined medical audit as 'a means of quality control for medical practice by which the profession shall regulate its activities with the intention of improving overall patient care'. Ahmed[10] emphasised for the first time that quality assurance depended upon patients' satisfaction as well as the doctors'.

Briefly, audit can be considered under three main headings:

1. *Structure*, which equates to resources found within the hospital. This means not only beds, but operating rooms, equipment, technology, staffing, investigations and administration of these resources.
2. *Process*, which equates to efficiency and the function of the staff, both by assessment of diagnosis and the treatment of patients and the utilisation of resources required for such a function.
3. *Outcome*, which concerns the patient, not only the patient's outcome from surgery, but also the surgeon's expectation, the patient's expectation, the community's expectation through community health councils and any legal means. Outcome is when quality of care becomes pre-eminent. However, outcome does vitally involve the patient's motivation, personality, determination, education and beliefs; how they can express outcome and how they see it. These attributes although very important, are equally very difficult to assess and to be given appropriate weight.

A model of structure and process

Orthopaedics in the UK was in the vanguard of surgical specialties in determining *structure* and *process*. In 1981 a working party was set up by the Secretary of State for Social Services to examine *Orthopaedic Services: Waiting Time for Outpatient Appointments and Inpatient Treatment*.[11] Its brief was to consider the organisation of orthopaedic services, its interreactions and related services and to recommend measures to eliminate excessive waiting times for out-patient appointments and in-patient treatment. Through the SBH#203 in-patient waiting list, numbers of all surgical specialties were obtained for a three year period, together with details of urgency on waiting lists. Orthopaedic surgery was analysed for

Table 2.1 *Waiting times in weeks for out-patient appointments:*
orthopaedic surgery: South East Thames Region: 1979

District	Hospital	Waiting time (weeks)	District	Hospital	Waiting time (weeks)
A	1	6–10	F	18	9–13
	2	6		19	22
	3	7		20	15
B	4	16	G	21	8–35
	5	8–12		22	2–3
C	6	14–24	H	23	18
	7	4		24	17
	8	2		25	5
				26	8
D	9	1		27	16
	10	8		28	1
	11	4–19			
	12	5	J	29	4–13
				30	3–4
E	13	3–22			
	14	22	K	31	6
	15	8		32	4
	16	12		33	16
	17	11		34	6–7
				35	8

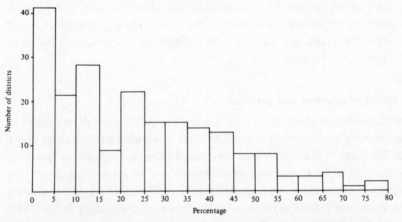

Fig. 2.1. Percentage of orthopaedic surgery non-urgent cases waiting over one year,
analysed for districts in England, 1977. (By permission; source SBH 203.)

Table 2.2 *Number of consultants in orthopaedic surgery and in anaesthetics: whole-time equivalents: England and Wales: 1973, 1976 and 1978*

	All surgical specialties	Orthopaedic surgery	Anaesthetics
1973	2875	507	1255
1976	3131	547	1394
1978	3243	577	1448
% change 1973–1978	+13%	+14%	+15%

Source: Manpower returns

Table 2.3 *All NHS hospitals: orthopaedic surgery. Bed availability and usage: England and Wales, 1969–1978*

	1969	1973	1978
Average available beds (daily)	19400	21637	22312
Beds per 1000 population	0.40	0.44	0.45
Discharges and deaths	386531	423193	472484
Discharges and deaths per available bed	19.9	19.6	21.2
Discharges and deaths per 1000 population	7.92	8.61	9.62
Average duration of stay in days	16	14.7	13.7
Waiting list	67176	79374	129073

Source: SH3

the 12 English regions for the non-urgent cases on the waiting list and the percentage of non-urgent cases waiting more than a year (Figure 2.1). This was examined further by looking at how long it was before the patients were being seen as out-patients in each district and hospital, particularly involving the South-East Thames Region (Table 2.1). Such information was important in order to delineate why there were lengthening queues for orthopaedic services. These had resulted from the growing imbalance between the demands on the service and its capacity to meet them, particularly when one considered the average number of beds available for all surgical specialties, and the number of staff, e.g. surgeons and anaesthetists, available (Table 2.2). Because of the changes in population structure, the development and use of new procedures, such as total joint replacements, spinal surgery and micro-surgery, and the survival of the

Table 2.4 *Inter-regional comparison of resource levels and resource utilisation in orthopaedic surgery: England and Wales: 1972*

Region	Average no. beds per million managed population	No. consultants per million managed population (whole time equivalents)	Discharges and deaths per available bed (throughput)	Number on waiting list per million population	Median waiting time in weeks
Northern	481	13.2	18.2	1746	11.5
Yorkshire	494	13.4	21.1	1578	10.2
Trent	375	9.1	21.2	2686	13.5
East Anglia	363	12.0	22.8	2272	11.9
N.W. Thames	393	10.5	23.8	1983	12.3
N.E. Thames	434	12.8	18.7	1862	9.5
S.E. Thames	456	10.3	22.1	2525	12.7
S.W. Thames	444	10.2	22.3	1794	8.8
Wessex	424	11.6	25.8	2321	12.6
Oxford	435	9.6	28.8	2720	11.7
S. Western	425	10.1	21.7	2195	10.6
W. Midlands	455	11.0	22.3	2477	12.2
Mersey	525	10.7	16.0	2222	9.3
N. Western	469	12.6	20.0	2531	12.3
Wales	521	10.7	21.1	2097	9.6
England[1]	450	11.4	21.4	2247	11.4
England and Wales[1]	454	11.4	21.4	2238	11.3

[1]Including Boards of Governors.
Source: SH3, Manpower Returns, HIPE.

elderly population, including after major injury, greater numbers of patients were requiring treatment. Bed availability and usage were clearly stated and the mean duration of stay by age-groups, discharge by deaths and ordinary discharge were studied (Table 2.3). Inter-regional comparison of resource levels and resource utilisation in orthopaedic services (Table 2.4) was obvious. This was related to the throughput, i.e. discharges and deaths per available bed, for each district in two regions (Figure 2.2). Further breakdown took place by analysing district performance against demand in certain units by observing length of stay and turnover intervals (Figure 2.3). From this it was possible to work out staffing and bed requirements for units (i.e. structure). General conclusions were drawn from such statistical audits and it emerged that the most damaging factors were always strike action and changes in work practice. Such activities always resulted in an increase in the waiting list and waiting times for all. Indeed they were always more important than the loss of operating sessions by the compulsory bank and statutory holidays, anaesthetist shortages, etc.

From such work the inadequacy of good hospital data became more and more evident. The Murrison Report of 1979 from the Royal Commission

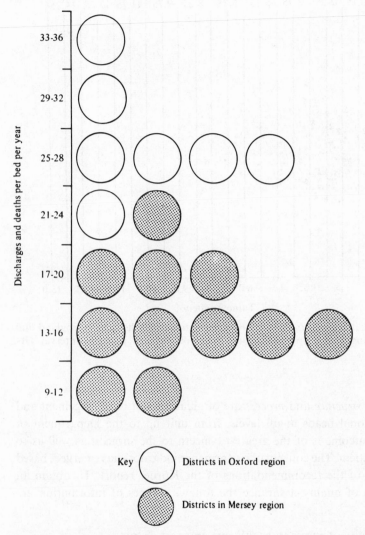

Fig. 2.2. Throughput (deaths and discharges per available bed) for each district in two regions, 1977. (By permission; source SH3.)

on the National Health Service also pointed out how it lacked relative information, especially when it depended upon the hospital activity analysis figures (HAA). In 1980 Mrs Edith Körner set up and chaired a very important *Steering Group on Health Services Information*. Its main concern was to obtain information for health services management, rather than for the work of the professional staff or for any analysis of outcome down to the individual patient level.

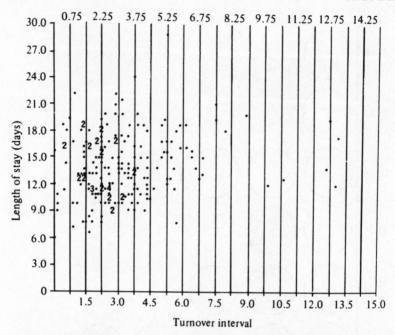

Fig. 2.3. Scattergram to show local performance of all districts in England and Wales against two simple indicators, length of stay and turnover interval. (By permission.)

Outcome

Although *structure* and *process* are of great interest to management and organisational heads at all levels, from unit up to the Department of Health, outcome is of the greatest concern to the surgeon as well as to his/her patient. The concept of performance indicators has emerged, based upon one of the recommendations of the Körner report. To obtain an indication of quality assurance the following types of information are required:

1. the quality of access to health care amongst districts,
2. the number of actual operations of a specific nature carried out, and
3. the various hospital activity analyses such as expected length of stay, throughput, operating theatre usages and avoidable deaths.

However, assessment of outcome is very difficult. It depends upon measuring professional competence based upon knowledge of audit. It requires study of individuals over significant lengths of time and of obtaining sufficient numbers for statistical analysis but, more importantly, having the experience and methods to carry out such studies accurately and promptly. The significant period of time for reporting back on the results of audit should not be too long otherwise the learning momentum has gone out of the exercise. Important features to be part of any audit are mortality rates versus the degree of pathology; the difficulty in achieving numbers; any associated morbidities; the validity and power of the statistical analysis required; and the psycho-social mixes and motivations of the patients, as well as of the nursing and doctoring staff. Grimley Evans,[12] in an analysis of outcome following treatment of patients with fractured neck of femur in two hospitals, has demonstrated that survival and discharge depend upon the number of nurses caring for these patients and the patients' psycho-social category. Death alone is not a good performance indicator, unless one includes classifications of what is termed *quorum* morbidity and the use of scoring techniques. Surgical skills and their exploitation and the one who carries them out also strongly determine outcome as do lengths of postoperative stay. The appropriate operation, the knowledge, experience and the caring attitudes of the surgeon, the degree of supervision and fitness for particular operative procedures are of the utmost importance. This has recently been highlighted by the NCEPOD report, which was a national audit of surgical deaths in Britain.[13] Their results and conclusions dealt with such things as the storage, movement and retrieval of patient notes, particularly of deceased patients, and the failure to carry out regular audits and to determine outcomes. Shaw[14] has written on clinical outcome indicators, and pointed out that the determination of such indications is limited by lack of agreement on standards or on the objectives to be achieved, especially when one measures such secondary outcomes as complications. He emphasises that measures of outcome should relate to success or avoidance of failure. Risk factors should be determined and balanced within homogeneous cohorts of patients with a 'tracer' condition. Tracers can indicate process and outcome. He defines an ideal tracer condition as having high incidence/prevalence, early and definitive diagnosis, limited co-morbidity and adequate indicators.

Medical audit is a strong educational tool for doctors to educate themselves about their clinical practice and to compare it with others. However, for this to be functional and ongoing it must be prospective as well as retrospective and the immediacy of the availability of data and analysis is paramount. This will become a very significant feature in the British system of higher surgical training because of the rapid changeover of the junior house staff (registrars every six months, etc.). It requires a peer review understanding of surgical techniques and their outcome and this necessitates careful consultation, and agreement on the measurement of outcome and the subsequent commitment. Most surgeons are determined to improve quality of care, but some may well feel threatened by the actual technique required to achieve this.

Donabedian,[15] has thrown a new light into distinguishing between 'research' of various technologies and 'audit' which he defines as quality assessment. Research into techniques determines the relationship between outcome and structure or process, whereas audit uses outcome as indirect evidence as to whether structure and process are being provided appropriately or not. He simplifies it by stating that research is the performance of instruments, whereas audit is the performance by practitioners and systems. He believes that studying the methods of research should be by mathematical and statistical modelling and epidemiological studies and controlled trials, whereas in studying audit simple yes/no measures using consensus and reliable indicators are often the most helpful. The Wessex *Guide to Medical Audit*[16] has defined audit as being 'an evaluation of the quality of patient care based upon explicit and measurable indicators of quality'. This guide describes the 'observance' of the 'practitioner and performance systems'. Roberts and Prevost[17] describe how to determine outcome indicators in order to evaluate quality of care by considering the patient, the degree of symptom relief, the level of function and improvement, and the responsiveness to care. The degree to which care meets the professional standards and current technical state of the art, and the degree of freedom to act in the full interest of the patients, are the indicators of prime importance. The purchaser is examined for how efficiently they use available funds for care; the appropriateness of the use of resources for health care is examined, as is the extent of the contribution of health care to reducing the loss of the patients' contribution to society.

Dixon (1989)[16] pointed out the strategies for measuring audit by observing practice and establishing measurements of patient care – patient records, diagnosis and surgical procedures, intervention, specialty, looking for positives and negatives of outcome. She emphasised that these can be found from a case notes review, an education review, a numerical review or an epidemiological review. She warned that formal medical audit should *not* be considered medical research, a cost-benefit analysis requiring a database, or staff or computers, but should be based upon peer review.

The future

In the future, audit systems will have to be based upon an integrated hospital information system with a central database with all hospital staff and facilities involved. It will be based upon interface schemes, rather than isolated medical audit systems, and probably will only be found in those hospitals with adequate computer resource management and hospital information systems. In brief, medical audit developments will involve individual requirements, statistical analysis, wordprocessing, a database, a standard coding classification, the ability to recode out-patient/in-patient data and adverse events, and an adequate and sensible classification of diseases and disorders.

Much of the input and impact of computers has been in storing personal records of diagnosis, some statistical analysis and some retrieval. Statistical packages are being developed but there are still difficulties and problems to be solved, such as vertical integration of computer records within hospitals. Gough and colleagues[18] introduced a system called the 'Oxford Surgical Department System C4 Limited', which allows medical secretaries to enter their data from the patient's case notes during their normal work routine. As well as surgical audits there is a pharmacy module in the USA called MEDITAKE, which is comprehensive for in-hospital patient care and for financial management requirements. It is a realtime inter-reactive computer audit system for processing orders, checking drug interactions, maintaining inventory levels, etc. With this system patients' demographic data is available on-line to give accurate analysis, and most importantly, knowledge of the 'medicine trail' throughout the hospital from receiving the drug in the hospital to the patient's use of it.

Another American system, about which the author is concerned, is the CareSys Company system based upon the so-called '*rivers of care*' exception base philosophy. At present in the USA it is only being applied to workmen's compensation injuries. The main advantage of this expert system approach is in computerising patients' standard of care for analysis, where it maintains flexibility by having a specific rule base that is established by a physician review panel. If the patient with his diagnosis and reasonable investigations and treatment falls outside acceptable standards, a 'red flag' brings in the expert specialist. The hardware for the system consists of enhanced Apple MacIntosh 2CX work stations. An expert system case analysis is implemented by a common LISP/OPS5 industrial standard artificial intelligence platform. The medical expert system has been developed by involving multi-disciplinary specialists such as orthopaedists, neurosurgeons and neurologists to develop the rule base, which has been focused on musculo-skeletal injuries and programmed in OPS5. This system is now being developed for use in the orthopaedic field. Although the system is only functioning in the United States it signals the way forward, especially if it can be utilised not only for musculo-skeletal injuries, but for designated orthopaedic conditions, such as arthritis, congenital malformations, etc. It will be particularly valuable in continuing educational programmes both for postgraduates and their teachers.

Orthopaedic surgeons must improve patient care and the quality assurance of what they do, rather than going down the American road of improvement by peer review under American Medical Association (AMA) regulations or by litigation or by the economic control of practice. Economic determination through the diagnostic related group systems is being attempted by classifying patients according to the severity of their pathology.[19] It was set up to control the costs of many classes of disease and injury using length of hospital stay and various diagnostic categories. Probably politicians and management would prefer to take *this* particular road, but we in the profession must be concerned with outcome and hence quality of care. The profession can no longer hold privileges against both public and patient criticism without demonstrating clearly that we have the capacity to be critical of our practice, of our teaching and of the prevention of errors or inadequacies in our performance.

References

1. Pollock, A. & Evans, M. (1989). *Surgical Audit*. London: Butterworths.
2. Burdett, H. C. (1882). The relative mortality, after amputations, of large and small hospitals and the influence of the antiseptic (listerian) system upon mortality. *Journal of the Statistical Society*, **45**, 444–483.
3. Hey Groves, E. W. (1908). Surgical statistics: a plea for a uniform registration of operation results. *British Medical Journal*, **2**, 1008–1009.
4. Roberts, F. H. (1969). Joseph Bell – The origins of paediatric surgery in Edinburgh. *Journal of the Royal College of Surgeons of Edinburgh*, **14**, 304–307.
5. Sir James Learmonth (1946). Personal communication.
6. Guidelines to Clinical Audit in Surgical Practice (1989). The Royal College of Surgeons of England.
7. Buck, N., Devlin, H. B. & Lunn, J. N. (1987). *The Report of a Confidential Enquiry into Perioperative Deaths*, Nuffield Provincial Hospitals Trust, London. The Royal College of Surgeons of England and The College of Anaesthetists.
8. *Medical Audit in the Hospital and Community Health Services* (1991). Department of Health Circular.
9. Johnson, R. (1991). *The Purpose and Conduct of Medical Audit – an educational perspective*. Director of Postgraduate Medical Education and Training, Oxford University and Region.

10. Ahmed, A. (1981). *Review and Practice in Medical Care – Steps for Quality Assurance.* London: George McLaughlan, Nuffield Press Hospital Trust.
11. *Orthopaedic Services: Waiting time for outpatient appointments and inpatient treatment* (1981). Report of Working Party to the Secretary of State for Social Services. DHSS. Her Majesty's Stationery Office (Chairman Professor R. B. Duthie).
12. Grimley Evans, J. (1984). Fractured proximal femur in Newcastle upon Tyne. *Age and Aging,* **6**, 16–24.
13. Association of Surgeons and the Association of Anaesthetists of Great Britain and Ireland (1990). *National Confidential Enquiry into Perioperative Deaths.*
14. Shaw, C. D. (1989). Clinical outcome indicators. *Health Trends,* **21**, 37–40.
15. Donabedian, A. (1988). The assessment of technology and quality. A comparative study of certainties and ambiguities. *International Journal of Technology Assessment in Health Care,* **4**, 487–496.
16. Dixon, N. (1989). *Guide to Medical Audit* (2nd edn). *The Quest for Healthcare (UK) Limited.*
17. Roberts, J. S. & Prevost, J. A. (1987). Using outcome indicators to evaluate quality of care. The interest in health policy in practice. *American Society of Internal Medicine.*
18. Gough, M. H., Kettlewell, M. G. W., Marks, C. O., Holmes, S. J. K. & Holderness, J. (1980). Audit: an annual assessment of the work and performance of a surgical firm in a regional teaching hospital. *British Medical Journal,* **281**, 913–920.
19. Fetter, R. B. (1987). Introduction: In *DRGs and Health Care. The Management of CareSys.* ed. M. Bardsley, J. Cole & L. Jenkins, pp. 5–10. London: King Edward's Hospital Fund.

3

Audit philosophy

CHARLES D. SHAW

Introduction

There is now general agreement among the medical profession, health care managers, the public and the Government that the measurement by doctors of medical performance is an essential element of service. A growing requirement by the Royal Colleges for more formal audit in the middle 1980s was accelerated by publication of the *Confidential Enquiry into Perioperative Deaths* (CEPOD) in 1987[1] and the Government White Paper in 1989[2]. The CEPOD report made very clear and public a number of areas in which clinical work (and patients) would benefit from more rigorous scrutiny. The White Paper required formal audit to be established in hospitals in the NHS by April 1991. There remain concerns that the general principles of audit are agreed but the details of implementation may differ in the eyes of managers and clinicians. It is therefore worth emphasising the stated view of the English Royal Colleges of Physicians and of Surgeons that the purpose of audit is primarily the quality of medical care, second, standards of medical training and education and third, the effective use of resources. Although the use of resources is primarily a management concern, it is notable that it was expressly included as a subsidiary goal by these two colleges.

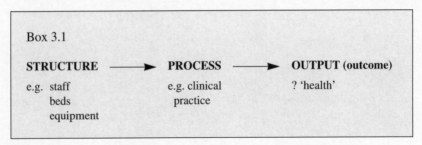

Box 3.1

STRUCTURE ⟶ PROCESS ⟶ OUTPUT (outcome)

e.g. staff   e.g. clinical   ? 'health'
     beds   practice
     equipment

Principles of measurement

Traditionally, health services have been measured in terms of the input or the resources they use (Box 3.1). The impact of the service on the population or the individual was an implicit assumption not only because such outcomes were hard to measure, but also because the resources used were more readily enumerated and had the most immediate political impact. The growing interest in clinical outcomes is seeking to differentiate between '*output*' in terms of volume of throughput as opposed to benefits in terms of health care ('*outcome*'). But since, in many clinical circumstances, the final outcomes are either hard to define or take many years to become apparent there is a legitimate case for examining instead the *process* of medical care that is provided to individual cases, assuming there is sound evidence to associate that process with the required outcomes. Process audit is commonly criticised on the grounds that in many areas of common clinical practice there is no research-based evidence of appropriateness; on the other hand, there is also evidence that what has been established to be sound clinical practice is not universally put into effect. It may also be a service to the development of medical research to identify priorities among the commonplace and significant issues rather than the esoteric fields of endeavour.

Whichever of these points ('*structure*', process or outcome) is used for measurement, any evaluation must imply an explicit statement of what is the expected standard against which any service will be measured. In reality, the expectations of the public, the managers or even the clinicians are frequently not agreed or made sufficiently clear to provide a basis for such measurement either at individual or at population level. One interesting by-product of the introduction of service contracts is a need to clarify explicitly what are the objectives of the service and the criteria by which their achievement will be measured. The second challenge in the measurement of performance is how to quantify current practice against the agreed standards and it is at this stage that data systems may provide a generous contribution. The least information that clinicians require for internal audit is the means to identify patients who have in common either procedures, diagnoses, or complications that may be the subject of detailed review in audit. The capacity of many British hospitals to produce accurately even this limited information is unfortunately rare. The third element and challenge of audit is to make the appropriate response in terms of changing clinical or managerial practice in order to improve the quality of care. Unless participants are willing and able to make this change there is little point of embarking on audit; it is this behavioural issue which far outweighs the technical problems of computers and data in the introduction of medical audit.

Characteristics of effective audit

Research and practical experience suggest that clinical practice is not easily influenced by published information alone. It appears that, to effect change, audit must have a number of key characteristics including:

1. Explicit criteria for good clinical practice: This does not require prescriptive protocols that do not allow for clinical variation but does imply general policies based on proven experience and published literature.
2. Objective measurement of patterns of current practice: This involves the analysis of representative samples rather than individual case presentations and demands substantial resources in terms of data and time.
3. Comparison of results among peers: Analysis of individual performance is a more cogent agent of change than individual results aggregated by hospital or district, but it is these results that are most sensitive and should remain confidential until the participating clinicians are satisfied that they are sufficiently accurate and representative for any further dissemination.
4. Explicit identification of corrective action: Conclusion of audit discussions must be translated into explicit policies and revised targets for future audit.
5. Documentation of procedure and results: A basic record should be maintained for the purpose of identifying the existence of audit both for the purposes of accreditation by the Royal College of Surgeons, and for advising managers and clinical colleagues of progress and implications for other departments. This record should include participants, general topics discussed, general conclusions reached, action to be taken and when the audit will be repeated.

Organisation of audit

The introduction of effective audit in any specialty will have ramifications for other specialties and other groups of staff, both managerial and clinical. It is therefore essential that the medical staff as a whole accept formal responsibility for overseeing the process of audit and ensuring that its conclusions are put into practice. For most purposes, at least three consultant firms would be necessary to form a critical mass; smaller and more isolated units may therefore have to form larger groups, which may require further resources for organisation and travel. The audit group must, therefore, have clear links not only with the local medical audit committee, but also with the relevant regional specialty committee whose contribution may include the sharing of methods and results of audit and the definition of common criteria for data capture.[3] Links at local level will depend on the subject under discussion but should include any relevant specialty, for example, audit in the surgical specialties should be linked to audit by the anaesthetists.

Methods

Examination and discussion of individual cases, although less effective, may provide a convenient starting point. For example, the installation of video recording in the resuscitation room of the accident unit has proven valuable in some hospitals. Individual records taken at random and reviewed by a third party can also generate a useful discussion.[4,5]

There are two broad approaches to the objective measurement of medical performance: The first is generic and includes 100% of all caseload; the second is specific and focuses on an agreed subset of patients with a common problem, investigation, treatment or outcome. Such topics may be selected by virtue of their high volume, high risk, high cost or variation of local practice or other reasons or concerns.

Generic monitoring of medical performance tends to be a fishing expedition; expected levels of performance are not generally defined in advance but examination of trends and variations may lead to defined targets and to corrective action if and when this appears appropriate.[6] Each audit group could review on a regular basis routinely collected data such as:

1. Workload and case mix.
2. Appropriateness of care (e.g. operations out of hours by unsupervised juniors).
3. Access to care (e.g. waiting times, non-attendance at out-patients, refusal of admission due to lack of beds).
4. Outcomes of care (e.g. return to full function, failure of implants, wound infections).
5. Quality of records (e.g. delay in sending discharge summaries to general practitioners, patients discharged without full diagnosis).

6. Efficiency (e.g. use of diagnostic investigations, prescribing, the attendance at clinics).

This approach to monitoring and measurement would be extremely time consuming if the data capture and linkage were not computer assisted. Much of this should be available through existing patient administration systems together with pathology, radiology and pharmacy information.

Review of selected topics may be triggered by such generic screening but is otherwise less reliant on computer data, except for identification of index cases, and resorts ultimately to the patients' medical records for clinical details.[7] One model for the review of the individual clinical topics involves the definition of the explicit criteria against which a non-medical assistant may screen an agreed number of patient records to determine whether or not essential elements are appropriately recorded.

These elements may refer to:

1. The referral procedure (e.g. how soon the patient was seen, and by whom).
2. Diagnosis (e.g. key points in the history, examination and investigation).
3. Treatment (e.g. the timing, extent and duration of therapy).
4. Follow-up (e.g. monitoring by investigations, frequency and duration of outpatient follow-up).
5. Outcome (e.g. return to function, satisfactory placement of implants).
6. Communication (e.g. information given to GP and to patient).

Using these criteria a non-medical audit assistant can screen large numbers of records to develop a quantified profile of current management for further discussion by the clinicians as well as identifying cases that differ significantly from the criteria and may require further individual reviews.

Sadly, most successful examples of audit in Britain have in the past relied on avoiding existing hospital data systems; but the opportunity for improving the latter rests largely with the clinicians concerned. Substantial errors arise from the traditional practice of using often inadequate and incomplete discharge summaries as a basis for data abstraction. More direct involvement by consultants in verifying the accuracy and completeness of clinical data recorded on discharge before entry into the hospital data system would dramatically improve the quality of the routinely available data even without involving surgeons directly in clinical computing. Clearly there are major benefits in terms of patient management and clinical administration in having dedicated computer systems,

Table 3.1 *Examples of health service indicators*

Screen	Number	HS1 code[1]	Indicator
Trauma/orthop	30	CL67	Out-patient referrals per population
	39	LS4	Standardised average stay
	45	HA63	% day cases, 15–64 years
	70	WL44	% elective admissions waiting 12 + days
	75	CL51	% out-patient Did Not Attend
	82	TH41	% theatre sessions cancelled
	83	TH52	% theatre cases out of hours
Access by condition	1	HR48	Hip replacement rate, by age
	5	HR48	Knee replacement rate, by age
Policy tracers	91	WL41	Waiting, hip replacement
	94	LS43	Average stay, hip replacement
	103	WL41	Waiting, knee replacement
	106	LS43	Average stay, knee replacement

[1]Health service indicator

but the basic indices required for audit could be provided by a well-tended data capture system that forms part of the routine hospital database.

Health service indicators (formerly known as performance indicators) remain of doubtful accuracy and relevance to clinical practice but they are improving and may provide a useful and interesting starting point for examining variations in access to care and the process to care. Indicators that are available for districts in England and Wales and which may be of particular relevance include those listed in Table 3.1.

Practical problems

The measurement of medical performance faces challenges many of which will not, despite the enthusiasm of many technological devotees, be resolved by computing alone. Broadly these issues are in the realms of policy, organisation, and technical areas of computing.

The first problem for clinicians, managers or anyone else who seeks to measure performance is to define what should be measured and what standards are expected. This requires explicit service objectives, agreed standards of performance, common data sets and common definitions to permit comparisons between and among individuals. Guidelines must be defined both locally, regionally and preferably nationally using the networks of national specialty organisations.

The second problem is in the organisation and management of patient information systems. Most systematic review of hospital medical practice rapidly reveals gross inadequacy both in the clinical and administrative aspects of patient records, in methods of clinical data capture, in data validation and in retrieval of clinical records themselves. To this confusion of traditional data capture systems (based on the vagaries of the discharge summary) should be added the general absence of casemix data on out-patients, who comprise an increasing proportion of clinical practice. These examples alone suggest it is time for a radical revision of traditional values and methods in the handling of clinical data, with a significantly increased investment in the grading and training of staff as well as in technology itself.

The third problem relates partly to the inadequacy of current technology and partly to the failure of computer system designers to allow for the legitimate requirements of secondary users. For example, many pathology and radiology systems, though well orientated towards the individual departments, give little or no support to other legitimate users, such as in providing profiles used by individual clinicians. The inability of many micro-computer systems to link with hospital patient administration systems (PAS) leads to gross inefficiency in duplication of data entry and transfer between the clinical systems run by doctors and the main hospital administration systems. A further problem is that even if out-patient data capture were undertaken, the currently standard ICD-9 (International Classification of Diseases, 9th revision) and OPCS (Office of Population, Censuses and Surveys classification of operations) classifications do not allow for the coding of non-specific conditions and symptoms which represent the problems of many patients who have not been fully investigated.

Conclusions

The introduction of more formal and effective audit need not be held up on the grounds of inadequate computing systems. The essential elements are a state of mind, and the will to examine and change clinical practice where indicated. Although cases for review may be identified with computer-generated indices, detailed audit of selected samples relies primarily on the original patient record. Even without major capital investment, existing hospital data systems could be substantially improved if clinicians check the accuracy and completeness of the clinical information in the discharge summaries on which these data systems feed.

References

1. Buck, N., Devlin, H. B. & Lunn, J. N. (1987). *Report of a Confidential Enquiry into Perioperative Deaths*. London: Nuffield Provincial Hospitals Trust/King's Fund.
2. Department of Health, *Working for Patients* (1989). HMSO: London.
3. Collins, C. D. (1990). Contribution of regional specialty subcommittees to organising audit. *British Medical Journal*, **300**, 94–95.
4. Heath, D. A. (1990). Random review of hospital patient records. *British Medical Journal*, **300**, 651–652.
5. Williams, J. G., Kingham, M. J., Morgan, J. M. & Davies, A. B. (1990). Retrospective review of hospital patient records. *British Medical Journal*, **300,** 991–993.
6. Bennett, J. & Walshe, K. (1990). Occurrence screening as a method of audit. *British Medical Journal*, **300**, 1248–1251.
7. Shaw, C. D. (1990). Criterion based audit. *British Medical Journal*, **300**, 649–651.

4

Medical audit: a view from the centre

DUNCAN MacPHERSON

Introduction

In March 1988 the Prime Minister announced that there would be a
fundamental review by ministers of the way in which the National Health
Service was organised and financed. The Government's intentions were
announced in January 1989. The main proposals as expressed in the NHS
review White Paper 'Working for Patients'[1] were:

- To make the Health Service more responsive to the needs of patients by
  devolving as much power and responsibility as possible to a local level.
- To establish independent self-governing hospital trusts that would
  operate within the framework of the NHS.
- To reimburse providers of health care according to the services they
  render rather than the population they serve. The money for health care
  should follow the patient.
- To increase consultant posts in order to reduce waiting lists and help cut
  long hours worked by some junior medical staff.
- To enable large general practices to become budget holders, with the
  responsibility of purchasing some elements of health care on behalf of
  their patients.
- To reduce the size of health authorities, and to reform them along
  business lines by the appointment of executives and non-executive
  directors.
- To audit more rigorously the performance of health services to ensure
  optimum quality and value for money.

A theme running throughout these proposals was the need to improve
the quality of care that the NHS delivers to its patients. It was perceived
that there were two major areas in which the quality of service provided

was being questioned and criticised – customer services and quality of care.

Customer services

The NHS was often criticised as being too impersonal and too inflexible. Long waiting times, poor communications, dingy buildings, unhelpful staff and poor food were criticisms that were frequently made.

The noun 'patient', is defined in the Oxford English Dictionary in two ways:

A person showing calm endurance of pain or of any provocation; perseverance; forbearance; quiet and self-possessed waiting for something.
A person under medical, dental or psychiatric treatment.

It was widely perceived that the two uses of the word were too closely associated to be acceptable in contemporary society. The Health Service should become more aware of not only the basic clinical 'needs' of its patients, but also of their 'wants'. Some of the concepts of customer care and quality management should be adopted from private industry.

Quality of clinical care

There are many articles published in medical journals describing variations in clinical practice and outcome of treatment. Often, these are subsequently reported more widely, and come to the attention of the general public and politicians. A stark example of international variation in clinical practice is the different rates of coronary artery by-pass grafts in the USA and the UK. In 1985 the rate per million population was 1000 in the USA and 210 in the UK. This was not simply a reflection on the difference between the means and amount of funding in the different countries, because when two panels of doctors, one from the USA and one from the UK, were asked to make judgements about appropriateness of surgery, with respect to possible benefit to patients, regardless of the facilities available, there were wide variations in the perceptions of the two panels.[2]

Clinicians working within this country are aware of wide variations between consultant practice – often within the same units. How often do junior medical staff, when making decisions about patient management ask the question 'Which consultant am I working for tonight?' This variation in practice has been quantified recently with regard to decisions to perform caesarian sections for foetal distress. A retrospective audit in a large NHS maternity unit suggested that 30% of caesarian sections were unnecessary. Furthermore, there was significant disagreement between auditors on the decision whether to do a caesarian section or not, and even when the same obstetrician was faced with the same information on two different occasions, there was inconsistency in the decision reached in 25% of cases.[3]

On a population level, geographical variations in mortality between health authorities in England and Wales, using routinely collected data, have been examined. Variations in mortality from conditions amenable to medical intervention have been clearly demonstrated even after adjustment for social factors.[4]

Although the criticism by the general public of the standards of clinical care are less common than those of the 'customer services', some patients, politicians and health professionals were becoming increasingly aware of, and concerned about, the wide variations in the ways patients were being treated, and the outcome of that treatment. Journal articles such as those described above written for a professional audience were considered newsworthy by the media, who highlighted the apparent failures of the National Health Service. The clinical decisions made by individual doctors were being criticised in the courts with increasing frequency.

The Government recognised that doctors were concerned about these variations, and that there was a desire among the profession for more self-evaluation of the way patients were treated and the outcome of that treatment. The medical Royal Colleges and faculties were taking an increasing interest in audit, and some had made participation in audit an essential prerequisite to accreditation of training posts, but major problems existed. For those who wished to participate, there were few consistently recorded data on interventions and even fewer on outcomes that could be analysed and compared.

Various *quality control* mechanisms already exist. These include the General Medical Council disciplinary procedures, accreditation of training posts by the medical Royal Colleges, and the law. These are, however, threatening top down mechanisms, designed to weed out the grossly aberrant performers. There were also existing professional audits such as the Confidential Enquiry into Maternal Deaths and the Confidential Enquiry into Perioperative Deaths, the Health Advisory Service, many local audits and informal clinical meetings. These were often low key non-threatening exercises covering only small areas of clinical practice and without any power, and with little influence on subsequent practice. Moreover, despite increasing interest among doctors there remained many who did not see participation in medical audit as a relevant or necessary part of their professional work. It was likely that it was this group of doctors who had the most to gain from a medical audit programme.

It was the Government's view that they should act, to ensure that the poorly co-ordinated and sporadic self-evaluations of clinical work in which many doctors were becoming interested should become part of normal professional practice for all doctors. The expectation that all doctors should participate in medical audit was therefore included in the NHS Review White Paper.

Medical audit policy in the NHS Review White Paper

Medical audit was defined in the White Paper as:

A systematic critical analysis of the quality of medical care, including the procedures used for diagnosis and treatment, the use of resources and the resulting outcome for patients.

Hospital-based care

This definition of medical audit has become widely accepted in hospital-based care, although some have questioned the reference to the use of resources. Consideration of resources is not, and should never be the prime purpose of audit; however, it is inevitable that they should be considered if optimum care is to be given to a population within resources that will always be finite. Cries have been heard from the stalwart defenders of professional independence '*What is happening to clinical freedom?*' The answer must be that clinical freedom has always been restricted by availability of resources, and that doctors working in a publicly funded health service that attempts to provide comprehensive and equitable care to the population it serves have a duty to provide the highest possible standards of care within the available resources. This argument was fully examined by the President of the Royal College of Physicians, Sir Raymond Hoffenburg, in his Rock Carling Lecture in 1986.[5]

The White Paper requirements for medical audit in the Hospital and Community Health Services (HCHS) are that:

- Every consultant should participate in a form of medical audit agreed between management and the profession locally.
- The system should be medically led with the local medical audit advisory committee chaired by a senior clinician.
- The district management should be responsible for ensuring that an

effective system of medical audit is in place and also that the work of each medical team is reviewed at whatever regular frequent intervals are agreed locally.

– Peer review findings in individual cases should be confidential, but the general results of medical audit should be available to management locally and lessons learned published more widely.

– Management should be able to initiate an independent professional audit; for example, where there is cause to question the quality or cost effectiveness of a service.

Primary care

Medical audit in primary care is less well developed than audit in the hospital service, and many difficulties are recognised. Care is delivered in more places; periods of treatment and diagnosis are less well defined; medical records may be less detailed; outcomes may only become apparent many years after treatment commences. Whilst recognising these difficulties the Government made similar recommendations for audit in general practice to those for the hospital service. Family Health Service Authorities in co-operation with local medical committees have established *Medical Audit Advisory Groups* (MAAGs), to direct, co-ordinate and monitor medical audit activities within all general medical practices in their area.[6]

Implementation of the policy

For medical audit to become a useful means of improving standards of clinical practice, doctors must themselves be convinced of its value both as an educational tool, and as a means of activating appropriate and equitable allocation of resources. It must be non-threatening to the participants (except possibly to the small minority whose practice differs widely from standards deemed acceptable by peers). Wherever possible, the obstacles to (or excuses for) not performing audit should be removed. The removal of these obstacles may be primarily the responsibility of management or of the profession, but in most cases close co-operation between the two is necessary. Table 4.1 outlines some of the perceived obstacles, and routes to resolution.

Table 4.1 *Perceived obstacles to medical audit*

Perceived obstacle to audit	Management responsibilities	Professional responsibilities
No data	Improve or provide data collection	Decide what data need to be collected. Complete clinical records in such a way as to allow collection.
No criteria		Accept corporate responsibility for developing criteria.
No standards	Standards achieved in relation to criteria may depend on resources made available to clinicians.	What are 'acceptable' standards?
No time	Job plans should be discussed with consultants, including, where possible, necessary sessional time for audit.	Is time currently being well used – including that spent on management and postgraduate educational activity? Will dropping some clinical work in order to analyse what you are doing lead to improved efficiency and effectiveness?
No support staff	Provision of high quality, well-trained support staff will reduce medical staff time spent on audit.	Acceptance of 'non-medical' help with audit. Training support staff. Widening responsibilities and interest of existing support staff.

Local and central co-operation

There are two strands to the development of audit which must interweave – local activity and central support.

Local activity

Medical audit must be done primarily at a local level. This is where data are collected, and where most doctors will compare their performance in terms of process and outcome with that of their immediate peers. All units providing services to the NHS are expected to have arrangements whereby all doctors are enabled to participate in medical audit, and for there to be a medical audit committee on which all major specialties are represented. The committee should agree audit work programmes with management locally, to whom they will also make regular reports on the general results of audit. Such reports should not identify individual patients or doctors, but need to be sufficiently detailed to inform managers and those with whom they are making contracts that proper quality assurance pro-grammes for clinical performance are in place. Furthermore, managers need to know what recommendations come from audit committees that have cost consequences, to enable them to make informed decisions about resource allocations.

In 1990/91 £24 million was allocated to Regional Health Authorities and Special Health Authorities for implementation of medical audit – funding was not released until the Department of Health approved *Medical Audit Implementation Plans* (MAIPs), which had to include:

- An overall strategy for the development of audit including the balance of responsibilities between regions, districts and units.
- Requirements for information and information technology that would enable integration with resource management to be developed.
- Manpower requirements including sessional appointments for key clinicians at regional and district level.
- Training programmes for doctors and support staff.

Although ear-marked funding is necessary for medical audit in its developmental phase, the costs of medical audit will eventually be absorbed into general costs of provision of health care and will be taken into account in the pricing of contracts.

Central support and co-ordination

The local activity described in the preceding paragraph needs national support and co-ordination to:

1. develop widely agreed criteria against which local standards can be set and performance can be audited;
2. organise audit of rare but important events (e.g. perioperative deaths) or audit in unusual specialties;
3. develop audit that compares performance across districts and regions (global audit).

The medical Royal Colleges and faculties are the bodies with responsibility for standards within their speciality groups. It is therefore primarily through these bodies that the Department of Health works to develop nationally applicable audit methodologies, criteria and recommended standards. Financial support for audit units carrying out this work has been agreed with all of the colleges and faculties. Although the Government has a legitimate interest in influencing those areas of clinical practice that they believe should be considered by professional bodies, such as those of high cost, or of particular public concern, the establishment of acceptable clinical criteria and treatment protocols remains a matter for the profession. It is in the interest of all concerned with the delivery of health care that the criteria against which the delivery of health care is judged should be widely agreed, and the standards to be achieved when making judgements against those criteria should be realistic.

Sharing of audit information

For medical audit to be effective it must be carried out in an atmosphere of mutual trust and respect, if it is to achieve its primary aim of improving, through self education or peer-group education, the quality of clinical care provided by doctors. Doctors are likely to be most frank in their discussions of patient management if those discussions are kept completely confidential.

There is, however, a dilemma. Others have a legitimate interest in the quality of work of doctors, and the quality of work performed by doctors is dependent upon others. Medical audit cannot therefore be entirely confidential to the medical profession. Clearly, it may be unsatisfactory for doctors to discuss the ways in which doctors treat patients without others present, who influence the clinical outcome for the patient. Nurses, physiotherapists, radiographers, psychotherapists, clinical psychologists and others all have a legitimate interest in how patients are treated, and should, where appropriate, be involved in multi-disciplinary clinical audit. Indeed, there is a case for having direct representation of the patients' views when auditing performance.

And yet we should not underestimate the difficulties of having a frank and constructive discussion about the way patients are treated, when outcome, including death or major disability, is being considered. If inclusion of non-medically qualified health professionals or 'consumer representatives' are going to inhibit that discussion, they should be excluded. Equally, the discussion of nurses' clinical management of their patients may be inhibited by the presence of a senior consultant. Professional groups should develop their own audit among themselves and only come together for multi-disciplinary audit when this is deemed appropriate by all concerned. How quickly this happens will vary from specialty to specialty. Some are already well used to managing patients in multi-disciplinary terms.

I have suggested that the general results of audit should be made available to management locally. *How general is general?* This remains for local determination, but as confidence in the audit process grows, and expertise develops, I believe that doctors will want to be increasingly specific in their audit reports to management, if only to strengthen their argument for more resources, or to ensure the renewal of a contract. We need, however, to be aware of the danger that results of audit could become subject to commercial manipulation. The easiest way to lower your microbiologically proven wound infection rate is to take fewer swabs!

Audit data and disclosure in the courts

The issue of confidentiality is one that concerns many doctors, in particular the possibility that audit data would be subject to subpoena and used to help the prosecution case when medical negligence is being considered.

The main guarantee of confidentiality lies in the adoption of local policies and protocols that ensure that any permanent record of medical audit does not contain details identifying individual doctors or patients. Nevertheless, it is possible that damaging inferences could be drawn even from 'anonymised' reports.

Additional protection may be possible by resisting disclosure of individual audit results as part of medico-legal actions, on the grounds that this is not in the public interest, as such disclosure would be likely to lead to the cessation of medical audit.

A claim for public interest immunity can be raised at any time in respect of evidence in court proceedings. The court then adjudicates on the claim, balancing the public interest in full disclosure for the proper administration of justice, which is the norm, against the claim for protection from disclosure in the public interest.

In the past the Department of Health has undertaken to enter a plea for immunity with regard to the Confidential Enquiry into Maternal Deaths, and, with appropriate caveats, has offered similar protection to the National Confidential Enquiry into Perioperative Deaths. The justification is twofold:

– That without such guarantees clinicians would not participate in these enquiries.
– That such national enquiries produce national benefits.

The adoption of such an approach to local audit is likely to be less clear cut, and has not been tested. It will be harder to argue 'public interest' related to a small local audit as opposed to a major national enquiry, although the general argument that a single use of audit results in a medico-legal action would be likely to diminish substantially participation in effective audit still stands.

When discussing the dangers of audit data being used by the courts to substantiate claims for medical negligence, consideration should also be given to the possible protection that participating in audit might afford. It may demonstrate in the eyes of the court that a doctor is taking proper steps to ensure that he is monitoring the quality of care he or she is giving. Conversely, he may be culpable if he or she does not participate in audit.

Future developments

The enthusiasm for audit is widespread. Doctors are increasingly accepting the notion that they cannot work in isolation, concerning themselves only with patients under their immediate care, but that they should take corporate responsibilities for the quality of clinical care that the organisation within which they work delivers to its patients.

Managers are reassured that formal mechanisms are being established whereby they can be reassured that clinical standards are regularly reviewed, by their professional staff.

The conclusion of the South West Thames Regional Health Authority's excellent document '*A Plan for Implementation of Medical Audit*' uses the quotation:

The truth is, hardly any of us have ethical energy enough for more than one really inflexible point of honour.
(*G. B. Shaw, Preface to The Doctor's Dilemma, A Tragedy*, 1906).

and they make the following commentary on the quotation:

Medical audit is widely seen as fundamental to any attempt to assure an adequate standard throughout the reformed health service. The medical profession has enthusiastically agreed to invest its 'ethical energy'. If the Government does not match this investment with adequate resources, we will soon find the ethical energy of the profession being dissipated by frustration and disillusionment. Effectiveness will succumb to many different and conflicting concepts of efficiency, and no amount of money invested elsewhere in the service will ensure an adequate quality of care for patients.

Resources are being put into the development of medical audit, but the intellectual investment is also necessary if audit is to be effective. This must come from the medical profession itself. It is clinicians who must agree clinical criteria, and acceptable standards. Managers have a role in data collection and feedback of information, but before they can make a useful contribution to medical audit they must know what needs to be recorded. Sensible decisions can then be made about the extent to which data collection for audit can be integrated into resource management and patient administration system.

Agreement on the type and form of data recording will be reached most rapidly at a local level, and such agreements are vital. To obtain maximum benefit from audit, nationwide comparison of performance is desirable, but needs for national agreement should not hold up local developments.

References
1. Department of Health (1989). *Working for Patients*. London: HMSO.
2. Brook, R. H., Kosecoff, J. B., Park, R. E., Chassin, M. R., Winslow, C. M. & Hampton, J. R. (1988). Diagnosis and treatment of coronary disease: comparison of doctors attitudes in the USA and UK. *The Lancet*, **i**, 750–753.
3. Barrett, J. F. R., Jarvis, G. J., MacDonald, H. N., Buchan, P. C., Tyrell, S. N. & Lilford, R. J. (1990). Inconsistencies in clinical decisions in Obstetrics. *The Lancet*, **336**, 549–581.
4. Charlton, J. R. H., Hartley, R. M., Silver, R. & Holland, W. W. (1983). Geographical variations in mortality from conditions amenable to medical intervention in England and Wales. *The Lancet*, **i**, 691–696.
5. Hoffenburg, Sir R. (1987). *Clinical Freedom*. Nuffield Provincial Hospital Trust.
6. Department of Health (1990). *Audit in Primary Care*. HC(FP)(90).8. London: HMSO.

5

Audit: a view from the Royal College of Surgeons of England

H. BRENDAN DEVLIN

Introduction

The Royal College of Surgeons of England (RCS) derives its authority for the training of surgeons and the regulation of surgery from the charter given by George III under the Great Seal of England on 22nd March 1800. A further charter bestowed by Victoria in 1843 empowered the RCS to make by-laws concerning the activities of its fellows. Since then the RCS has constantly sought to improve the selection and training of surgeons and the standards of surgery in England and Wales. The scope of the RCS remit has recently been increased and refined by the changes in medical practice that will flow from the Government White Paper '*Working for Patients*'. These changes, enacted as law from 1st April 1991, and the National Health Service and Community Care Act 1990, delegate to the Royal Colleges a central role in quality assurance. For surgery this task falls to the RCS in respect of surgical care in England and Wales.

The RCS has always conducted examinations for surgeons, indeed possession of the FRCS diploma is a prerequisite for autonomous practice as a surgeon in the National Health Service. As an extension of these examinations the RCS has prescribed conditions for apprenticeship and training. The RCS inspects and approves training posts in hospitals in England and Wales and has developed tight criteria that training posts must meet. Each training hospital is inspected every five years, or more frequently if doubts arise. This inspection is crucial to ensuring good surgical training and good practice. Removal of approval for surgical training is the most powerful sanction the RCS possesses in its pursuit of high surgical standards.

The training role is also encompassed by the courses and lectures the RCS organises in London and throughout England and Wales. The RCS training reaches into every hospital in England and Wales through the agency of its tutors who are appointed to guide and counsel young surgeons. The regulating, standard-setting role is performed nowadays in each region by the college advisers (in general surgery, orthopaedic surgery, and otolaryngology), who vet job descriptions, attend appointment committees and advise health authorities about many facets of day-to-day surgical practice. The RCS council regularly visits throughout England and Wales and thereby hopes to keep in touch with and to reflect vigorously the views of surgeons both locally and nationally.

The RCS encourages surgical research, promotes good practice and campaigns for improved facilities to enable surgeons to employ new techniques and to develop new modes of delivery of surgical care. The RCS, with the surgical specialty associations, therefore, publishes authoritative advice on surgical topics. This advice sets standards and prompts the Government and others to improvements in surgery. Three recent documents are relevant to the discussion of audit – the *Report on Day Surgery* (1985); the *Report of the Working Party on the Composition of a Surgical Team in General Surgery, Orthopaedics and Otolaryngology* (1988); and the *Report on Consultant Responsibility in Invasive Surgical Procedures* (1990). Currently the RCS wishes to facilitate the development of surgical audit in hospitals in England and Wales.

The Audit Commission

Another change in the statutory situation of hospital medicine occurred in 1990 when the Audit Commission for England and Wales had its remit extended to include the National Health Service. The commission pursues quality in the public sector – perhaps it should be renamed the 'Quality Commission' – and within the Health Service it acts in concert and in consultation with the Royal Colleges; its recent report on *Day Case Surgery* was developed with advisers nominated by the RCS. The Audit Commission has statutory powers that allow it access to documents, including hospital records and operating room registers. It can require evidence from individuals. So far, its influence throughout local government has been catalytic and beneficial in helping develop better services for customers. It is bringing this successful record to the NHS.

Audit, continuing education and research

Audit of clinical practice is not a new idea; audit, integrity and service to patients are the bedrock of the western medical ethic. Now that more formalised audit has been introduced into our practice it is forgotten that it has always been there. By audit we mean the systematic review of our work so that we can improve our activities. The wide variation in current clinical practice and the consumerist philosophy have combined in a new agenda for medicine; high on this agenda is the achieving of uniform, high-quality, clinical care. Audit is a responsible reaction by our profession. But audit alone is unlikely to remedy all the problems we face; we must have the means to re-educate ourselves in the new technologies and in the new attitudes that are demanded of us in the emerging health care culture. Hand in hand with the audit explosion there must be an offensive in continuing medical education. The apprenticeship system, which has served generations of British surgeons, today needs to be supplemented by structured educational input throughout our professional lives.

Adding the dimension of continuing education immediately describes how audit and quality assurance differ from research. Audit and quality assurance endeavour to improve good practice equitably to the care of each patient. Research sets out to find new knowledge and therapies. When these are found and tested they can then be applied to clinical practice; audit and quality assurance will then be needed to ensure they are applied correctly.

The audit cycle

Audit is a biofeedback mechanism. Standards and clinical guidelines are set, practice observed, variation of practice from standard assessed and then action taken to improve the clinical practice (if it falls short) or to alter the standards if they prove incorrect in use.

A first stage is to set the standard. A standard may be set by an independent agency charged with regulation, the General Medical Council or the RCS for instance – or, when things go badly awry, by Her Majesty's Judiciary! More usually, standards for clinical audit are set within our profession by expert groups of surgeons reviewing the relevant research literature, by consensus among colleagues, or by more formal consensus conferences which then write a standard of practice.

RCS guidelines are derived by a mixture of these methods, expert advice, conferences and seminars, working parties, and then finally all RCS guidelines travel through the RCS committee system. RCS guidelines are always fully debated by, and in their final form, approved by, council. RCS guidelines are ideals of clinical practice that every surgeon can achieve;

they do not replace clinical judgment and are not substitutes for knowledge and textbooks. RCS guidelines, like the RCS regulations for training posts, are constantly under review and are updated for changed circumstances; for example, the RCS *Guidelines for Day Surgery* has recently been rewritten and the new edition circulated to college fellows.

Stage two of audit is applying the standard to everyday clinical activity and measuring how practice varies from the standard.

Stage three is closing the audit loop – 'feedback'. Direct feedback to each individual surgeon is clearly the ideal, an ideal that is probably logistically impossible to every surgeon on each and every detail of practice. Feedback, particularly feedback of adverse comment, has to be achieved confidentially if it is to be helpful and constructive. The aim of audit is to improve clinical practices, not alienate colleagues. Due consideration must always be given to the confidentiality and legal implications of any audit feedback.

Finally, as part of the feedback there is the 'Hawthorne effect'.* Just reviewing practices encourages practitioners to try harder and reach higher standards.

All these effects of audit are to do with improving the clinical care of patients. That is what audit is all about.

How should surgeons audit?

The RCS perceives audit as an essential component of every surgeon's practice. Regular audit is a pre-condition for the approval of posts for training purposes. The college insists that the equivalent to one-half day a week is devoted to audit and the consequent continuing education. Every consultant is now required to participate in clinical audit.

Audit may be a local, a regional, a specialty or a national initiative. Local audit is a time-honoured and very traditional British surgical activity. The surgical firm – the dressers and the chief, the sister and nurses, and the almoners – making a ward round and then discussing the patients and their problems over coffee, is the antique audit traditional in teaching hospitals. This processional audit was, for many years, an adequate safeguard to good surgical care. It was perfection when surgery was employed only as a last resort to prevent death, when the calculus was death or an operation; it sufficed when surgery became safe in the early part of this century but when patients still needed extended post-operative

---

* Hawthorne, Illinois, USA: An Electric Lamp Company – a classic study of work practice; just reviewing the operatives improved their output!

stays to recover from the insult of the anaesthetic and an operation. It is no longer adequate because so much surgery is out-patient, day care and short stay. These patients will not be considered by a traditional ward round.

Deaths and complications meetings are also a very successful and time-honoured form of surgical behaviour. Such meetings are important to review the clinical practice that preceded a death or a serious complication. Reviews of deaths of surgical patients should be undertaken regularly in every department. Similarly, complications need to be reviewed. Lessons must be learned and new management protocols devised and written down for all to follow.

Writing down the lessons from audit is an important discipline; the audit is only successful when changed clinical practice prevents an adverse event in the future. A written record is the only way to assess progress and change.

Today, surgery is performed for disability rather than as an alternative to death, and the crude mortality for all types of surgery in the UK is 0.7%, while some specialties have a zero mortality, ophthalmology and oral surgery, for instance. Despite the low overall surgical mortality rate, deaths due to surgical failure or errors by surgeons still occur at a rate of one in 2860 operations. Anaesthetist failure is much less frequent than surgeon failure – one death for every 185 056 anaesthetics administered. The long history of anaesthetic audit clearly has contributed to the safety of modern anaesthesia. Hence, if quality control and audit of surgery is to be successful, regular local reviews of all surgery must be the norm.

Information needs of audit

All the current audit initiatives are hampered by information short-comings. These shortcomings occur at each stage of the medical process – data about demography, admission and discharge are often poorly collected; diagnostic and operation coding is given a low priority; data about complications, outcome, re-admissions etc., are similarly often unavailable. The RCS has published guidelines to medical records that address these issues and set out a minimum data set to be collected for each patient. The RCS now inspects patient records as part of its hospital inspection programme.

The RCS has published guidelines to computing for clinicians, which indicate how the individual clinician can use a computer to develop correct information on his or her practice. However, unless clinicians personally take an interest in data acquisition, the appalling state of NHS data will remain. Each clinician must ensure that data about his or her own practice are collected and adequately validated by him or herself; unless this is done criticism of practice will continue to be derived from dodgy sources. Unfortunately, criticism from outside the profession is easy and can be damaging. It is for each surgeon to make sure that all data about his or her practice is honest and timely. Only when this is so will audit be able to show beyond doubt that British surgeons deliver high-quality care.

Developing better diagnostic coding than the current ICD-9 CM is an issue that is being addressed, but this is a fairly long-term venture because of the national and international perspectives that coding conventions must fit. In the short term, to get the current coding right and on time would enable more valid statistics on surgical activity to be presented. Similarly, the operation codings OPCS-4 need revising and updating to reflect the rapidly moving horizons of modern surgery, but if what was coded was correct it would help in the short term. All the recent initiatives in audit and quality improvement have been hampered by the data shortfall; surgeons must give data collection a higher priority. We must stress that the RCS does not intend surgeons to do the coding themselves, but they must ensure it is done and validated. Every surgeon makes the diagnosis and does the operation; coding is no more than a numerical description of these and nowadays if the diagnosis and operation are written into patient care plans and discharge summaries, a computer can code this directly.

Confidentiality

Audit must be confidential. Audit should comply with the time-honoured conventions of confidentiality in clinical practice. This confidentiality is to protect the patient and his or her interests. The patient gives the doctor information in trust, in trust that this information will only be given to another doctor or member of the health care family in furtherance of that patient's well-being.

Audit is a technique to improve the care of all patients; relevant anonymised patient data can be used for audit purposes without any breach of medical confidentiality occurring. Audit uses confidential information ethically and in the patient's interest.

Doctors are rightly concerned about their own reputations if audit discovers their professional shortcomings. The confidentiality of medical audit is a proper concern of clinicians. Before discussing the confidentiality of medical audit, it is well to rehearse the current situation regarding 'confidential' information about the care of patients. All information contained in the patient's notes is the property of the Health Authority and could be subject to subpoena in the courts were it required. Similarly, clinical information held upon computer is subject to subpoena in accordance with the Data Protection Act. Demographic, numeric and clinical information collected routinely as part of hospital activity analysis and similar statistics is already available and published as a public record. No ground for claiming privilege or confidentiality can be advanced in respect of it. So far as factual information on patient care is concerned, it is all, therefore, already available to a court of law. The situation of the Audit Commission, a statutory agency, has already been addressed.

Data obtained by the National Confidential Enquiry into Perioperative Deaths (NCEPOD) (and the Confidential Enquiry into Maternal Deaths) is protected by the courts by the Secretary of State, who has given an undertaking that should any attempt be made to subpoena that information, the Crown would claim the principle of public interest in order to protect those data from disclosure. This situation has been confirmed by the Department of Health in writing to NCEPOD. It is perhaps worth noting, however, that NCEPOD does not collect any opinion and that NCEPOD shreds all the data it receives as soon as they have been considered and transferred to computer. All the data held on computer by NCEPOD are anonymous and no record is kept of the original data. Linkage of data cannot be advanced as part of a prosecution in the courts in the United Kingdom and this is a further safeguard to NCEPOD data. Indeed, unless a legal challenge were mounted and subpoena delivered prior to NCEPOD shredding data (within two weeks of NCEPOD receiving it) there would be nothing to subpoena. NCEPOD is absolutely strict and indeed paranoid about preserving the anonymity and confidentiality of its activities. Therefore, NCEPOD is very different from all the other current initiatives.

The burning question is 'what is the legal status of comment on patient care raised in district and regional audit committees?' Clearly, such comment could be subpoenaed at present if it were written down and the patient's identity to it recorded. No-one recommends making such a patient-specific record of audit proceedings. Indeed, the *Guidelines for Audit* published by the RCS and similar guidelines published by other bodies specifically state that records of audit meetings should not contain details of patient identity. Records of audit meetings are not privileged and could always be obtained by a court on subpoena by calling a witness to it, e.g. someone participating in an audit meeting. Of course, if that happened, a court would then have the right to cross-examine and challenge the witness. Undoubtedly this would seriously qualify the value of any such comment!

Although the Department of Health assures the profession that such subpoena of audit records is unlikely, this whole area of confidentiality of comment in audit meetings is unclear in the legal sense. The Department of Health has been struggling with this problem. Hopefully, in the near future, this will be clarified and then the Department of Health and the Conference of Royal Colleges will be able to issue some very explicit guidance for this disputed area. Currently, the RCS does not see a problem if only general-conclusion orientated records are made of audit meetings. Ministers and the Department of Health have given general reassurances about the confidentiality of clinical audit meetings. Because Government sets great store by audit, these official reassurances must be accepted by the medical profession. Audit is no more than an extension of traditional clinical care, a sedentary rather than an antique processional process. That is how we should regard it and as no more.

Resources for audit

Resources are needed if audit is to be successful and worthwhile. The critical resource is an attitude of mind. Audit will not achieve the hoped-for improvement in surgical practice unless surgeons adopt an open approach to reviewing their work collectively and unless there is a corporate intention to change and improve practice. No mortal surgeon is always perfect; audit is about decreasing our imperfections. The variations in clinical practice are available for all to see; we must address this issue ourselves rather than letting others, the managers, regulate our clinical practice. This is our problem.

Apart from the mental attitude, other more material considerations of resources are relevant. Time is needed for audit; this will mean not doing something else – a clinic or a ward round or an operating list will need to be cancelled. So that the burden of cancellation is spread, either a rolling programme of audit meetings on different days each week could be arranged, or a complete shut-down of the department at a stated time each week. The audit meetings of anaesthesia and all surgical disciplines interact. Clearly, there needs to be a co-ordinated response if resources are not to be squandered. Perhaps a 'clinical and academic afternoon' is what every hospital should have, with an integrated audit and educational programme for all disciplines. While the clinical staff learn, the routine maintenance of operating rooms and clinics can take place, a strategy that will save resources currently spent on expensive weekend and out of hours maintenance.

Using doctors' time for audit and cancelling clinical activities will have an effect on throughput; more consultants will be needed. This is acknowledged already and more consultant posts have been sanctioned. So far, probably not enough additional surgical posts have been created and the RCS is constantly pressing for more.

Other non-medical resources required if audit is to be wholly successful include clerical support; 'audit assistants' are popular persons to have, and while they undoubtedly have a role, they are not immediately necessary to make audit a reality. Similarly, computers are not indispensable. If you have one in the department, it is most useful for aggregating data and number crunching (and for doing many other humdrum repetitive secretarial tasks). The RCS *Guidelines to Computing* set out what can be expected of a computer system and should guide the decision whether or not to go computerised. Ultimately, however, data are so crucial that some local data acquisition and analysis will be mandatory. Most importantly, it is vital that the computer system is common to all the consultants and that it can communicate with the hospital patient administration system.

The components of health care

For convenience, we can divide health care into three components – structure, process and outcome. It is important to dissect clinical activity in this way to enable us to study, and to audit, each component.

1. *Structure* includes the multitude of factors that enable the patient to be treated, the availability of resources, the physical amenities of the clinic or hospital, the accessibility of care in both its geographical and financial sense. Everything, in fact, that enables the patient to consult with a doctor.
2. *Process* is started at the first consultation. It includes the history taking and clinical examination, confirmatory tests that enable a diagnosis to be reached, the design of a care plan (treatment plan) for the patient, the discussion of the care plan with the patient and his or her consent to it, carrying through the care plan, including the various operations and therapies, and then aftercare and any necessary rehabilitation for the patient.
3. *Outcome* is the end result. The old adage 'First do no harm' must be reiterated here. The outcome should leave the patient physically,

psychologically and socially improved when his or her status is compared with his or her pre-therapy state. Today, the majority of surgical patients enjoy measurably better health after treatment than before.

The ultimate measure of clinical intervention is patient satisfaction. Patient satisfaction in clinical practice is the 'bottom line' similar to the customer satisfaction so embraced by industry. However, medical care is not quite like other goods and services that are traded in today's markets; few patient choose to be ill, and when they are ill, they have the choice of therapies restricted by their pathology. There is no choice between a hip replacement and a heart transplant, and without this choice the forces of a completely free market can never operate. Our professional ethic is one of the regulators of this quasi-market. Clinical audit of patient satisfaction is a mainstay of this regulatory process.

Structure, process and outcome can, and often are, regarded mechanistically as components of health care, and perhaps surgeons are most likely to adopt a production line stance when faced with the repetitive operation, but we must beware this factory floor posture and work ethic. We are apt to forget the behavioural aspects of surgical care because we tend to be enchanted by and so enjoy operating. Yet clinical surgery has a human side to it; there is the patient at one end of the scalpel, and at the other end there is the surgeon. Empathy with the patients and their relatives, civility and punctuality and the many other facets of good professional behaviour are each legitimate items for us to audit. Audit is not only about throughput and number crunching; it is all about delivering high-quality care to the patient.

RCS requirements for audit

The RCS has a minimum requirement for audit; each consultant surgical team must devote one half day a week to audit activities. This is also a contractual obligation for all consultants since the NHS changes in April 1990.

The college tutor has a pivotal role in surgical audit. He or she must ensure that a record of audit meetings is kept, that global results and conclusions are recorded, and that action is taken as a result of audit meetings. The record must also be signed by each of the attendees. The RCS requires this record to be produced for inspection when accreditation for teaching is renewed. Such a record must also be available to the district audit committee. Adequate data are essential for local audit and have become even more vital since the NHS purchaser/provider split and contracting has become the norm since 1st April 1991. This point bears repetition: consultants must ensure that correct data on their practice are available and coded; the RCS guidelines set a minimum standard for surgical notes.

Local audit meetings need a chairman and someone to organise them. The RCS tutor may be appropriate to both these roles but a system of rotating chairmanship will probably suit local circumstances better and keep the freshness of meetings. All the consultants and all the trainees in the speciality should attend these audit meetings. They should review diagnoses, pathology, X-rays, etc. and all other areas of clinical endeavour. Resource utilisation is an important measure of the quality of care both to the individual patient and to the community served. Regular reviews of resource management are important; the RCS believes consultants have a responsibility to teach their juniors the skills required to manage resources efficiently.

However audit is arranged locally, it must be constructive and collaborative between surgical teams. There is a great benefit in varying the format of meetings, in combining with different specialties to review particular topics – for instance, the management of diabetes may involve physicians in an audit meeting with orthopaedic surgeons. Collaboration is the keynote of local audit meetings. The chairman must ensure this collaboration and that the meetings are productive and constructive; they should be geared to improving the service, not to discerning faults.

Whether nursing staff should attend local audit meetings must vary from place to place and time to time. Similarly, other groups, such as physiotherapists and occupational therapists, may be a vital ingredient of an audit meeting, but their attendance must be a local decision. While managers have a duty to know that audit is happening and what the key findings are, they should not expect to attend by right, though it may be appropriate to invite them from time to time. These are local issues that must be decided by those on the spot. It must be remembered that, in the sense of this book, audit is a medical activity whereby doctors are striving to improve their performance.

RCS audit initiatives

Clearly, because death and major complications are so rare in contemporary surgical practice, large samples of patients and surgeons are needed to set standards and compare and improve outcomes. Above all, because surgery is so complex and highly technical, the specialists' opinion of good practice needs to be heard. For these reasons, the RCS places great store on the role of specialist associations in developing and encouraging audit.

For example, during 1991–1992 the RCS undertook an audit of ankle fractures with the crucial direction of the audit being given by the British Orthopaedic Association. The audit reviewed the diagnosis and management of ankle fractures. The intention was to describe what was happening during the period of study, and then derive some guidelines for the future. Guidelines will have to cover the structure of care, who should treat ankle fractures and where they should be treated, the process of care, what X-rays and investigations are needed to make an adequate assessment, and then what treatment, operative or otherwise, is correct and, finally, the outcome. Outcome is a particularly difficult parameter to measure. There are both short- and long-term clinical outcomes and then there are patient perceptions of outcome. Patients were specifically questioned about their degree of satisfaction and their responses may give us a new insight into the choice of treatment for ankle fractures. Patient satisfaction is the bottom line!

The RCS is currently, with the appropriate specialist associations, leading other audit projects in England and Wales. These include audits of upper intestinal endoscopy (jointly with the Royal College of Physicians, British Society of Gastroenterology and the Association of Surgeons of Great Britain and Ireland), of the management of cleft lip and palate (jointly with the Faculty of Dental Surgery, the British Association of Plastic Surgeons, the British Otolaryngology Society and the British Association of Plastic Surgeons), of prostatectomy (with the British Association of Urologists and the Association of Surgeons), and of colorectal cancer surgery (with the Coloproctology Society and the Association of Surgeons).

The college philosophy is to spread these initiatives throughout England and Wales and to involve all the specialties of surgery. The college hopes that the general awareness of these audits and the specific topics addressed will enable surgeons to achieve better results, and if there are resource or logistic shortcomings, to identify these so that the RCS can press the National Health Service to facilitate improvements.

A most important audit enterprise is the RCS *Patient Satisfaction Study*. This is a relatively long-term project to develop methods for measuring patient satisfaction with surgical services and surgeons. This project is involving much fundamental work with the basic sciences of psychology and sociology, adapting the methodologies derived from the customer satisfaction ratings used in marketing to the surgical scene. It is hoped this project will produce guidelines that will enable surgeons to measure and monitor their own 'customer ratings' and, hence, keep the activity of their own units under review.

Patient satisfaction is closely related to the information needs of patients: What are they told and what do they comprehend? Are alternative strategies adequately explored with patients? We all recognise good bedside manner and the contribution a good bedside manner makes to patient recovery. The RCS *Patient Satisfaction Study* will analyse and quantify this. The relevance of patients' own assessment of their health, both before and after surgery, is an important focus of our attention. Surgeons' perceptions of a good outcome after surgery is often at variance with patients' opinions; this study will explore this variance, which is a significant cause of complaints. The first of these studies to report will be the orthopaedic ankle injury project.

RCS confidential comparative audit service

The college believes audit embraces all these technical (clinical) and behavioural aspects of surgical care, that audit is concerned with the quality of surgery rather than just an arithmetic exercise concerned with throughput and numbers, but while we emphasise the quality of care, we cannot ignore problems of volume of care delivered. For this reason the RCS has established a database and computing clearing house. This clearing house, with its own computer analyst and accompanying staff, offers to surgeons in England and Wales facilities for comparative audit of their own performances. So far, the college has hosted three meetings to carry through comparative audit in general surgery and urology. By December 1991 this facility had been extended to orthopaedic surgery. To do this comparative audit, the RCS specifies to participating surgeons a data set they could produce either from their own computerised data or manual records. These data are aggregated and ranges and norms calculated for each variable for the whole sample by us at the RCS. Each surgeon is then given, in confidence, his own figures. The RCS will protect the anonymity and confidentiality of the analysis. A meeting of all participants is then held and the group data discussed. This is peer-group assessment and feedback, but accomplished in an anonymous, confidential and non-threatening way. This strategy improves surgeons' performances. The technique was developed first in the Large Bowel Cancer Project in the

1970s and 1980s. Students of audit and the value of feedback can usefully study this project, which involved a self-selected cohort of 'the best' colorectal surgeons in the UK. One year into this audit, quite surprising variations in surgeons' operative outcomes were identified. The leak rate for colonic anastomoses varied from 0.5% to 30%, the 30-day death rate (peri-operative death rate) varied between surgeons from 11% to 31%. When these data were first received by the participants at a general meeting, they were astonished. But the meeting and the feedback did cause rapid change. After a further year of the project, there was an abrupt improvement in the surgeons with high leak rates and high mortalities – showing that surgeons learn by their mistakes (perhaps!), but confirming the value of audit. The long-term outcome data emerging from this project are even more enticing to the enthusiast. In the long-term, better short-term values, low peak and sepsis rates correlate with longer survival times. Hugh Dudley, commenting on these data, coined the useful phrase 'surgeon-related variables' – leak rates, sepsis rates, durations of stay, death rates, recurrence rates and survival times. Translating the conse-quences of these 'surgeon-related variables' into economic and sociologic values (quality of life) gives yet more dimensions to the measuring of surgeons' performance debate and the need for audit.

National Confidential Enquiry into Perioperative Deaths

Another activity to which the RCS is committed, along with other medical colleges and faculties, is the National Confidential Enquiry into Peri-operative Deaths. This enquiry was initiated in 1982 by the Association of Surgeons and of Anaesthetists. Currently, NCEPOD reviews samples of perioperative deaths occurring in England, Wales and Northern Ireland and in the Channel Islands, Isle of Man and defence establishments. NCEPOD covers approximately 70% of the private sector, too. NCEPOD uses the technique of peer review – panels of assessors are chosen each year (and changed each year) after recommendations have been sought from the specialist associations. This is peer review of surgery, gynaecology and anaesthesia by doctors. The whole process is totally anonymous and confidential with the confidentiality specifically protected by the Secretary of State. It follows the long tradition of the Confidential Enquiry into Maternal Mortality in insisting on clear legal and logistic protocols for confidentiality.

As well as a rolling programme of sampling and reviewing deaths related to anaesthesia and surgery and scrutinising the management of the patients who died, NCEPOD is attempting to compare the management of the patient who died with that of similar patients who have survived similar surgery. The identification of these survivors (controls) is proving very difficult. Additionally, NCEPOD is randomly sampling all surgical activity (index patients) to develop annual pictures of surgical care in England and Wales.

The first (then) CEPOD report identified clear examples of failed surgical practice – operations being performed by inappropriate persons, surgeons operating outside their specialty, juniors operating on cases beyond their competence, inappropriate supervision and delegation. Apart from these lapses, there were clear examples of failure by surgeons to apply their skills correctly – operating on the wrong side of the body, administering regional anaesthesia and sedation without monitoring or due regard, and inappropriate surgery – the radical mastectomy on the woman already dying of metastatic breast disease is one example that caught the imagination. Problems in orthopaedic surgery, for long known about anecdotally, were highlighted – the epidemic of fractured necks of the femur in the elderly with multiple co-morbidities and the shortage of orthopaedic consultants and junior doctors to cope came out clearly. This report was followed initially by shock, but then the data produced led the profession and the public to acknowledge that more orthopaedic surgeons at all grades were needed if better outcomes were to be achieved. Orthopaedic surgery is now the fastest growing specialty in British surgery. While this is not entirely a consequence of CEPOD this audit did, for the first time quantify and delineate the problems of orthopaedic surgery and gave all concerned facts to campaign with.

The downside

'Audit fatigue' is a new syndrome that may spread epidemically in the UK unless we identify the early signs and prevent too much antibody developing. If audit degenerates into no more than a number-chasing exercise, and if no benefits are seen to come from it, 'audit fatigue' will set in. Locally, audit meetings need to be varied to fit the kaleidoscope of surgical practice.

Nationally, we need to involve all surgeons at different times and to vary the menu of audits. The RCS is endeavouring to do this by doing different audit studies in different locations, by spreading our initiatives through the specialties and most importantly by bringing all the surgeons in England and Wales into the action. Because the RCS is charged with audit in

England and Wales, it is our intention to give all surgeons the opportunity to join in and most importantly to invite them to be members of peer assessment programmes and working parties designing audit programmes. NCEPOD, an independent agent of the colleges, is following an identical embracing policy.

Continuing education: the feedback loop

No view of audit from a medical Royal College would be complete without a mention of the handmaiden of audit: continuing medical education. If the lessons of audit are to be learned and applied, optimum educational activities must be available to the consultant surgeon throughout his/her working life. This means good courses at good locations and generous study leave arrangements. Clearly the specialist associations will have a major input into this. The RCS puts the provision of adequate continuing medical education top of the new agenda. It is not surprising that other highly technical professions from which the public expect high standards go in for more formal audit of performance and provide continuous updating of professional skills. In our sister profession, law, the time scales for change are much longer than in a science-based profession like surgery. Hence, the law has not embarked as we have on audit and continuous education. In contradistinction, airline pilots, who can be compared to surgeons, have regular reviews and re-skilling.

Performance review and well-remunerated new training opportunities are needed urgently in surgery. We will need explicit methods of putting the findings of audit into practice if it is to be worthwhile; much better educational facilities for established surgeons remain a top priority. Some 15% of consultants in England and Wales take no annual study leave and most average only seven or eight days study time in each year. Yet surgery changes; without study leave, and sabbaticals, how can we keep up to date over a 25-year consultant career?

Hospital Accreditation UK: The King's Fund Initiative

Good surgical care can only be delivered in an adequate environment. This concept of environment embraces structures, out-patients, wards and operating rooms, the organisational aspects, medical records, catering, portering and administration, the supplies function, etc. These might be thought of as the stage set and the stage hands of the surgical pantomime – why else do we call operating rooms 'theatres' in the UK? Audit of these functions and the maintenance of standards for all these functions is as necessary to patient well-being and to the well-being of medical and paramedical staff as our audit of clinical activity. As part of the current drive to quality health care, the King's Fund has set up an organisational audit, 'Hospital Accreditation UK'. This initiative is led by a council which includes representatives of all the nursing, administrative and health authority bodies and also includes three representatives of the Conference of Medical Royal Colleges. Hospital Accreditation UK is setting explicit standards for the myriad of non-clinical and non-teaching functions of hospitals: it is inspecting hospitals and then advising hospitals on how they measure up to these explicit standards. This is an exciting project that should do much to improve British hospitals and, for the first time, provide an independent measure of hospital standards. This accreditation is not concerned with clinical or medical educational standards and is separate from the hospital inspection (for educational and clinical standards), which is the prerogative of the universities and medical Royal Colleges.

Conclusion

The patient comes first and last in every paradigm of surgical activity. We must empower the surgical patient to know more about his or her treatment and enable him or her to make rational choices about surgical care. The patient is the focus of a surgeon's activity; for this reason within the RCS audit initiatives we have included patient representatives on our audit working parties. At the local level some patient representation could usefully be brought into the audit programme, though audit must remain a professional activity to improve patient care. Surgical audit must remain the property of surgeons. The Royal College of Surgeons is created to ensure the delivery of this high-quality surgery to patients: audit and quality assurance are the quantification of surgical success.

References and further reading

1. Devlin, H. B. (1988). Professional audit: quality control: keeping up to date. *Bailliere's Clinical Anaesthesiology*, **2**, 299–324.
2. Devlin, H. B. (1990): Audit and the quality of clinical care. *Annals of the Royal College of Surgeons of England*, **72**, Supplement, 3–14.

These articles review the literature of audit in anaesthesia and surgery and are both exhaustively referenced.

College of Surgeons publications:

1985 – *Guidelines for Day Case Surgery*.

1988 – *Report of the Working Party on the Composition of a Surgical Team – General Surgery, Orthopaedics and Otolaryngology*.

54 *H. B. Devlin*

1989 – *Guidelines to Clinical Audit in Surgical Practice.*
1990 – *Guidelines for Clinicians on Medical Records and Notes.*
1990 – *Consultant Responsibility in Invasive Surgical Procedures.*
1991 – *Guidelines for Surgical Audit by Computer.*
1991 – *Guidelines for Clinicians on the Maintenance of Waiting Lists.*
1992 – *Guidelines for Day Case Surgery,* revised edition.

6

The regional viewpoint

IAN BOWNS

The general role of Regional Health Authorities

The National Health Service in England has 14 Regional Health Authorities (RHAs) and around 190 District Health Authorities (DHAs). Each RHA covers several million people, the average DHA has a population of around a quarter of a million people, though there is considerable variation in the size of each type of authority.

Managerial accountability

DHAs are accountable for their performance to their RHA, which are, in turn, accountable to the Department of Health (DoH). The RHAs have a number of roles, predominantly related to strategic planning and the monitoring of districts' performance. They have a general leadership role, and have traditionally managed specific services that are too small or specialised to be run cost effectively by districts. Thus, RHAs set the broad context for services and their development, leaving detailed plans to be developed by districts. Regions then assess the achievements of DHAs in achieving both broad and detailed plans.

The new role of health authorities

In the past, DHAs have been responsible for the provision of the health services situated within their boundaries. With the changes outlined in the NHS White Paper, *Working for Patients*,[1] now enacted as law in the National Health Service and Community Care Act, 1990,[2] they have become responsible for the health and health care of their resident populations.

DHAs, and Family Health Services Authorities (FHSAs, previously

Family Practitioner Committees), have become explicitly responsible for ensuring that the health needs, however defined, of their resident populations are met. The services are purchased from a series of 'providers', e.g. hospitals within the district, hospitals in other districts, regional teaching hospitals, community units, and mental illness units. In this context, the term 'unit' refers to a unit of management, usually corresponding to a hospital or group of hospitals, and not the clinical unit, such as a medical unit or an intensive care unit.

Health services, quality and medical audit

Quality is one of three major, and wholly legitimate concerns of health authorities, namely: volume, how many people are treated; quality, how well treatment is delivered; and cost, the sacrifice of scarce resources to achieve these objectives. All attempts to alter this balance are based on the assumption that there is an optimal compromise between quantity and quality, for any fixed level of resources. It must always be remembered that the relationship between these three factors can be complex. Sometimes there is a trade-off between quality and volume, governed by the inevitable scarcity of resources. Often, however, high quality is less costly, enabling more patients to be treated with fixed resources. For example, it is frequently the case that cases with iatrogenic complications are more costly to treat than simple cases and, therefore, the avoidance of complications is a large area where high quality costs less.

In the Government's plans for the NHS, great store has been placed on quality. Health authorities are attempting to develop *total quality management* (TQM), where a constant effort is made to improve the quality of all the activities of those working in the NHS. The overall goal is one taken from manufacturing and service industries, namely perfection in performance. This has so far concentrated upon simple, though important, issues such as waiting times and the quality of the environment in hospitals. However, health authorities see the introduction of medical audit as a major opportunity to improve the quality of medical services.

Medical audit has been defined by the Government[1] as:

The systematic and critical analysis of the quality of medical care, including the procedures used for diagnosis and treatment, the use of resources, and the resulting outcome and quality of life for the patient.

This definition initially caused some concern amongst the medical profession, some of whom felt, indeed some still feel, that doctors should have no concern other than for the quality of care. However, the Royal

Colleges[3] have also included reference to the efficient use of resources in their documents on medical audit, and the inclusion of some notion of economic efficiency is now broadly accepted. Medical audit is essentially that part of overall quality assurance that relates to the professional practice of medical practitioners. Clinicians, including doctors, increasingly have managerial responsibilities; the review of these activities is not generally seen as part of medical audit.

Most, if not all, contracts for health services will include reference to the presence of appropriate medical audit within the units concerned. Initially, this will only refer to the presence of adequate processes for carrying out audit. Later, this may expand, with commissioning authorities, usually DHAs, requesting audit groups and committees to consider various quality issues. Units and authorities will depend upon reports from appropriate audit groups and committees to satisfy themselves of the adequacy of the arrangements, and the results of specific audit investigations.

There has been little research into the benefits and costs of such comprehensive medical audit, but it is hoped that major improvements in quality can be achieved by the peer review of professional activity by groups of doctors, nurses, etc., working in isolation from each other. Indeed, much may be done by a specialty alone, although audit of most medical work benefits from the contribution of other specialties, such as the contributions of anaesthetists to surgical audit, and of the laboratory specialties to the audit of investigations.

Although single professions can improve their performance by these methods, it is equally certain that some improvements will depend on the eventual development of clinical audit, with multi-disciplinary professional groups. This has already been recognised by some specialties, and such audit has been carried out for several years in many units. It is important to foster these links, so that common concerns about the quality of care can be adequately addressed.

In some ways, these systems of professional quality assurance are seen as a counterbalance to potential pressures within the process of contracting that could place downward pressures on costs. If there is also pressure to increase the numbers of cases treated, this may only be achievable at the expense of service quality. A clear medical audit process that points out the effects of such pressures on the quality of care would be a significant mechanism for maintaining balance.

Medical audit: the region's responsibilities

The RHAs are uniformly of the opinion that audit must be led by the professional group concerned, in this case doctors. This is largely based on the belief that the group that is most aware of uncertainties about treatments is doctors, and that open discussion of differences of opinion and practice is only really possible in a somewhat protected environment. The broad aim of all health authorities is, therefore, to create an environment in which the medical profession is able, indeed enthusiastic, to carry out medical audit. In this regard, RHAs have a more strategic role than DHAs, although their interests are broadly similar.

The region's formal responsibilities

The basic, formal responsibilities of RHAs in relation to audit were outlined in the Draft Health Circular on Medical Audit in the Hospital and Community Health Services (HCHS), announced under cover of an executive letter from the DoH, EL(90)P/28.[4] These are:

- Strategic planning
- Monitoring DHAs arrangements for medical audit
- Advice and support
- Coordination of supra-district audit
- Facilitation of collaboration between DHAs and FHSAs.

Indeed, the RHAs had been given specific instructions in an earlier executive letter[5] released in December 1989. This was a letter of considerable importance, as it announced the allocation of £24 million to RHAs for audit in the HCHS for the financial year 1990–91. This was the first time that such a central, earmarked allocation had been made for medical audit in the HCHS, although it was expected that others would follow, probably for two further financial years. It was even hoped that the allocations over the next two years would be greater, partly because the current allocations were only expected to become available part-way into the financial year and, therefore, constitute only part-year funding. However, funding is negotiated each year between the DoH and the Treasury, and medical audit funds were allocated non-recurrently; that is, with no formal guarantee that they will continue in following years.

Allocations to regions were based on the current number of consultant staff, expressed as whole-time equivalents (WTE), working within each region. This calculation included academics and researchers holding honorary contracts, in recognition of the need for them to carry out audit of their NHS work.

The allocation for each RHA was dependent upon the submission to the DoH, by the end of April 1990, of a satisfactory *Medical Audit Implementation Plan* (MAIP). In this way, the executive letter gave RHAs a set of specific tasks to be addressed. These MAIPs are available from the RHA, by contacting the nominated officer that each RHA was asked to identify by the DoH.

Plans include reference to the following specific issues, as requested by the DoH:

Overall strategy

Regions were charged with the task of developing an overall strategy to ensure the willing involvement of every doctor working in the HCHS in medical audit by the end of April 1991. This includes those doctors in the training grades, who stand to benefit greatly from the educational process of audit. This comprehensive involvement is the short-term objective set out in Working Paper 6, on medical audit.[6] The MAIPs should cover the allocation of funds to districts, the intended formal organisation, links with postgraduate medical education, information and information technology developments, and the training and educational requirements to carry out audit.

It was difficult for regions to develop this strategy in great detail, as they remained unclear about future financial allocations and the costs of staff and information technology to support medical audit were, and still are, difficult to estimate.

Financial allocation to DHAs

Part of the MAIP had to relate to the method of allocation of these funds to districts, and the conditions which DHAs would have to meet to receive these funds. This usually involved the submission of a district plan, to be approved by the RHA. RHAs have generally allocated the great majority of funds to districts, retaining variable amounts, generally between 5% and 15%, for use on development work, on region-wide audits, or on regional and small specialties. Funds have been allocated in this way only until 1993; after this the funds will simply be included in the overall allocation of funds; the 'revenue' and 'capital' allocations to each RHA.

The funds from the DoH have been allocated to RHAs on the basis of the number of whole time equivalent consultants, including honorary contract holders, working within each region. Generally, regions have used a similar method to allocate funds to districts. In most instances, regions have allocated the bulk of funds directly to DHAs. Such allocations have often depended, in turn, on the production of an adequate district plan (and MAIP) from each DHA, which generally address the same issues as regional MAIPs.

It is likely, though not certain, that earmarked financial allocations for medical audit will come to an end. However, the Department of Health, RHAs and DHAs will all intend that medical audit will continue. This poses a major question, how will audit be funded when earmarked allocations are no longer present in the system? The answer is essentially simple; the cost of audit must be included in the price of the service. Thus, within the new 'commissioning framework', each contract must include clauses which include the presence of an effective audit scheme, and must also include the resources to support the audit activity. This is the simplest solution and it is not too early to open discussions about how it can be achieved. In particular, the transition to a situation where audit is, in some form, funded from 'general' NHS funds will be difficult. The arrangements may have to differ from service to service, particularly between designated 'regional' specialties (such as cardiothoracic surgery and neurosurgery) and small specialties, and the more common, 'general acute' services.

Regional organisation

A range of different formal advisory and collaborative structures have been put in place by the different RHAs. This partly reflects their different sizes and geography, but their managerial approach has been a far more significant influence. Some regions have relied on their existing medical advisory machinery, with its network of advisory committees based on the major specialties. The exact names of these committees vary slightly between regions. Other RHAs have developed separate audit committees at regional, district and, occasionally, unit levels. Most employ a pragmatic mixture, depending upon the size and dispersion of the specialties concerned. Most regions have adopted a structure that includes a regional audit committee, district audit committees, and less fixed mechanisms for the specialties to have an influence, both locally and regionally.

The draft circular[4] made firm recommendations regarding the constitution of 'local audit committees'. It was suggested that groups should be relatively small, and be drawn principally from those doctors who had enthusiasm for medical audit. It was judged to be important to include representatives of postgraduate medical education, such as deans or clinical tutors, in view of the educational nature of audit. In order to foster collaboration, local audit committees should have at least one GP member, preferably nominated by the medical audit advisory group of an appropriate FHSA. Furthermore, it was stated that, where possible, a Public Health consultant should be a member, largely because of their skills in assessing audit methods and results.

A particular problem that has not yet been adequately addressed is the involvement of NHS hospital trusts in the audit machinery. While it is clear that they will want to demonstrate the adequacy of their audit mechanisms, how they will relate to district and regional audit committees is not clear. At the moment, their accountability will be to the Department of Health for their financial viability, and to the purchasers of services only through the contracting process. How they will be represented on local audit committees, obtain specific audit funds, and report the results of their audit to health authorities is not clear. Regions expect the DoH to clarify these issues in due course.

Information and information technology (IT) requirements

There appear to be emerging two levels for audit, broadly defined as 'manual' and 'computerised'. In addition, the consensus, among clinicians and managers alike, is that the introduction of simple, 'manual' audit is the initial objective. Computerisation is not an essential prerequisite for effective medical audit, although it can assist in data collection, particularly for the more complicated audit techniques.

Medical audit is only one of a number of legitimate reasons for introducing more computers into medical care. Computers can improve clerical and administrative tasks, they can collect audit data, management data and resource management data, and they can include 'expert systems', which can assist the clinician in arriving at a diagnosis and deciding on the appropriate treatment. Where computerisation is introduced, it is sensible to fulfil as many of the organisation's information needs as possible using one computer system.

Here again the managerial culture in the regions has had a large influence over the involvement of RHAs in technical developments. Until recently, much of the NHS's information technology and computer skills were concentrated in RHAs. This is no longer the case. Districts and units are increasing their own, 'in-house', IT staff, and regions are increasingly divesting themselves of their computer departments. Without debating the wisdom of this trend, it clearly affects the involvement of RHAs in IT developments. This varies from region to region, with some RHAs taking a centralist stance and developing 'audit systems' for each specialty on a regionwide basis, others devolving almost all IT decisions to DHAs and units. The overall trend is to devolution.

There are already a variety of audit systems on the market. Most work on personal computers (PCs), although some are less tied to a single type of machine. Most are 'stand-alone' systems, which do not, or cannot, be linked to other systems, such as a hospital's patient administration system (PAS).

It is important to be clear that the information requirements are the important issues. It is all too easy to get involved with the computer system, which is, after all, only a means to an end; a tool to collect, manipulate, and present the data to the user. The most important decisions are about the information requirements, not about systems. The questions that should be considered most carefully relate to:

What information do we want?
What goes into an information system depends on what you want out of it.
What specific data items does this represent?
How are they to be coded in the system?
When is the information required?
How will data be collected?
Will they be accurate?
How should data be stored and how long for?
How will data be manipulated?
How will data be presented – tables or graphs, on paper, on screen or on disk?

If groups of clinicians want to compare their results in treating a particular disease, the important consideration is that they measure success in a clearly defined and agreed way. There are important functions for Royal Colleges, faculties, and specialist associations and societies, in deciding criteria by which to judge success, in defining measurement and coding systems, and in promoting such methods to the relevant professional groups. As long as groups of clinicians use such methods, it is much less relevant how they collect the data and which computer system they use.

Issues of comparability are of particular importance where there are relatively few clinicians in a specialty present on any one site. The so-called 'minorologies', a very misleading term, have particular difficulties in carrying out meaningful peer review. They can, however, gain much from audit with a related, parent specialty, such as general medicine or general surgery, but there are limitations. There is a need for such specialists to carry out audit on a multi-district, even a regional basis. This will obviously involve more travel to agree methods, and to meet to carry out audit. There are potential difficulties in obtaining funds to support such audit from any single district as this may be seen as a regional responsibility, particularly as this is laid down in the executive letter.

Regions have taken a range of approaches to the development and purchase of clinical information systems (CISs), a generic term for systems containing clinical information, which perform a mixture of functions, usually including simple administrative functions, such as the production of discharge summaries, data collection for audit and managerial purposes, and the generation of standard statistical returns.

Some regions have drawn together groups of specialists to develop a single system for that specialty across their region. An early example of this approach is the development of a system for general surgery in the Oxford region. Other regions have adopted a common computer package, including software and hardware, as a 'regional standard'. In some regions a belief in managerial devolution, and the importance of placing the development of audit firmly in the hands of the medical profession, has led to almost complete freedom of choice for each specialty on each site.

These differing approaches have their strengths and weaknesses. The 'centralist' approach probably keeps the costs of developing systems low, and ensures that comparable data will be available for all consultants in any specialty. It is, however, less flexible to local wishes, and is not 'owned' by every user. Devolution, while scoring highly on local ownership and flexibility, can be costly and lead to a proliferation of computer systems, which do not produce comparable information, and are not capable of communication with other types of system, or each other. It is important, when considering the need for comparable information from different hospitals, to remember that the important step is to agree on common definitions for the information required. This could, certainly in theory, be collected using different computer software and hardware.

Regions are also somewhat divided in their view of the overall value of computerised data collection for audit purposes. Whilst many leaders in the audit field stress the importance of establishing simpler methods of peer review and improving the quality of manual data collection, others believe that it is important to proceed quickly to more technological solutions. This question is more about the pace of development than its direction. There is the additional complication that the hands of audit leaders are being forced by the allocation of considerable sums from the Department of Health as capital. Approximately half of the 1990–91 allocation was capital, around £1 million in the larger regions. The DoH generally expected that the bulk would be spent on computer systems and, although there was some flexibility on timing, money had to be spent relatively quickly.

Links with the resource management initiative

The final matter considered in this area is the relationship between the *Resource Management Initiative* (RMI) and medical audit. The RMI is a central initiative, begun before the publication of the White Paper. However, *Working for Patients* included the introduction of the RMI to some 260 acute hospitals among its main proposals. This was in spite of an agreement with the profession that the initial six pilot sites would be evaluated before further implementations commenced. Fortunately, many clinicians are supportive of the RMI, both for the better information it should produce and the opportunity to have greater influence in the management of their units.

One of the central parts of the RMI is the introduction of a casemix management system (CMM). This is the name given to a large, computerised database, comprising individual patient records, relating the diagnoses and operative procedures carried out to the resources used. It is intended that this information is used to inform decisions about the use of the hospital's resources, in a new managerial context, where doctors, and other clinicians, are more directly involved in the discussions.

The two developments of RM and medical audit are funded separately, and have their own formal organisation and informal networks. As with most White Paper developments, they are operating to their own timetables, with little regard for the timetables of other, related activities. At several levels of the organisation there is cross-representation, to improve the co-ordination between activities.

Co-ordination between RM and audit is important because of the common information requirements. While not identical, the processes of managing resources and assuring quality are very similar and so, consequently, are their information needs. For example, managers, including doctors, will want to know about the use of laboratory tests. An important topic for audit will be the appropriate use of tests and, possibly, whether or not the results are acted upon. In addition, it is important for the care of the patient that there is a record of the actual results of tests, particularly if information systems are to be used to produce discharge letters and summaries.

Medical audit is different from, and complementary to, research. Research is, generally, about discovering what the best treatment is for patients with a particular problem. Audit is completing the circle, by checking whether we are applying that knowledge. This is not to say that the NHS can provide every service that might benefit patients, resources are limited and choices about priorities must be made. However, once a treatment policy has been decided upon, medical audit checks that it has been implemented and maintained. Audit can give clues on the effectiveness of treatments, but cannot replace the controlled trial and a variety of other techniques for assessing treatment efficacy. It can however, confirm whether the results in routine practice are living up to the promise first shown in the specialised centre. This is called the effectiveness (does it work), to distinguish it from efficacy (can it work).

A specific function of CMM systems is to monitor the extent to which intended patterns of care for groups of similar patients are actually achieved. A good CMM system can check that general patterns of investigation and care, e.g. the use of electro-cardiograms, X-rays, cardiac enzymes, analgesics, and thrombolytic drugs for patients with suspected myocardial infarction can be monitored. Clearly this information is very useful for audit and managerial purposes. It provides basic material for discussions about the quality of medical care and future service developments.

It seems self-evident that it is important to avoid duplication in the collection and storage of information held in NHS computers. There are many involved in medical audit and the RMI who are very concerned about the potential for such duplication, when two projects with such similar information requirements are proceeding with many problems of co-ordination. Again the influence of each region's management culture is evident. Some RHAs have taken a more centralist approach to the purchase of computer systems for RM, others have left decisions on the purchase of CMM systems almost entirely to each hospital. The advantages and disadvantages of these approaches are similar for RM and medical audit. Clearly the methods needed to co-ordinate the introduction of computers are different between regions adopting such varied approaches. Where regional control is strong, the region has more work to do, but the job is relatively simple. Where decisions are generally devolved, co-ordination must be achieved more by persuasion, and is managerially more difficult to attain.

At the specific request of the DoH, MAIPs should address these difficulties explicitly, even if they cannot state clearly the solutions to be adopted locally. Fortunately, the problems are being increasingly recognised, both at the Department of Health and within hospitals.

Manpower requirements

It is clearly recognised that the introduction of universal medical audit will have considerable resource implications. The most important of these relate to staffing, both the increased demands in scarce medical time, and the need for staff to support audit work.

A distinction must be drawn between the time required for those leading audit and the greater number who will simply participate. Leadership may require a specific sessional commitment, recognised in job plans. Participation will become another call upon scarce clinical time and it seems inevitable that some of this will be at the expense of clinical work. However, the adverse effects on patient care can be minimised if the current rate of consultant expansion continues and patient care is improved by the audit process. This has been one of the most difficult areas for RHAs, as the time requirements for audit vary dramatically between the different approaches to audit.

The requirement for support from audit assistants has been equally difficult to gauge. Perhaps two grades of staff are needed, one fulfilling very basic administrative and clerical duties, under specific guidance, the other having more detailed knowledge and expertise in data collection techniques, statistics and computing. Initially, the priority will be for the more basic grade of staff to support the manual types of audit. Even with this simplified requirement, estimates of need range from 0.05 WTE per consultant team to 0.5 WTE – a difference of a factor of ten. This partly, though not exclusively, relates to differing perceptions of the methods of audit. The lower estimate can probably be funded from the DoH allocations, the higher estimate cannot.

Training and educational implications

Under new arrangements, RHAs will be responsible for commissioning services for postgraduate medical education, with the regional postgraduate deans playing a major role. This places RHAs in an important position to improve the educational input to audit activities, and the use of medical audit techniques to identify particular training requirements for postgraduate doctors.

Important training issues remain to be solved, and health authorities have particular responsibilities in these areas. There are several key groups in relation to audit; medical undergraduates, who will require some basic training in the aims and methods of audit; clinicians who are not yet practising audit, who may need varying amounts of basic training in audit methods; clinicians leading audit, who may require training in managing change; and audit assistants, a new breed of staff, of varying grades and skills, who will need training in areas ranging from basic data collection techniques to advanced information technology. This forms a considerable challenge and the range and volume of training required is far from clear.

Other specific responsibilities

It is difficult to carry out peer review if you have no peers. Smaller specialties, particularly designated regional specialties, which are funded by Regional Health Authorities rather than districts, may only have one or two consultants on any one site. They are often characterised as 'high-cost, low-volume' services and, therefore, have only small numbers of cases to compare. This implies that region-wide audit activities might be important for these specialists and the doctors training in these fields. This can only be carried out after considerable discussion. Meetings will probably be less frequent than those for the more general specialties because of the travelling involved. RHAs have specific responsibilities to encourage, indeed 'ensure', that audit is introduced in designated regional specialties.

RHAs have been given, in DoH circular EL(89)MB/224, specific responsibilities in relation to designated regional specialties and small specialties. The exact definition of regional specialties varies considerably from region to region, and there is no precise definition of a 'small' specialty. In addition, the responsibility to ensure that audit takes place is open to differing interpretation.

Other responsibilities

It is important to recognise that RHAs also perceive other responsibilities not placed upon them by the DoH. They also act to some extent as representatives of the service to the DoH. This means that they can act as a channel to the centre for the concerns of those implementing medical audit. This could conceivably be on any matter, although the most frequent concern they have addressed so far related to audit has been about issues of confidentiality and concerns over the possibilities of litigation.

Audit in primary care

Until April 1991 FHSAs were accountable to the Department of Health. The FHSAs were given responsibility for encouraging audit in general practice. This situation changed in April 1991 when FHSAs became accountable to RHA. A final health circular concerning medical audit in general practice was issued.[7] This outlined formal arrangements for the introduction of comprehensive audit. In particular it recommended the establishment of *Medical Audit Advisory Groups* (MAAGs), comprising practitioners with experience in audit and representatives of those involved in medical education. Although practical experience of audit was probably more advanced in this sector than in the HCHS, the administrative arrangements were less well developed.

Co-operation was furthered by two developments: first, the cross-representation between members of local audit committees and MAAGs; secondly, the change in accountability from the DoH to the regional health authorities. This should improve the possibilities of co-ordinating activities and investments to make the most of activities in both sectors.

The rights of health authorities

Regional Health Authorities will have, as part of their redefined role, a responsibility to monitor the appropriateness of DHA's contracts with providers. Both types of authority will, therefore, have a legitimate interest in the volume, quality, and cost of services provided under contracts. As I have already outlined, medical audit is concerned with the quality of medical care. It is also a professional, educational exercise. However, there may be conflicting perceptions between clinicians and some managers, regarding the rights of unit managers, district and regional health authorities, to audit information, even if it is highly aggregated and cannot be used to identify either individual patients or doctors.

The DoH's circular is quite clear on these issues, and provides a way forward that provides an atmosphere of broad confidentiality for audit data, which should enable open, critical review of care by the medical profession, while allowing managers and authorities access to aggregated data about the quality of care. In practice, this will be achieved by regular reports to managers and authorities, outlining statistical data about the quality of care, and giving some information about the audit activity undertaken and the improvements in care brought about as a result of the audit work.

The DoH has stated that one of the functions of the medical audit machinery is to give managers the opportunity to refer matters of managerial or public concern to the profession for consideration. This will obviously be a mechanism to encourage the profession to tackle such controversy internally, by peer review. This type of issue would be referred to a district or regional audit committee. It is likely that the first issues to be considered in this way will relate to the quality of outcome in relation to the degree of specialisation of the clinician. For example, concerns have been raised over the quality of lower limb amputations when they are carried out by surgeons who do very few operations of this nature. This matter is potentially amenable to an audit of outcome, which would address the issue of volume without criticising individual consultants.

Conclusion

The success of the implementation of medical audit rests locally, in DHAs and, increasingly, in units. Regional Health Authorities have an important role in ensuring that the environment created can encourage this development. RHAs have very important, though basic, functions in relation to resource allocation. They also have a general leadership role in relation to medical audit, and may assume specific functions in relation to training, manpower planning, information systems development, the audit of regional and small specialties, and the co-ordination of large, region-wide audit activities.

The immediate aim is to create an organisational climate where all doctors can confidently begin, or continue, medical audit activities. Longer-term challenges are to establish audit throughout the service, to increase collaboration between the two main health care sectors, and to strike a balance between the resource and time going into audit and its effectiveness. Medical audit will be judged primarily by its effects on patient care.

References

1. Department of Health (1989). *Working for Patients*. London: HMSO.
2. NHS and Community Care Act, 1990.
3. Royal College of Physicians (1989). *Medical Audit: a first report, what, why and how?*
4. Department of Health (1990). *Medical Audit in the Hospital and Community Health Services*. Draft Health Circular EL(90)P/28.
5. Department of Health (1989). *Implementation of Medical Audit: Allocation of Funds for the Support of Medical Audit*. EL(89)MB/224.
6. Department of Health (1989). *Working for Patients, Working Paper 6, Medical Audit*. London: HMSO.
7. Department of Health (1990). *Health Service Developments – Working for Patients – Medical Audit in the Family Practitioner Services*. HC(FP)(90)8.

7

Medical audit: the needs of the District Health Authorities

HARRY W. PURSER AND JONATHAN SECKER-WALKER

Background

The publication of *Working for Patients*[1] in January 1989 and subsequently *Working Paper* 6[2] on medical audit confirmed the central role that professional audit would play in the new-style NHS. The separation within the Health Service of the *purchaser* and *provider* functions is aimed at developing a more consumer-responsive approach to the delivery of health care services whilst ensuring that such services represent good value for money. In the new environment of *managed competition* purchasers, through their *service specifications*, will exert considerable influence over the practice of such providers as directly managed units (DMUs), NHS trusts and the private sector. One of the central issues in the contracting process will be balancing the range and quality of care required by purchasers with the provider unit's capacity to deliver appropriate and cost-effective services. If the standard of service delivery becomes drowned in the noise of commerce then the National Health Service is likely to suffer a serious crisis of confidence in the coming years. The contracting process therefore, needs to be steered carefully along a fine line between obtaining the best value for money in a competitive environment whilst maintaining consistent standards of medical care. Medical audit is seen as playing a key role in ensuring that this balance is maintained in the short term and consolidated in the longer term.

Although the primary responsibilities of District Health Authorities after April 1991 are mainly concerned with assessing local health needs, devising appropriate service specifications to meet these needs and contracting with suitable providers to deliver the required services to local residents, there will be a continuing responsibility for the corporate management and performance review of all directly managed units. In time, as the NHS reforms gather pace, it is anticipated that virtually all DMUs will eventually become self-governing NHS trusts, and thus the arm's length management role of the DHAs will gradually disappear. However, until the NHS trust movement attains critical mass the majority of DHAs, in addition to performing their purchaser role, will need to retain a close interest in the contracting and financial performance of their directly managed provider units. In order to discharge this latter responsibility the key enabling force will be *better information* about the volume and casemix of the clinical activity, the resources employed in delivering services and the costs associated with providing such care under contract. Unless this information base is readily available neither the DMUs nor their parent DHAs will be able to relate income generated through contracts to the expenditure associated with the provision of health care services. The track record of the NHS in generating this type of information is not good, but with the advent of the contracting process a very major effort will now have to be made to devise appropriate information systems for the service and ensure they are consistently maintained by health care providers.

This dual DHA purchaser–provider manager role will require very careful implementation over the next five years. For the majority of health authorities up and down the country the volume of service generated by local provider units and the health care needs of resident populations are likely to form a fairly close match. Where demand exceeds capacity it will be for the health care purchasers to steer their providers towards more efficient and more effective ways of providing care whilst remaining within the cash limit available to the purchaser. There will of course inevitably be some relatively small cross-boundary flows of patients between DHAs, which reflect both traditional geographical associations between primary and secondary care and the historical development of regional specialty services, which tend to be concentrated at particular hospital sites. As time goes by it will be for DHA purchasers to determine whether they continue to fund such cross-boundary flows through contracts, or whether, in relation to regional specialties, they would wish to see the development of a more comprehensive local service covering all specialty areas. Such a shift in emphasis may prove expensive for any single DHA and it is more likely that purchasing *consortia* will develop in future to contract for highly specialist services. However, the typical contracting situation becomes considerably more complex in the metropolitan teaching health authorities.

Like many other metropolitan teaching authorities Bloomsbury and

Islington* has traditionally drawn a significant proportion of its acute services patients from well outside its own resident population. In 1989/90 some 73 % of the acute hospital in-patient episodes in Bloomsbury involved patients from neighbouring and distant DHAs. This volume of out-of-district workload presents formidable challenges for those involved in provider contracting. In order to cover 95 % of the acute services clinical activity that took place in 1989/90 contracts will need to be agreed with some 67 DHA purchasers around the country. To cover 100 % of the activity would mean negotiating with over 200 health care purchasers in England, Wales, Scotland and Ireland. The implications for Bloomsbury and Islington of this range of service uptake are far reaching under the *NHS and Community Care Act*.[3]

As a DHA purchaser we will have to live with the fact that our major provider units, who also happen by and large to be our local DMUs, will need to forge contractual relations with 66 other DHA purchasers in order to maintain their historical revenue base in the coming years. This range of relations could well compromise the amount of leverage the local DHA purchaser can apply to achieve the kind of service required by local residents. As a DHA with management responsibilities for its provider units and a continuing commitment to support high-quality medical education, it is a matter of considerable concern that nearly three quarters of the acute services activity in the DMUs is dependent on external contractual relationships, many of which could change quite dramatically over the next five years. This scenario is of course of equal concern to our strategic partners, the University College and Middlesex School of Medicine.

It remains to be seen whether the traditional patient flows from neighbouring and distant health authorities will continue in the same volume and casemix in future as the contracting process begins to take effect. Even marginal variations in overall referrals to the London teaching hospitals could have quite catastrophic effects on the viability of some hospital specialties, with consequent impact on the quality and continuity of service, medical education and research. It is Bloomsbury and Islington's belief that the key to managing the changes that will impact on the NHS over the coming years is the pursuit of high-quality value for money services. As both *purchaser* and *provider* of health care services we are interested in working with the DMUs to the point where they can

---

* Bloomsbury and Islington Health Authority came into existence on the 17th September 1990 following the merger of the former Bloomsbury Health Authority and the Islington Health Authority. The majority of the work described in this chapter was undertaken in the predecessor Bloomsbury Health Authority.

demonstrate unequivocally the *value* of the services they provide, not simply in terms of bed throughput for cash, but rather in terms of the quality of the *process* of care and, in particular, the effectiveness of the *outcomes* that can be achieved for patients. Medical audit is one of the central planks in our emerging strategy for quality in the Bloomsbury and Islington provider units and this chapter aims to explore the relationship between medical audit and the purchaser–provider arms of the new district health authorities.

Introducing medical audit

In April 1988, some nine months before the publication of the Government's NHS review, Bloomsbury Health Authority took a strategic decision to pursue the introduction of the principles of medical and clinical audit throughout its clinical services. This decision was stimulated by several factors, though at the time none of them anticipated the radical changes to the Health Service that were later to be unveiled in *Working for Patients*. The pursuit of the medical audit initiative was set against a background of chronic year on year overspending in the acute services amounting to several million pounds. This cycle of overspending led to a spiral of service reductions and deteriorating staff morale. It was evident that better management of the available resources was urgently needed, but the key to such action lay in the availability of timely and accurate information to support any joint clinical and management action, and such information was hard to find in Bloomsbury at that time.

The shift towards developing medical audit systems emerged in the early stages of work to develop an *information strategy*[4,5] for Bloomsbury Health Authority. Our existing operational information systems fell far short of being able to deliver the kind of information required for concerted action to address service and financial pressures. These first-generation information systems had been designed largely to support the administrative needs of the district for supplying central returns to the Regional Health Authority and the Department of Health. They had very little to offer clinicians and frontline service managers struggling at the sharp end to balance the inexorably increasing demand for service with a dwindling resource base. The clinicians, when asked to review their workload and identify where new service pressures were occurring, were consistently disappointed with the available information. Key patient-based data, on source of referral, diagnosis and treatment, were often either non-existent or inaccurately recorded on the main operational systems. This led to a loss of credibility in the basic activity information that was not conducive to any joint clinical–management action programmes. It became abundantly clear that a major initiative was needed to address these shortcomings. The development of a comprehensive information strategy was seen as the first step towards launching such an initiative.

Following a period of systematic study of the information requirements of both clinicians and service managers it became obvious that the key to better information lay in a two-pronged attack aimed at improving the existing administrative infrastructure and procedures coupled with a shift in the focus for recording key clinical information towards the clinical workface. This emphasis on delegating information management responsibilities to individual clinical firms was also consistent with the wishes of the majority of clinicians who were keen to develop on-line computerised databases to support their clinical and research activities and underpin the systematic audit of their professional practice.

Set against a background of highly centralised information systems largely servicing the top levels of the organisation, the proposal to devolve responsibility for key information management to individual service units and clinical firms seemed radical in the extreme. There were many misgivings expressed by the information systems community that the loss of central control over key data items would result in chaos. However, given the fact that the policy of centralisation seemed to have already created its own fair share of chaos, the risk of any further deterioration seemed to be minimal. Moreover, given the resource constraints then in force, it was simply not feasible to do anything other than pursue a gradual approach to this decentralisation of the information function. The tangible dangers inherent in any *big bang* approach to this strategic shift were simply not in evidence because there was not the cash to achieve it.

The overall thrust of the information strategy was therefore to improve both the quantity and the quality of patient-based information available to the organisation that would then support clinicians in their practice, audit and research activities. A subset of this information could then be used to enable unit-based resource management practices resulting in accurate patient episode costing and other service management benefits. Thus a partnership was formed between the clinicians and their service managers to invest in patient-level information systems that would be mutually beneficial both to those delivering clinical care and to those with a responsibility for maintaining budgetary control. A project was rapidly established to design and implement six experimental *medical audit workstations*[6] within Bloomsbury Health Authority that would be capable of capturing detailed patient information at the level of the individual clinical firm. Further, these systems were designed in a way that would allow them to be directly interfaced to the main operational and financial systems within the authority,[7] and ultimately become the feeder systems of a comprehensive *resource management*[8] system.

Work began in September 1989 to develop the first generation of *medical audit workstations* and as *Working for Patients* began arriving on manager's desks a number of clinical firms were already well advanced in recording their work for audit purposes on personal computer-based systems. The plans unveiled in *Working for Patients* further reinforced our strategy of devolving the information function and improving patient-level information. Some two years on we found ourselves in a position to begin bringing our medical audit systems in from the information periphery and integrating them into the core of new systems that have arisen from the implementation of the *NHS and Community Care Act* and the *resource management programme*.

Medical audit and the provider function

The operation of medical audit systems within the acute hospital services brings many advantages at provider unit level. Even where the introduction of audit systems is not the centrepiece of a modern information strategy aimed at improving the quality of patient-level information there is still a raft of tangible benefits to be gained. In this section we address *three* main advantages that the existence of an operational medical audit capability brings to the health care provider. Perhaps one of the most important benefits is the support of the *quality assurance* and *medico-legal* dimension of modern medical practice. In addition however, audit brings powerful support to the *business planning process*, and can act as an organisation-wide *diagnostic function*, capable of highlighting issues of efficiency and inter-disciplinary co-operation in the delivery of health care services. Each of these areas is explored in more detail below.

Quality assurance and risk management

Purchasers of health care will look to their providers in future for indices of quality of care which, up until the present time, have seldom been routinely collected within hospital practice. Medical audit plays a central role in any overall quality-assurance programme. Whilst the main thrust of audit is aimed at the systematic analysis of clinical care carried out through the peer review process with the objective of enhancing the quality of patient care, there can be little doubt that the effects of audit are more diffuse and pervasive. Although there has been little cost–benefit analysis undertaken to date of the value of introducing audit programmes we are sure that the very act of introducing audit programmes can have far-reaching effects. At the same time audit clearly has considerable educational value, and because in a cash-limited environment profligate use of resources deprives many patients of access to care, medical audit should identify efficiency, or the lack of it, in modern medical practice. The fundamental principle of medical audit is to set standards against which practice can be measured, to ensure that practice is altered to achieve the set standard, and then to maintain those standards consistently. Standards can be set by the clinicians concerned, specified by purchasers, or through the adoption of nationally agreed guidelines and protocols. The latter are likely to become increasingly common as the national specialist bodies[9] or Royal Colleges[10] develop and publish professional practice guidelines.

We have taken the view that there are two methods of collecting information related to medical audit and quality. The first is to provide medical firms with computer systems that allow them to collect data on individual patients. The second method is to congregate and synthesise data that are already collected within the district and to feed this information back to clinicians and at the same time build a picture to see whether there is any pattern to adverse events such as incidents to patients or patient complaints.

The data gathered through the audit workstations satisfy several quality requirements. Demographic details should allow accurate identification of the age/sex/ethnic group of patients receiving care and thus examine equity of access to the service. Clinical details include the admission diagnosis together with details of the various clinical investigations undertaken during the diagnostic work-up. At later stages during the episode the interventions that have been performed and the complications that have occurred are accurately recorded. At the end of the episode a final diagnosis is entered prior to discharge, and some clinical firms include a coded prognosis which can later be tested through follow-up out-patient assessment or through primary care feedback. This information describes the *process* of medical care and highlights the investigative and treatment protocols followed by clinical staff during an individual episode of care. Any adverse reactions, complications or other unexpected phenomena are carefully logged into the system allowing periodic cumulative reviews to be undertaken on the database that may reveal patterns of adverse effects that are not always discernible at the level of the individual case. This type of cumulative analysis is a central pillar of the quality-assurance and risk-management programme. When undertaken on a unit-wide basis it can highlight areas where changes in clinical practice may be desirable. Further quality issues such as the length of time between decision to admit and admission, the grade of staff carrying out operations and their degree of supervision should of course form part of the core audit dataset. Some index of the severity of sickness of the patient, such as the ASA scale,[11] will allow the provider to classify patients accepted for treatment more accurately than a simple diagnostic code might suggest. A patient with angina, chronic bronchitis, and a duodenal ulcer who requires an inguinal hernia repair is likely to require considerably more care, and ultimately to result in a more expensive episode, than a fit 25-year-old suffering from the same problem.

Relating diagnosis, length of stay, and complications to particular treatment protocols allows some index of the relative success of different treatment to be established. Adding data about the individual *outcomes*[12] of such treatment protocols generates a much more interesting matrix. Yet whilst length of stay and complications are relatively easy to measure, outcomes, with the exception of death and major disability, are notoriously more difficult, particularly if the intention is to examine every single patient episode. Further, the successful measurement of patient outcomes by doctors, nurses or paramedical staff requires additional resources. It does not come cheap. However, advances are being made in the development of subjective (by the patient) outcomes measurement devices which could make the routine assessment of individual patient outcomes at the end of an episode a routine procedure.[13,14]

Collecting district-wide indices of quality, such as complaints, deaths, patient incidents and hospital acquired infections, is extremely worthwhile. Not only is it useful to feed back to clinicians for discussion at audit meetings, but also it allows the creation of a unit-level database from which to start the process of risk management. In January 1990 the responsibility for settling adverse litigation against medical staff transferred from the medical defence societies and settled firmly on the shoulders of the provider units. Liability for settling cases brought against doctors out of unit budgets is further compromised by the Department of Health ruling that insurance agreements set by provider units against malpractice are not allowable. This effectively means that provider units will have to borrow from a central contingency reserve to pay the plaintiff, and then repay the money out of their operating revenue. This process will inevitably put an extra cost on each case treated by the unit, and those that are particularly prone to such litigation will eventually lose out to their competitors.

Provider units therefore have a clear need to identify areas of potential risk, and then actively pursue strategies to minimise any adverse outcomes. Plotting such events as complaints, patient incidents, hospital acquired infection, readmission within five days of discharge, unplanned return to the operating theatre and other indices of care that indicate where a patient episode has apparently not gone according to plan allows the provider to build a picture of where and when particular clusters of adverse events are occurring. These are often due to lack of protocols or operational procedure manuals, or simply lack of understanding and training. There are many types of incidents that are in fact precipitated by organisational failures resulting in human error. Medical audit therefore represents an important component of any unit-based risk management programmes.

A further consequence arising from the change in financial responsibility for adverse medical litigation is the relationship between doctor and employing authority. When the defence societies were responsible for settling the awards and costs of cases, the doctor had little or no professional accountability to his employer. Rather, the doctor saw accountability being to the patient and the GMC. Now that the employer pays the cost of litigation, the relationship between doctor and employer must change to include professional accountability. This will lead to the employer insisting on its chosen standards being met by all clinical staff. No doubt the audit process will be the mechanism to set the initial standards, and having done so, will probably do much to protect the organisation against the advice of expert witnesses acting for the plaintiff, as long as the local standards have been met.

We have no doubt that the existence of a well-developed medical audit function within provider units will go a long way to providing a comprehensive quality assurance programme and can become the vehicle to minimise the risks inherent in modern clinical practice.

Business planning

As the new world of purchaser–provider contracting unfolded during 1990–1991 an insidious cultural change swept over those involved in the delivery of health care services. Virtually every provider unit in the country had been engaged in the process of developing *business plans* for their services in preparation for April 1991 and beyond. Although the terminology of the business planning process had often jarred with the philosophies of caring for patients the majority of clinicians and service managers rose above this obstacle and ended up appreciating the value of the process in preparing their units for the challenges of the *managed competition* marketplace. One of the core components of the business planning process has been the SWOT analysis: each unit has tried to assess its Strengths and Weaknesses, and the Opportunities and Threats inherent in a competitive marketplace. Whilst for some units the threats have been to the fore it has become apparent to others that there are many real opportunities to develop services in the future that have, in the past, been thwarted by historical cash-limited budgets. Although under the new contracting arrangements patient referrals could no longer be guaranteed beyond April 1992, the possibility existed that some services might be able to develop and flourish if it was obvious that they represented high-quality care delivered in a cost-effective manner. The challenge was of course for the unit to reach a position where it could demonstrate quite unequivocally that this was the case. The ability to measure regularly the process of patient care and the outcomes achieved through treatment became a major advantage to any modern provider unit.

The business planning process in Bloomsbury and Islington has again highlighted the poor quality of the majority of the central information maintained by the health authority. Information on in-patient episodes, though probably correct in terms of overall volume, still lacks essential detail such as the patient's post-code (necessary to determine their DHA of residence, and hence who will pay for care in future), source of referral, and accurate diagnostic and surgical procedure coding. It was often difficult for particular clinical firms to arrive at an accurate analysis of patient flows and patterns of referral from primary care and other secondary providers. The questionable medical coding also made the interpretation of casemix analyses a process fraught with difficulties. If such an analysis can be properly carried out it becomes possible to determine how referral patterns may be affected in future by DHA purchasing policies, which will inevitably gravitate towards keeping relatively routine clinical work within local contracts. In the absence of such information it becomes little more than a matter of guesswork to estimate what proportion of a firm's clinical practice could be adversely affected as the contracting process unfolds.

The business planning process was however very different for those firms currently operating *medical audit workstations*. Here, the necessary information for business planning, and a good deal more besides, was readily available for analysis and led to the development of some very sophisticated business plans. In addition to supporting the SWOT analysis the medical audit systems were able to highlight the relationships with a variety of hospital functions, such as the diagnostic sciences and other clinical firms involved in joint care programmes. This information is of course also essential to the development of accurate costings for individual clinical services.

Such dramatic improvements in the information base available for business planning are a direct result of the efforts of the clinicians themselves in capturing the key items of information. Although each clinical specialty has its own particular information requirements for audit purposes, every clinical firm has a common core of data it has agreed to collect on every single referral. It is this common core data that can be used in the business planning process to arrive at the SWOT scenarios outlined above. Essential information on diagnoses and procedural interventions are entered directly by clinicians and ordered hierarchically to meet the requirements of the most popular casemix analysis tools, such as the HHS DRG grouper (Healthcare Knowledge Systems Diagnostic Related Groups).[15] It is this same information that is required for more global corporate analyses at District Health Authority level, and through the thoughtful application of modern information technology it is perfectly possible to draw off such essential information from the medical audit workstations for subsequent analysis within the corporate database. In this way the medical audit enterprise supports both the unit level business planning team and assists in the formulation of corporate strategy to meet the challenges of contracting.

The diagnostic function

The exponential improvement in the quality of clinical information that flows from the introduction of medical audit systems brings with it many unanticipated benefits. Not the least of these is a completely new set of data in NHS terms highlighting the key events and the reasons for any significant deviations in diagnostic and treatment protocols. For example, patients scheduled for theatre, but who in the event had their operation cancelled, have been a source of concern to hospital resource managers for some time. Existing Körner information systems merely record the fact that a cancellation has taken place. For audit purposes this information is wholly inadequate. It is important to record on the audit systems the precise reason for any unplanned cancellation. This information can be used to diagnose inefficiency, inadequate procedures and poor communications between departments within the hospital site.

Another example might be recording the point at which patients are considered medically fit for discharge, but for social reasons cannot be discharged at the present time. Such information highlights the inter-dependence between acute hospital services, community and primary care services, and social care services provided by local authorities. This is an all too common story throughout the NHS, but can become particularly acute in deprived inner city areas. Valuable bed days are lost each year through the failure of the various agencies to co-ordinate their efforts on behalf of patients.

For service and hospital managers this level of audit information highlights areas where better resource management is required, and subsequently provides the monitoring information needed to measure the effectiveness of any targeted action. The establishment of networked audit systems as a method of diagnosing organisational dysfunction should take firm hold in the hospital services over the next five years.

Medical audit and the purchasing function

The value of an organisation-wide programme of medical audit to purchasers, whether they be District Health Authorities or General Practice Fund Holders (GPFHs), is inestimable. These two sets of health care purchasers have quite distinct roles to play within the Act. DHAs have been charged with assessing the health status and health needs of their residents, and with developing an overall *health strategy* for the population with the emphasis very much upon maximising *health* rather than simply contracting for appropriate health care *services*. GPFHs, on the other hand, are not generally in a position to undertake such a comprehensive health needs assessment, but rather they are concerned with contracting for routine hospital services that are demonstrably responsive to their own patient's needs. Secondary care provider units therefore need to relate to these two groups of purchasers, and need to satisfy both that the highest standards of care are being achieved for patients within the agreed contractual arrangements.

All purchasers will need assurance that the *process* of clinical care meets the quality standards set out in their contracts with individual provider units. To date in the NHS the only indicators of *quality* that have been reasonably accessible have been *waiting times* and *readmission rates*, but neither has been easy to interpret. Given the considerable pressures the acute services have been under in recent years it has often been a matter of clinical judgement how long some patients requiring routine treatment have had to wait in relation to more urgent cases. The view can be advanced that waiting times may say more about the level of resources available to a particular service than anything about the *quality* of care that will eventually be received by the patient. Readmission rates can be equally misleading. Some patients do require a series of planned readmissions to complete their treatment, whilst for others the process of recovery is not linear and further intervention may well be required despite the best efforts of the staff involved.

As outlined above, establishing a programme of systematic medical audit within hospital units provides new opportunities to assess the quality of care, both in terms of process and indeed of the outcomes that are achieved for patients, which go far beyond the crude indicators that have been available to date. However, at the same time the operation of medical audit programmes raises some serious issues about the level of access purchasers may reasonably request to the available information. The current guidance makes reference to purchaser access to *the general results of the audit process* and clearly there will be a spectrum of arrangements struck between purchasers and providers around access to audit information as the contracting process takes hold. However, given that both purchasers and providers will be experiencing their own learning curves in relation to audit the issue of access to information may take some time to evolve.

In general, purchasers are more likely to place contracts for health care services with units where audit is firmly established and demonstrably operational. Since audit is seen as a key element in maintaining clinical standards through a period when clinical costs are likely to become very competitive it is reassuring to know that a programme of systematic case review undertaken by peers is in force. This is a powerful counterweight to the inevitable financial pressures and should ensure that standards in future do not fall victim to market pressures. Purchasers can also take comfort from the fact that the work of individual clinicians within a unit will be subject to regular peer review and any adverse findings will need to be addressed internally, in the interests of both the individual and the unit as a whole.

From these rather passive beginnings further forms of assurance are likely to flow. For example, within some provider units there may be a movement towards agreeing specific diagnostic and treatment protocols amongst groups of clinicians that enshrine good practice without sacrificing sensible efficiency. The introduction of such new protocols can be closely monitored through the audit process, and, if demonstrably successful, may be rapidly adopted by peers and ultimately lead on to the development of more efficient and cost-effective means of addressing particular health problems. These global effects of the audit programme may well be monitored over time by purchasers through such tangible indicators as reductions in length of stay. However, the very existence of an audit programme instills a greater sense of confidence in purchasers than might otherwise be the case. The availability of an annual audit report highlighting the progress, problems and innovations that have occurred during the year may be all that is necessary to satisfy purchasers in this area.

However, one of the key expectations of medical audit programmes that is likely to be held by all purchasers lies in the development of methodologies to assess the health *outcomes* achieved for patients. In the absence of any information on the overall effectiveness of medical interventions purchasers can do little more than contract for an estimated volume of service and attempt to negotiate a good price for that volume of care. If asked to choose between two provider units both offering the same range of services, but at different prices, it will be difficult for a purchaser to make a rational decision about which provider is offering the best value for money in the absence of any comparative *outcome* information.[16] Rather than simply contracting on the basis of *episodes for the buck* most purchasers would prefer to contract on the basis of *outcomes for the buck*. Unless medical audit addresses the issue of outcomes the fundamental issue of the quality and effectiveness of clinical care could easily become drowned in the noise of commerce.

The whole area of health care outcomes is of course infested with many traps for the unwary; given the inevitable pressures placed upon clinical services by the new environment it is perhaps high time that we abandon the search for the holy grail of an objective, reliable and scientific approach to outcomes measurement and take the plunge. One of the most salient questions here is of course who is in the best position to assess the outcomes of medical care? The answer, almost invariably, is that it all depends. It may well be the case that in the treatment of malignant disease the clinician and his pathology colleagues are in the best position to assess the eventual outcome, but the orthopaedic surgeon may well prefer to have the success of his hip replacement procedure carried out by his physiotherapy colleagues and his patient's GP. There are many conditions where the view that counts is the patient's own subjective experience of better health. Further, at what point should an outcome be measured? For many health problems the recovery period extends far beyond the completion of the hospital episode, and it may be several months before recovery plateaus and a valid measurement of final adjustment can be obtained. Despite these very real problems there can be little doubt that purchasers would prefer to have *some* indication of outcome, even if perfection cannot be attained in the near future.

Conclusion

This chapter has attempted to explore some of the relationships between medical audit and the District Health Authority, both as a *purchaser* of healthcare services for its local population, and as a manager of local *provider* units. It has been argued that medical audit plays a central role in maintaining the *quality assurance* function within hospitals that will become a key requirement of all health care purchasers in future. This function also moves some way toward the development of *risk management* systems within units, and this is an important benefit given the recent changes in liability for adverse outcomes.

The development of medical audit systems can also support what amounts to a quantum leap in both the quantity and the quality of the clinical activity information that is required for effective *business planning* and efficient *resource management*. Over the next five years it is our expectation that audit will evolve into a vehicle for the measurement of health outcome. These measures will inform clinicians, service managers, purchasers, GPs and indeed patients of the *value* of particular programmes of health care and allow the NHS to move away from its current myopic view of health care in purely financial terms. Clearly it is in the interests of purchasers, providers and indeed patients that the growth of the medical audit movement in the UK is swift and decisive.

References

1. Department of Health (1989). *Working for Patients*. London: HMSO.
2. Department of Health (1989). *Working Paper* 6: *Medical Audit*. London: HMSO.
3. The NHS and Community Care Act (1990).
4. *A National Strategic Framework for Information Management in the Hospital and Community Health Services* (1986). NHS Management Board, London.
5. *Guidance for Information Strategies* (1987). NHS Management Board, London.
6. Purser, H. & Secker-Walker, J. (1989). Exploring Medical Audit in Bloomsbury. *British Journal of Healthcare Computing*, **6**, 11–15.
7. Foundation for Information Technology in Local Government (1989). *The Model T Computer and Beyond*. London: FITLOG.
8. Department of Health (1989). *Resource Management*. London: HMSO.
9. British Thoracic Society, The Royal College of Physicians (1990). Guidelines for management of asthma in adults: II – acute severe asthma. *British Medical Journal*, **301**, 797–800.

10. Guidelines for clinicians on medical records and notes (1990). Royal College of Surgeons of England, London.
11. Saklad, M. (1941). Grading of patients for surgical procedures. *Anesthesiology*, **2**, 281.
12. Ellwood, P. M. (1988). Shattuck Lecture – Outcomes measurement. *New England Journal of Medicine*, **318**, 1549–1556.
13. Kind, P. (1988). The design and construction of quality of life measures. Discussion Paper No 43. York Centre for Health Economics.
14. Stewart, A. L., Hays, R. D., Ware, J. E. (1988). The MOS short-form general health survey. *Medical Care*, **26**, 724–735.
15. Healthcare Knowledge Systems (1989). *Yale Diagnostic Related Groups*. London: HKS.
16. Maynard, A. (1990). Whither the National Health Service? Upjohn Lecture, London: Royal Society.

8

Resource management and budget holding

AUDREY BRADFORD AND MICHAEL
DINSMORE

Introduction

Resource management was an initiative introduced into the Health Service
in November 1986 by Health Notice HN(86)34 and followed from the
earlier Griffiths Inquiry (DHSS 1983) which introduced general management into hospitals recommending that ' ... each unit develops management budgets, which involve clinicians and relate workload and service
objectives to financial and manpower allocations'.[1] Resource management
(RM) was a departure from earlier experiments focusing on clinical
budgeting, which demonstrated that whilst important, understanding how
much things cost is only one aspect of the resources needed to deliver high-
quality, cost-effective care and treatment.

Resource management is concerned with involving doctors and nurses
in management of clinical services. In an organisation whose core business
is the provision of health care, it is the decisions doctors and nurses make
about the treatment and care of patients that commit resources. It is often
said the most expensive piece of equipment in any hospital is the pen of the
doctor or nurse. To be effective any new management arrangements must
be capable of keeping the pen under control! What better way to do this
than having those using them actively involved in the management process
and accountable for the consequences of their decisions. Balancing the
unlimited demand for health care against a limited budget requires difficult
and complex decisions. Since the nature of those decisions will inevitably
impact on services to patients it is critical that doctors, nurses and other
health care professionals are involved in the management process.

Resource management

Resource management and the Community Care Act 1990

The NHS and Community Care Act 1990 introduced the concept of an internal market for the provision of health care and services. Funds within the NHS will flow through contracts agreed between purchasing health authorities and GP fundholders and provider hospitals.

The advent of the contracting process directly links income to the quality and volume of service delivered reinforcing the importance of involving those who provide the services in the management process. This development has introduced a new critical dimension to the management arrangements of all hospitals and one could be forgiven for thinking that whoever drafted the statement of principles in HN(86)34 did so in the knowledge of the reforms enacted from 1st April 1991.

The six pilot sites

Six acute hospital pilot sites were identified to develop the resource management initiative (Huddersfield Royal Infirmary, Freeman Hospital Newcastle, Pilgrim Hospital Boston, Royal Hampshire Winchester, Guy's Hospital and Arrowe Park in the Wirral). During 1989 a preliminary evaluation of the progress of the six sites was published.[2] The report suggested that:

1. Resource management gave the best opportunity to solve the knowledge gap on lack of information about treatment costs.
2. Resource management would encourage the active involvement of service providers in management.
3. Resource management would improve the limited confidence of those providing the service in the clinical activity data.

The evaluation also revealed that although a common feature of resource management developments was a 'bottom-up' approach to organisational development the detailed management arrangements in each of the pilot sites were different, reflecting the local cultures, problems and objectives and different starting points in relation to information systems and the involvement of doctors and nurses in management. These factors had also influenced the rate of progress within each site. It is significant that after three years each of the sites acknowledged that there remained a significant proportion of organisational and information system development to be undertaken, clearly demonstrating the scale and complexity of the programme of change required.

Based on the conclusions of the 1989 preliminary evaluation and in view of the information and organisational developments necessary for hospitals, to plan, negotiate, monitor and deliver service agreements, the Department of Health accelerated its plan to 'roll-out' the resource management initiative. The roll out would end when resource management had been implemented in most sizeable acute hospitals, subject to the continuing availability of centrally provided project funds.

Resource management – an opportunity not to be missed

The development and implementation of RM should be regarded by every hospital as a major opportunity to achieve improved patient services. Designation as a RM site does not automatically lead to improved services, nor does the installation of computer systems. Whilst the supporting information systems (casemix and nursing information) are a key feature, it is fundamental to recognise that the primary aim of the development is to bring about organisational change resulting in the greater involvement of doctors and nurses in management. This represents a major cultural change. Unlike previous health service re-organisations, resource management is the first change mainly concerned with service providers.

In common with all change, individuals, professional groups and managers from all levels within the organisation may feel threatened by and be resistant to the changes. This should be recognised and all aspects of the change process require careful planning over a realistic timescale with each stage skilfully managed. There is no right or wrong solution to implementing resource management. A set of management arrangements that are right for one hospital may not be appropriate for another. What is important is that the new management arrangements have the commitment from those involved and enable the hospital to achieve its objectives effectively and efficiently.

Significant benefits will be gained through the inclusion of those who are expected to be involved in the future management of the unit in the development of the new arrangements. From the clinician's point of view this involvement will, at the earliest stage of the implementation of resource management, raise the issue of the loss of clinical time. This is a real issue and cannot be avoided. Some possible remedies are discussed later in the chapter.

Clinical directorates

Whilst it is important that each hospital develops its own approach to resource management implementation there are certain characteristics common to all models. One such characteristic is the division of the hospital into management units based on clinical activity. These 'units' may be known as *clinical directorates* and are normally headed by a consultant from within the specialty, although there are examples of nurses who have taken on this role.

The introduction of service contracts for each clinical specialty will have a significant influence on the future shape and content of the clinical directorates, as they are now the business centres of the hospital through which the majority of revenue will be earned. The addition of this dimension to the pure RM role places the directorates in an even more crucial position and it is vital that the management arrangements and support are geared accordingly.

Impact of the internal market

Experience to date suggests that as the '*internal market*' matures, there will be a rapid progression from the basic block contract to the more closely defined cost and volume and cost per case contract. Consequently, there will be a separate set of contracts within each clinical specialty for individual procedures and conditions relating to purchasing health authorities and GP fundholders. The aggregate income of these contracts will form the base line budget for the specialty. It is logical, therefore, to structure the directorates to be co-terminus with the service contracts for each specialty. A large acute district general hospital may well have up to 15 'bed holding' directorates, e.g. general surgery, ENT, ophthalmology, general medicine, traumatic and orthopaedic surgery, etc. or several similar specialties may be grouped into one directorate, e.g. surgical specialties, obstetrics and child health.

Support services

A review of the relationships between the directorates and support departments is another important element of resource management implementation. The demands made by front-line clinical departments on physiotherapy, occupational therapy, medical physics, dietetics and hotel services amongst others need to be understood with an explicit agreement about the volume of service, quality and cost.

There are many services to be considered under this heading each with special features which influence where the department might feature within the revised management arrangements. For example, should theatres or intensive therapy units (ITUs) have their own management arrangements, be directorates, or be included within a surgical directorate? How should anaesthetics be organised – is it a service department or a clinical specialty? Should pathology be a single directorate or divided into the specialist areas? Should medical records be a central service or devolved to individual directorates? Should paramedical functions be included in directorates or managed separately?

The questions posed and solutions developed will vary from hospital to hospital. As with the grouping of the clinical specialties there is no right or wrong model. The most important characteristic is that the model is appropriate for the hospital concerned recognising its culture, strengths, weaknesses and the need to achieve organisational objectives efficiently and effectively.

Clinical directorates and corporate management

Having defined the structure at directorate/service department level, their links into the corporate management of the hospital must also be considered. Experience from the six pilot sites demonstrates the different approaches reinforcing the individuality of resource management arrangements. The starting point is that each directorate/service should have a recognised head, the Head of Department, Clinical Director, or Clinical Co-ordinator who must be involved in the top-level management board of the hospital. At this level each board member will be contributing to and influencing the future vision of the organisation, developing policy, determining strategic business planning in addition to playing their part in the resolution of operational problems. Following on from the principle that each clinical directorate will be co-terminus with a clinical service contract a possible pattern of organisation is depicted in Figure 8.1.

With this approach the size of the hospital management board, with potentially 20 plus members, is in classical management terms too large a meeting to manage and reach conclusions. Moreover, unless the diagnostic, paramedical, hotel and other support services are included in the clinical directorates they will not be an integral part of the top-level management process. This may pose problems for the 'ownership' of corporate strategy and policy and have a detrimental impact on the commitment of the whole organisation to their achievement. To deal with this, one solution would be

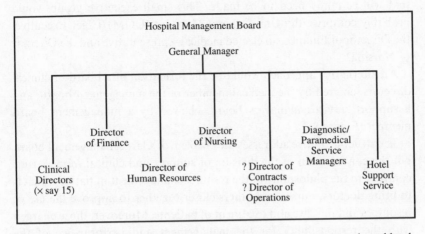

Fig. 8.1. Management arrangements to include clinical directorates at board level.

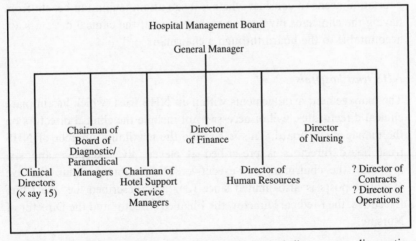

Fig. 8.2. Management arrangements to include clinical directorates, diagnostic, paramedical, hotel and other support services at board level.

to give directorate status to the support services either individually or grouped, with the director serving on the board (Figure 8.2).

Whilst the structure depicted in Figure 8.2 would exacerbate the numbers problem the advantages from having the 'full' involvement of the whole organisation at this management level may far outweigh the overhead of managing a large meeting. With either structure it is inevitable that a small number of board members will be empowered to take the 'quick decisions' that will certainly need to be made. This small executive group would probably comprise the Unit General Manager (UGM)/Chief Executive, the Director of Finance, an elected medical representative and the Director of Nursing.

An alternative approach would be the formation of a board of clinical directors, chaired by the medical member of the management board, and a support services managers board, chaired by a management board member (Figure 8.3).

The structure above addresses the problem of a large management board but the continuation of the division of support and clinical services runs contrary to the philosophy of the resource management initiative which is to bring doctors, nurses and others closer together to improve the use of resources and the care and treatment of patients. Moreover, those charged with the responsibility for the management and performance of the 'business centres' of the hospital will be one step removed from the body responsible for the corporate management. In this situation the organisation needs to consider whether it can attain maximum benefit from having the clinicians involved in management if the clinical directors are accountable to the board through a chairman.

NHS trust hospitals

The management arrangements within an NHS trust, which has in place clinical directorates, will of necessity not include the clinical directors on the management board. This is because the maximum number of NHS trust board directors is prescribed at eleven, five executive and six, including the chairman, non-executive. The flexibility within the five executive posts is also limited since four are prescribed, i.e. the Chief Executive, the Medical Director, the Finance Director and the Director of Nursing.

No right or wrong solutions

The final decision on the arrangements to be implemented will be particular to each hospital, reflecting its own culture and objectives. Once the organisational structure is agreed it is essential that the boundaries, scope and functional content of each directorate and support service department are clearly understood and defined. This will facilitate the development of a clear scheme of delegation, role specifications, job descriptions and a set of rules to deal with the relationships between directorates and support departments. These 'house rules' should be loose enough to enable an

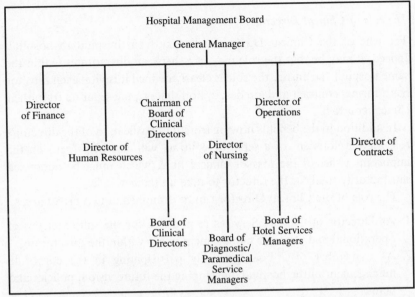

Fig. 8.3. Management arrangements with hospital board supported by a Board of Clinical Directors and a Board of Service Managers.

imaginative and innovative dimension to the organisational culture to develop and at the same time be tight enough to ensure objectives are achieved.

The continuation of the '*cogwheel*' advisory arrangements will inevitably be brought into question as it is probable there will be considerable duplication between the issues addressed within the clinical directorates and the specialty divisions.

Clinical Directors

Appointment of Clinical Directors

The role of Clinical Director is undoubtedly a difficult one. To have any prospect of succeeding the director must have the support of clinical colleagues and be acceptable to the General Manager.

Providing continuity for director appointments is also important. Contracts with varying tenure for the initial appointments will ensure clinical directors do not all step down at the same time. If possible the successor directors should be identified well in advance to allow a period of overlap and handover and for training and development needs to be identified and addressed.

The role of Clinical Director

The role of the Clinical Director will vary from hospital to hospital. Indeed, it may be that the role may vary between directorates within the same hospital. To ensure the role is clearly defined it is vital each director has a formal contract and job description that is quite separate from their clinical contract.

In addition to the benefits flowing from the clarification of the director's role the development of a separate contract will also help focus on the important issue, of the loss of clinical time, which must be addressed satisfactorily to allow the director to take up the new role.

The role of the Clinical Director can be examined in two broad areas:

1. As Director of Clinical Services responsible for the full spectrum of operational and strategic management issues within the directorate.
2. As a member of a board actively participating in the corporate management of the hospital, developing the future vision, policies and plans.

Each area of involvement will require different knowledge, skills and support. It is important that the training and development required to overcome knowledge and skill gaps are identified as soon as possible to enable the preparation of a tailored training and development plan. Training all groups of staff to work effectively in the new organisation requires considerable guidance and development. This was recognised as one of the weaknesses of early implementations and sites now have larger financial allocations to assist them and are encouraged to place a greater emphasis on training. Most project teams implementing resource management include a training specialist to advise and develop training programmes.

As the Director of Clinical Services:

The role as Director of Clinical Services will evolve over time reflecting the special characteristics of the hospital, the organisational objectives to be achieved and changes in the environment. Experience has shown the timescale involved is years rather than months and an evolutionary rather than a revolutionary approach will enable a smooth change with minimum trauma.

The areas of responsibility can be classified into:

1. Budgetary
2. Organisational

3. Management processes
4. Service/business planning
5. Contracts for clinical services
6. Communications
7. Quality, including medical audit

Against this demanding range of responsibilities the Clinical Director will have a limited amount of time to devote to the management of the Directorate. The NHS Management Executive publication *Personnel Issues* (July 1990) states that' … lead consultants spend the equivalent of one or two sessions a week on their management role and will expect further involvement when medical audit is firmly established'.[3]

Clearly the Director will need managerial and administrative support and many have a Business Manager and Nurse Manager both accountable to the Clinical Director. Alternatively both functions may be vested in one individual. Teamwork is critical to the success of any directorate. Ideally this should be built on the relationship between the Director, Business Manager and Nurse Manager.

Budgetary responsibilities

A key feature of RM is the devolution of budgetary responsibility. Traditionally, expenditure was managed centrally within functional budgets: nursing, pharmacy, pathology, radiology, medical records, etc., with no direct relationship to clinical activity.

Hospital managers were constantly struggling to balance their budgets without knowledge of changing levels of activity and casemix. The impact of financial constraints, imposed on functional budgets, often resulted in limitations on clinical activity that were both arbitrary and differential in their effect on individual specialties and support departments. For example, cuts in portering services, eliminating 'stand-by' time to provide a service geared to the average, reduces the flexibility to cope with peaks and troughs in activity or absence. This led to patients being transported late for theatre or X-ray, disrupting timetables, resulting in expensive resources standing idle and cancelled procedures.

One of the key objectives of resource management is the development of a better informed management framework within which the whole-hospital consequences of budget-related decisions, including those linked to service developments, can be understood and more effectively planned and executed. This will in turn allow the development of standards for patient services in terms of volume, quality and cost that can be planned and monitored.

In future, it seems inevitable that those involved in management within the NHS either as a purchaser or provider, will be faced with balancing an ever-increasing demand against a limited amount of cash. From 1st April 1991 the pressure to 'stretch' budgets even further, driving down unit costs, but at the same time maintaining and improving quality, increased as the 'internal market' began to operate. Successful provider hospitals will be those who develop innovative solutions to the cost, quality, volume equation, strengthening their position to retain and win contracts.

The driving force and expertise to identify and achieve these innovative solutions is most likely to emerge through clinical directorates. There is now a powerful incentive for Clinical Directors to examine the best way of organising their service since the contract income will flow to the clinical specialty and be a key determinant of the directorate budget.

For income or expenditure the long term aim should be that the Clinical Director will be accountable for the total directorate budget and associated workload. Budget reporting systems should be strengthened with information being both more timely and more accessible. The role of the Clinical Director as budget manager will be more effective if allowed to develop gradually over time. The early experiments with clinical budgeting demonstrated the difficulties in managing a budget without good-quality activity information to support it. A gradual development allows the supporting knowledge and information systems to be developed and ensures that the personal development needs of the Director can be met to allow him/her to carry out the budget manager role effectively. The pace at which accountability is devolved will depend on supporting information systems, the level of managerial support at directorate level, central support and the confidence of the Clinical Director and central management in the robustness of the new management arrangements.

From the outset it is important that the Clinical Director is involved in the formulation of each component of the budget and agrees the total sum and associated workload prior to accepting accountability. Initial budgets and related workloads will be based on the best available historic data and will be subject to adjustment in the light of experience and information.

The devolution of accountability and control should begin with the more straightforward 'direct' expenditure items, e.g. medical and nursing staff salaries, medical and surgical equipment, drugs and ward supplies. Building on knowledge gained through the devolution of the accountability and management of the 'direct' expenditure headings, other services can then be considered. This will embrace secretarial, professional and technical, administrative and ancillary salaries and wages as well as other non-staff items – printing and stationery, telephone charges, capital charges, depreciation and accommodation overheads. In addition to the direct expenditure incurred within the boundary of the directorate other expenditure, directly related to its clinical activity, will be generated in the diagnostic, paramedical and other support services. Is it realistic to have an open ended commitment from support services that have limited resources?

Consideration should be given to the development of a rudimentary set of internal contracts describing the base level of support service provided, with costs, for each directorate. Variations in clinical activity that impact on expenditure levels within the support departments would be negotiated and agreed between the director and departmental manager.

As the budget holder the Clinical Director is responsible for ensuring the delivery of an agreed level of activity, at an agreed standard within a specified sum. It could be argued that this is the most important and complex aspect of the Director's range of responsibilities. In reality, it should not be allowed to consume the majority of the limited time available to manage the directorate. Delegation of authority to the Business and Nurse Managers combined with short, carefully prepared monitoring reports focusing on variances, above or below agreed limits, will enable the Clinical Director to concentrate on issues that require their personal involvement and action. Achieving the budgetary objectives will inevitably involve an examination of the performance and activity of consultant colleagues to ensure agreed targets of activity, quality and costs are met. Contracts for clinical services, with income directly related to activity and quality adds a sharper more crucial dimension to this aspect of the Clinical Director's role.

Organisational responsibilities

As Clinical Director the individual will be the organisational head of the directorate with ultimate responsibility for both day-to-day and strategic management arrangements. Clinical Directors will want to develop an organisational structure for the directorate. It is important that any arrangements:

1. are within the context of the hospital policy and scheme of delegation;
2. are sensitive to any special characteristics of the directorate;
3. are effective to ensure delivery of objectives; and
4. allow individual flair and innovation to be encouraged.

A key feature of RM is the devolution of control, authority and decision making away from the centre. This carries a certain amount of risk, particularly in the area of corporate objectives. To minimise the risks RM hospitals will need policies and delegated limits within which the organisation will operate. These need to be tight enough to ensure corporate control but loose enough to offer incentives to stimulate innovation. Involvement of the Clinical Directors and departmental heads in the development of the policies and scheme of delegation will ensure the new arrangements are properly owned.

Although the Clinical Director will carry personal responsibility for the organisation of the Directorate, recognising the limited time available for 'management', in reality, a significant amount of this responsibility will be delegated. The majority will be delegated between the Nurse and Business Managers with perhaps other specialised aspects being delegated to other clinicians. The extent of delegated responsibility within the directorate should be agreed between those working within the directorate. Once individual boundaries of responsibilities have been agreed it is important that this information is known within the directorate and the rest of the hospital.

Setting management objectives for the Nurse and Business Managers and their subsequent performance appraisal is an area of work that should be personally undertaken by the Clinical Director. This is an extremely important aspect of the Director's role and, if done well, will do much to develop and strengthen the Directorate. Managing personal performance is a difficult area in which Clinical Directors may require training.

Responsibilities for the management processes

Again, although personal responsibility ultimately lies with the Clinical Director the majority of the work to set up and run the processes will be undertaken by the Nurse and Business Managers. Management processes include meetings and discussions with clinical and other directorate staff, to agree target activity levels, casemix, quality standards, and expenditure levels. These will be embodied in the directorate business plan, and require subsequent review and monitoring during the year.

The processes to agree and monitor clinical activity are now particularly important with the advent of service agreements. Within this area of work certain aspects will be difficult to delegate, particularly discussions with clinical colleagues relating to the volumes and casemix of activity undertaken. This may mean that within certain Directorates the time required from the director for this particular activity could be considerable.

To ensure the time taken is used effectively the process will need to be carefully planned and supported by accurate, timely and relevant information.

Responsibilities for business planning

Each clinical directorate will produce an annual business plan, for the period April to March, which will be aggregated into the hospital's corporate business plan. The Director is responsible for ensuring the directorate plan is prepared but the majority of the work is likely to be undertaken by the Business and Nurse Managers. The business plan should be understood and accepted by staff within the directorate to ensure its delivery. The business plan will normally be prepared on a rolling three year basis to coincide with the timescales of current service agreements. The first year will be described in detail and the second and third in outline.

Detail included in the business plan will describe the directorate aims and objectives, levels of activity, manpower profiles, quality standards, capital investment and associated capital charges, service developments, analysis of purchasers, budgeted expenditure, budgeted costs and prices, budgeted income, risks to income from other providers or internal factors that may impede delivery of contractual obligations, utilisation of support functions both clinical and hotel, opportunities for providing additional services, marketing strategy and teaching and research.

Once the business plan is agreed at corporate level, the budget and activity for the year is fixed and the Clinical Director is responsible for monitoring the directorate performance and securing delivery during the financial year. Since the business plans run from April to March each year, it is important to begin the review and planning cycle to ensure plans are agreed well enough in advance of the new financial year. The process is further complicated when it is linked with the timetable for the review and negotiation of contracts for clinical services with purchasing Health Authorities and GP fundholders.

Responsibilities for clinical service contracts

As 'business centres' of the organisation, it is through the activities of each directorate that hospitals will earn the income necessary to fund their total running costs. The achievement of contractual obligations will be a major responsibility of the Clinical Director, and a significant amount of support from the Business and Nurse Manager will be necessary to achieve this objective.

As contracts for services become more explicit, moving from block to cost and volume and cost per case, and purchasers become more specific about their requirements, the possible impact on individual clinical practice will become more of an issue. Clearly the degree to which purchasers are able to specify services will vary between specialties and will tend to focus on the non-emergency components. In the first instance those specialties with long waiting lists, e.g. ophthalmology, ENT, orthopaedics, general surgery and gynaecology are more likely to be targeted.

Given the nature of the unique relationship between the clinician and patient, the development of activity targets and costs may result in conflict between specialty objectives and clinical practice. The management and reconciliations of these tensions will be extremely difficult to achieve. Discussion with clinical colleagues, collectively or individually, in this particular area, will require the personal involvement of the Clinical Director and may be quite time consuming.

Contracts may be developed and negotiated by the directorate team or corporately by a senior manager within the hospital on behalf of all directorates based on an agreed volume of activity. Whichever model is adopted it is implicit that the level of contract activity and income to be negotiated is that described within the directorate business plan that has been agreed with the Chief Executive as incorporated into the hospital's corporate business plan. In addition to volume and price, quality is a key factor in contracts, and the delivery of specified standards is of equal importance as the more quantifiable volumes and costs. A clear strategy is required to satisfy purchasers. The provision of high-quality services will greatly influence a directorate's ability to attract additional work and revenue.

Responsibilities for communications

Effective communications for management purposes has traditionally been a problem within hospitals. Often this is a function of size and of hospitals providing a seven-day twenty-four-hour service. The creation of directorates goes some way to overcoming the size problem, which should make the task easier. Effective communications will undoubtedly enhance morale and strengthen the commitment of all staff. Key documents, such as the business plan, and key information, such as contract monitoring information, should be shared with all directorate staff. Good communication processes will ensure a two-way flow both to and from the centre. Directorate staff should feel they have a greater opportunity to shape and influence the pattern of service delivery and future plans, which should be regarded as a positive feature.

Responsibilities relating to quality and medical audit

As discussed within the section on contracts, in the market for health care, quality has assumed a high profile on the purchaser's agenda. If the market works effectively, providers who can demonstrate an innovative and positive approach to developing measurable standards and quality management processes will increase demand, benefitting from increased work and revenue.

Medical audit and quality are inextricably linked. The development of medical audit must be encouraged as a key integral component of the directorate quality strategy and action plan.

The quality agenda will broadly fall into three general areas:

1. Those aspects of patient care provided by clinicians. In addition to the elements of care that will be reviewed through medical audit, communications with relatives and general practitioners should also be considered.
2. Those aspects of patient care provided by nurses and other health care professions, including communications with relatives, community services and where appropriate social services.
3. All other, including the quality of hotel support services, the environment within which patients are cared for, the efficiency and effectiveness of appointment systems, and the 'user friendliness, softer side' of directorate activity.

The quality agenda is clearly enormous. Professional standards are the baseline with a great deal to be developed in addition to these. A great deal of the quality management function can be delegated by the director.

The role of the Clinical Director as a member of a board

Part of the answer to the question 'What's in it for doctors and nurses to become more involved in the management processes within the hospital?' is that it gives a real opportunity to participate actively in the corporate management of the hospital and influence its future policies and plans.

Whichever management model is in place, at some point there will be a board that brings together all Clinical Directors. This may be the top-level board of the hospital or a board feeding directly into the top-level board. Regardless of the position of the board within the organisation, the role of the Clinical Director should be identical and will be equally onerous. The role of board member will inevitably introduce new pressures into the relationship between the Clinical Director and others within the directorate. A key feature of the role is to represent the views of the directorate at the board.

The management processes established within the directorate should enable the Director effectively to bring together majority views and recommendations. It is essential that these processes are credible in the eyes of the directorate. Formulating a majority directorate position will inevitably involve ordering priorities and, in some cases, making difficult choices. Traditionally, these difficult choices have been made by 'the management'. As doctors become more involved in management there will be a shift of this tension into the Directorate which the Director may find uncomfortable at times.

Whilst achieving a majority directorate view is an important step, presenting and arguing the issues at board level will be equally if not even more demanding. The Business and Nurse Managers have a key responsibility to ensure the Director is well briefed not only on clinical issues but also on the 'business aspects' i.e. quality, price and volume.

Communication of the outcome of unpopular decisions made at the board may at some time present the Clinical Director with difficulties. The rationale behind the decision may need to be conveyed, which is important for ensuring that the motivation and morale of staff is maintained. The credibility of the Director and the board must also be ensured.

Whilst the board role can be described quite simply, the effective discharge of the role will require carefully planned management and communication processes, strong support from the Nurse and Business Managers and exceptional interpersonal and negotiating skills from the Clinical Director.

The time factor and remuneration

The position of Clinical Director will normally be part-time. The *Resource Management Process and Progress* report produced in June 1989 by The Health Economics Research Group at Brunel University stated that 'Directors generally report that they need to devote the time equivalent of two or three sessions a week to running the Directorate'.[2] This level of input was also suggested in the CCSC Guidance on Clinical Directorates produced in May 1990, which states 'The contract/job description should specify remuneration of the post, in terms of notional half days (NHDs).

Although it will vary from unit to unit and within units, it is suggested that an average of 2–3 NHDs per week be appropriate. Clinical Directors may (a) drop the same number of fixed clinical commitments as the NHD assessment, or (b) be paid for the additional NHDs as assessed, or (c) a combination of (a) and (b), i.e. drop some fixed clinical commitments and be paid for the remaining NHDs to make up the total assessment.'

It should be noted that at the time the above documents were produced, the impact of *Working For Patients* on the management time required at directorate level was difficult to assess. Early experience would suggest that the time necessary to develop and maintain the range of processes and systems to support operating within a market environment is significant. What can be done to enable the Director to discharge his/her role within the assessed time and keep the time lost to clinical care to an absolute minimum?

The Clinical Director's personal management agenda

The processes established within the directorate should be structured to deal with operational and strategic issues at directorate and corporate level, allowing the Clinical Director to concentrate on the corporate issues and provide the necessary leadership to formulate an agreed future vision and strategy for its attainment. Responsibility for concentrating on the delivery of the operational agenda within the directorate will be shared predominantly between the Business and Nurse Managers.

An analysis should be undertaken of the agenda to identify those issues that the director must, of necessity, be personally involved in, e.g. board meetings, directorate reviews, performance appraisal of the Business and Nurse Managers, and those that could be delegated. Clearly the quality of the business and nurse management support is of paramount importance.

Clear scheme of delegation

Having carefully analysed the management agenda, who has delegated responsibility for what needs to be clearly defined and understood by the individuals concerned and the organisation. This definition of delegated responsibility, and level of authority, will enable the setting of clear personal objectives against which performance can be reported and monitored.

Exception reporting

Traditionally, within the NHS, reporting on management issues has tended to be in the format of long complex computer print outs that the user has to flog through to determine whether or not any action is necessary. Following the theme that the Clinical Director must carefully plan the time invested in the management of the directorate, a scheme of delegation backed by an effective exception reporting system is required which should ensure operational objectives are delivered with input from the Director only when absolutely necessary.

The management processes should be structured to bring together the Director and the Business and Nurse Managers on a regular basis with reporting geared to drawing attention to variances, action taken, action required by the director with options, and a summary including an end-of-year prediction. The reporting will of necessity be both verbal and written and include quality, comparisons of budgeted activity and expenditure with actual, budgeted contract income compared with actual, extra-contractual referral activity and income, and a summary that should include an end-of-year projection.

The pressure on a Clinical Director's time will be similar to the pressure on the NHS – never ending. Strong support from the Business and Nurse Managers, careful agenda management, effective delegation and exception reporting will go a long way to enabling the director to focus the limited amount of management time available on corporate business and leading the directorate.

Information to support resource management

The resource management initiative has two main objectives. Firstly, to formally involve service providers in the management arrangements and secondly, to ' ... support clinicians and other managers to make better informed judgements about how the resources they control can be used to maximum effect' (HN(86)34).

Hospitals included in the Department of Health's resource management programme were provided with ring-fenced funding to purchase two separate information systems. The first, a nurse management system, is aimed at helping nursing staff organise nursing support to patients and to provide management information on the costs of the largest and most expensive staff resource within most hospitals. The other information system described as a 'casemix management' system, is a decision support tool to assist the management of clinical activity at directorate level.

Casemix management systems have evolved as the demands of managing clinical services have changed. Many systems currently available contain some form of contract monitoring facility and a number support clinical audit. The Department of Health issued a 'Core Specification'[4] describing the main elements of the type of casemix system hospitals should purchase.

One of the key lessons most hospitals learned from earlier information systems development is the importance of patient-attributable data for clinicians. Aggregate information on resource usage is of limited value unless it can be related to individual patients or groups of patients and the particular circumstances of their treatment. The Körner initiative was intended to stimulate information systems development.[5] For a variety of reasons many hospitals became slaves to the production of aggregate activity returns to Regional Health Authorities and The Department of Health, making the mistaken assumption that the provision of similar information to clinicians would be of value in managing their clinical practice.

Most hospitals have learned that such information is of little or no value to clinicians and are now developing information strategies that must be firmly rooted to the provision of operational clinical and support systems. Consequently, a casemix management system that will provide aggregate patient information extracted from operational and support systems will only be as good as the systems that support it. The need to improve the quality of information at every level is now well understood and is being tackled.

The key information requirements to support those responsible for managing clinical activity at specialty level are described in the Department of Health's *Core Information Requirements for Acute Resource Management* produced by the Information Management Group and Resource Management Directorate in January 1989.[6]

They are described as:

Patient identification and movement data usually supplied through patient administration systems.
Profiles of care used to compare actual treatment provided for individual patients against 'typical' treatment patterns for groups of patients. These should be specific to individual consultants.
Outcome measures, probably the area least addressed by most resource management implementations because of its close links to clinical audit and the difficulty of measuring outcome.
Clinical coding – the process by which all clinical activity is classified and which till relatively recently was implemented by a discrete group of staff

working within medical records departments and which must be regarded as the basic language for describing activity.

Casemix data – a mechanism of aggregating patient information into manageable groups.

Costs of individual procedures – information which in most cases has to be developed to support the implementation of casemix systems or more recently to support the development of cost and volume contracts.

Service utilisation or the use of supporting resources such as physiotherapy, radiology, nursing, etc.

Budgetary control is usually devolved to directorate or specialty level, linking the financial consequences of a particular volume and mix of clinical activity. The development of contracts means contract income will form the basis of specialty and directorate budgets.

Profiles of care, outcomes and clinical audit

It is difficult to distinguish precisely between the information requirements of audit and of resource management. Arguably, both sets of information requirements should be regarded as part of the same data set for managing clinical care. The debate about audit and clinical management information is, to date, still being held. Despite the fact that funding to support audit and resource management is routed through separate channels at national level, many sites are implementing systems that support both audit and resource management or are spending time developing a strategy that integrates audit and clinical management information.

Many resource management information system implementations have found difficulty in addressing outcome issues and logically this seems like a more appropriate activity for audit. Ensuring information systems developments meet the requirements of clinicians for audit also ensures that the data gathered are relevant to the way in which clinicians actually work. Any casemix system that purports to support audit must be clinically relevant, i.e. gather data relevant to the clinician and his specialty and provide the capacity to gather and analyse process and outcome information side by side. If the casemix system is unable to do this, audit and casemix should be developed as separate but linked developments.

Clinical coding

There are a number of clinical classification 'languages' – ICD-9, ICD-9-CM, SNOMED and Read. The medical term is the primary information carrier for all computerised clinical or clinical management information systems. Implementing any information system carrying clinical information must be done with the involvement and ownership of medical staff in the hospital. Within resource management casemix implementations one of the most important decisions medical staff should take responsibility for is the language for describing their clinical activity and the process for gathering the data. The process of coding the data once the classification system has been agreed becomes an organisational issue although clinicians are likely to want to play a part in ensuring the quality of the data.

The advantages of using a classification system like READ is its more expansive, clinically relevant language including synonyms, preferred terms, homonyms and deprecated terms or misnomers. Hospitals are still required to produce information in an ICD-9 format to allow regional and national comparison. However, adopting a more clinically relevant classification system within the hospital provides the basis of a more appropriate vehicle for planning and delivering clinical services and provides a rich data source for research.

Resource utilisation, costs, income and contracts

Managing a specialty budget means determining the level of service to be provided and the services required from support departments. Clinical Directors need information on which to make judgements about the support services required. Nursing, therapeutic and investigative departments have traditionally collected 'statistics' about their department's activity. The data they collect are in many cases being re-defined, ensuring that it is possible to define the costs of individual investigations or treatments. Clinicians should have access to information about the support services needed by individual and groups of patients. Most casemix implementations are supported by the development of computer links to departmental feeder systems. Information on the relative use of services coupled with costing information should allow clinicians and clinical directors to make informed judgements on how to invest the income earned from contracts.

Information staff and skills

Hospitals have had limited numbers of trained staff working within the information field. Medical records staff traditionally provided activity reports. However, the skills now required are more extensive. Information analysis and interpretation, management of accuracy and quality standards, and knowledge of software applications are some of the skills hospitals now need to be developing.

Clinical Directors are likely to have a number of these skills themselves but also need staff around them to carry out much of the analysis and presentation of information. The development of both the human and computerised aspects of information systems is likely to be one of the few areas of hospital activity expanding in the short term. It seems ironical but true that as funding becomes tighter hospitals need to make major improvements in information to help those who must decide how resources are committed.

References

1. Griffiths, R. (1983). NHS Management Inquiry. Letter to The Rt Hon N Fowler MP, Secretary of State, Department of Health, 6th October 1983.
2. Buxton, M., Packwood, T. & Keen, J. (1989). *Process and Progress*. Health Economics Research Group, Brunel University.
3. Chatfield, P. (1989). *Resource Management Programme*. Personnel Issues, Department of Health.
4. Resource Management Executive (1990). *Core Specification For a Case Mix Information System*.
5. Körner, E. (Chairman) (1982). *Report on the Collection and Use of Information About Hospital Clinical Practice Activity in the National Health Service*. London: HMSO.
6. Information Management Group (1989). *Core Information Requirements for Acute Resource Management*. Department of Health.

9

Unit and district information systems

MAURICE W. BEAVER AND TREVOR J. DYSON

Information systems for units and districts, are, in the terms of their functions, two different things. However, when looked at as a collection of data, they are only different aspects of a coherent interlocking of a number of systems, which deal with the same common set of data items. It is proposed therefore, in this chapter to discuss these two concepts as one, only defining a difference when this arises from a difference in use.

Information technology and its practical implementation is the 'art of the realisable'. The question is not 'can it be done?', but 'can it be done in good time without disproportionate cost?'. Current technology will allow complicated and extensive systems capable of serving any function or answering any question that an enthusiastic project board could conceive; however, most project boards work under constraints, of money if nothing else, so that systems as they are designed are a compromise in one or more aspects, e.g. functionality, performance, extent of implementation, etc.

Most systems are in existence as a response to a problem. They were not designed to solve that problem, they were retained for this purpose. The usual situation is that existing systems solved the last problem and have been adapted to deal with the present problems; with any luck they will do for the next set of problems.

This may appear illogical to a newcomer and certainly can be irritating to a would-be user. There are, however, good reasons why this situation should be accepted. It leads to 'bottom up' engineering, that is systems designed from tried and tested components, and it is a quicker, more economical and more flexible response to change. Much thought is given in the formulation of information technology strategies to the design of systems that can adapt to change and are capable of facing any challenge that may be forthcoming without the need to forecast what those challenges may be.

Hospital systems

A good starting point is to look at hospital systems. They have immediate relevance to medical audit for hospital-based medicine and they should serve as a feeder system for many of the systems associated with primary medical care. For example, a birth is the event that initiates a record in a child-care system.

Hospital systems have a comparatively long history going back nearly two decades. In North America they were developed as an instrument of financial control; in the United Kingdom the matching stimulus was the need to devise systems to relieve the clerical burden generated by the core hospital function of treating patients, and keeping track of this process and the consequent documentation. They also offered the promise of generating routine analyses or tabulations. This was seen as giving some promise of easing the burden of producing annual returns to the central government. In general, therefore, these systems had a strong bias toward performing a medical records function and as such they were considered as not only serving a bureaucratic function, but also satisfying a genuine clinical need. There is no doubt, however, that many involved in these projects saw a wider relevance. This relevance included clinical management, epidemiology, resource management and medical audit.

On the whole this promise was not fulfilled. The reasons for this were varied and included the perennial shortage of resources in the Health Service. The other important factor was the lack of the right technology. Computers were cumbersome and expensive. They were best suited to highly structured batch processes, an example being maintaining a patient master index, which they generally did well so that, where funds allowed, this sort of use became integrated into hospital management. In contrast, they were not very good at analytic tasks, particularly where the user wished to interrogate interactively the information held on computer. A few centres managed to overcome the limitations of the computer environment and persevered. As one would suspect these hospitals are now leaders in this field with well-established systems.[1]

Despite such examples, progress in the development of hospital systems was neither rapid nor general. The stimulus for their almost universal adoption did not come until the Government instructed health authorities to implement the Körner information system. The phrase 'Körner information system' is an omnibus term for the concepts embodied in a series of reports prepared by the 'Steering Group on Health Services Information', the chairman of which was Mrs E Körner. The first of these reports was issued in 1982 and the last, the sixth, in 1984.[2] Subsequently, the government took the decision to implement the proposals and issued an instruction to this effect (HCN(84)10) in April 1984. As the changes were quite fundamental, District Health Authorities were involved in far-reaching reforms of their information systems. It was quite clear that the proposals could not be implemented without using computer systems.

Fortunately, there were available a number of hospital systems as a result of the initiatives referred to above. As one would expect, and, in line with the principles discussed in the introduction, these did not completely solve the problems of Körner but they could be adapted to do a reasonable enough job. Such a hospital system had, by this time, come to be known by the collective term PAS (patient administration system).[3] This concept will be explored further in the next section.

During the last two decades, a number of other elements of a hospital information system have been developing, often quite separately. They can be summarised under two headings: diagnostic services and clinical support systems. Examples of the first are systems to manage the work of laboratories and of the second the so-called 'registers' which are far more complex than the title would suggest.[4] Implementation of such systems can be particularly extensive, especially in a large teaching hospital or group of teaching hospitals. Their development can easily become piecemeal if there is not an overriding comprehensive strategy and even if there is, it is sometimes difficult to acquire systems that are compatible.

Patient administration systems (PAS)

A PAS consists of a number of separable but integrated modules. The main components are as follows:

1. The patient master index
2. The in-patient module
3. The out-patient module
4. The elective admission module
5. The accident and emergency module.

As mentioned above, there are a number of commercially available packages with the above components that are in use in the United Kingdom. Most hospitals have some sort of system although there are many which have, for a variety of reasons, not implemented all the modules. In a large hospital a PAS is an expensive and complicated undertaking, both to install and to maintain. If the system is efficient and staff are well trained the PAS becomes an important and essential part of the hospital service. It is popular with medical records staff and makes a real, but often unappreciated, contribution to patient care. A recent, additional benefit has been that it has been possible to write software that interfaces with the PAS so as to produce data to manage and monitor the process of contracting, set out in the White Paper '*Working for Patients*', published in January 1989.[5]

The patient master index (PMI)

The PMI contains a record of patients who have received some sort of care that is recorded by any of the PAS modules, e.g. a hospital admission, an out-patient attendance, etc. Entry on the PMI will be initiated by such an item of service and if the patient is already recorded, new items of care can be added, that is, it contains a summary record of hospital care. If the diagnostic or clinical systems referred to above are interfaced to the PAS, then the PMI will, if required, record the existence of such events without going into detail. Also recorded in the PMI are such items as name and previous name, address and previous address, various hospital numbers and a district number, the National Health Service number, date of birth, family doctor, telephone numbers, post codes, etc.

The in-patient module

The in-patient module charts the progress of a patient through a hospital stay. It divides it into periods of care provided by different consultants and stays in different wards of a hospital. If the PAS is a true district one, it links together periods of contiguous care in different hospitals. During a hospital stay a patient can be located by making an inquiry of the system. The in-patient module is almost a 'real-time' system. Provided there is a robust and accurate method of recording discharges and admissions, the computer (or computers) will give a picture that is correct to within an hour during the day and within a few hours at night.

At the end of the period of care under a particular consultant, the usual practice is for the coding clerks in the medical records department to take the discharge summary and enter, in coded form, the diagnoses and procedures that have been carried out. The codes used for diagnoses are those in the *International Classification of Disease*, currently the ninth revision, and for procedures, the classification provided by the *Office of Population Census and Surveys*, currently the fourth revision. The process of coding is assisted by the PAS, which holds, as computer files, copies of both these coding systems.

The out-patient module

Originally this module was designed as a scheduling appointments system, capable of producing simple aggregate statistics. It was adapted to meet the Körner requirements and, currently, there have been the additional needs of contracting. Contracting requires the person who receives an item of service to be identified and for the cost to be allocated to a particular contract. It is important, therefore, that the patient is correctly and unambiguously identified, that his/her permanent address, including post-code, is known and that there is an up-to-date record of the patient's general practitioner. The details of the general practitioner should include the identity of the practice so that there should be no confusion should the patient be referred by another doctor in the practice or by a locum.

The NHS current policy is that in 1993 some clinical details should be added to the out-patient computer record. This will be quite a difficult undertaking. At present there is no clear doctrine on what should be recorded: it can be argued, for example, that people come to out-patient departments with a 'problem' not a 'diagnosis'.

As these systems were not designed for contracting, some thought has had to be given to how data can be extracted for this purpose. This question will be returned to below in the section on systems for contracting.

The elective admissions module

This system was designed to maintain waiting lists for in-patients and day cases. In principle this is not a difficult matter although the software design needs careful attention to detail. There are a number of packages available that fulfil this criterion. However, they have not been adopted as universally as other modules because of the differing arrangement for maintaining these lists in different hospitals and even within the same hospital. Although this is not insurmountable it has deterred hospital managers from implementing such systems. Another similar problem is that where consultants wish to keep their own lists, the system can be cumbersome unless they and their secretaries have ready access to a terminal. Although such a step is highly desirable, in many hospitals it would be an extremely expensive undertaking.

Again, contracting introduces an element of *force majeure* and, expensive or not, elective admissions systems will have to be implemented. Such systems will be necessary to give an analysis by contract and by reason for hospital admission. This can be done using file cards and pencil and paper but the demands of managing contracts will make such an arrangement impractical.

Accident and emergency module

The need for a computer system for Accident and Emergency (A&E) departments has been well established for over a decade. The actual functionality of such systems has been, nevertheless, a matter for continued discussion. There is a clear need for a system to deal with the onerous tasks of registration and recording attendances. This requirement has tended to dominate system design and, though most packages are capable of recording clinical details, the facilities for analysis are on the whole, fairly simple. This can be frustrating for clinical directors of A&E departments as they often wish to carry out more complex analyses for investigations, which have an epidemiological or operational research purpose. Attempts have been made to solve this problem by introducing general inquiry packages using some sort of inquiry language.

It is important to note that A&E modules should be fully integrated with the rest of the PAS. The so-called 'demographic' details, i.e. the name and address, etc., are already in the system if the patient has attended the hospital before, and only have to be checked for changes.

Attendances, like other episodes, will be entered in the summary record in the patient master index.

Other hospital systems

As described above, the other threads in the development of hospital information systems are those where the initiative came from clinicians. There are two main divisions to this group: (1) systems associated with the management of diagnostic departments and (2) systems that assist the process of the clinical care of patients divided into a clinical support system, a system to support pre-symptomatic screening programmes and a nursing system.

Diagnostic departments

It could be said that information technology in hospital started out in departments of pathology. Certainly, pathologists were amongst the pioneers and the reasons are quite obvious. In such departments, there is a lot of 'paper-work' which can be automated, there is a lot of machine-minding that can be delegated to another machine and there are a lot of repetitive calculations to be done that are best done by a computer. These functions, which are extremely manifest in departments of clinical chemistry, have their counterparts in other departments. It is not surprising, therefore, to find systems available for all types of pathological investigations.

Although there are common components, clearly there are bound to be substantial differences, and it is not surprising therefore to find a number of different systems on the market. This choice can be of benefit to the user, but it is important to ensure that any system that is acquired can be linked to and is compatible with the PAS. It should be noted that these systems can be quite large and in such cases, although they need a committed system manager in the department itself, they also require professional support by information technology staff.

The other field in which computer systems are beginning to be regarded as indispensable is that of medical imaging. The function within such a department is to automate the process of recording the patients who attend and the work carried out. Such systems lend themselves to the recording and analysis of the usage of resources. Again, they should be linked to and integrated into the PAS. Attendance at a department of diagnostic radiology can be entered into the patient summary on the patient master index. These systems can be very large and necessitate skilled management. Should digital imaging and computerised picture archiving be introduced then the two aspects should be integrated. A system constructed in this way is a major installation and should only be attempted after careful research and detailed planning.

Clinical support systems

These systems also have a long history. It is possible to discern two distinct concepts. The first is the idea of a 'register'. This is the situation where a clinician cares for a group of patients who need long-term follow-up and require standardised documentation. An example of this is a diabetic register.[4] This is a form of standardised medical care and the principles can, of course, be extended to other clinical groups and generalised to all care given by a clinician, i.e. the system generates standard letters and maintains a database for easy recall and for research. Again, it is most important that these systems are integrated with the PAS, that is the information which the PAS has is a subset of that which the clinician uses. The clinician can add to the patient record but there should not be two sets of the basic information. If this were the case they would inevitably get out of step with the possibility of subsequent arguments as to the accuracy of the data.

There are quite a number of systems of this sort available, but there is no general standardisation and there is little sign of it happening. The advent of medical audit has made the position more obscure. There is no doubt that clinicians are seeking more and more facilities in the systems and there is a desperate rush by software houses to produce attractive packages that will capture the market. The desire also for refinement in presentation, with colour graphics and sophisticated printers, adds to the cost and makes it increasingly difficult to find the resources for a rational development programme.

The other type of clinical care system is where there is an ongoing process that is recorded on computer as close in time as possible to the actual event. The archetype of this is the maternity system. Not only does such a system encompass the events of the ante-natal and the post-natal period but it is also used to record the progress of labour and its clinical features.

Another example of a situation that needs a 'real-time' solution is the recording of the activity in operating theatres. In a busy complex clinical situation, capture of data must be as simple as possible. In the system developed and in use in Nottingham each patient has a bar-coded card which is 'read' by staff using light pens situated at critical points of the patients passage through the operating theatre suite.

Systems to support pre-symptomatic screening programmes

The main developments of such services at present are those for detecting cervical pathology and breast cancer. These can be seen as an amalgam of register-type systems and systems that support diagnostic departments. They have facilities for generating recall letters and giving appointments automatically. It is very important that at-risk women are not missed by some quirk of circumstances or oversight and the system design should cater for any eventuality. It should not allow, for example, an individual to be deleted from follow-up without the explicit approval of the responsible clinician.

It is highly desirable that these systems are integrated into the PAS. There are many instances where such a design feature is extremely useful. An elementary example is the avoidance of giving someone an appointment at a screening clinic when they already have an appointment on the same day in another out-patient department.

Nursing systems

Something that is very similar in concept to clinical care systems is those designed for nursing care. Several packages are commercially available for this purpose. As the name implies, they are used to record the nursing care given to a patient. Some of the available packages are quite elaborate. There are perhaps two main components. The first derives from systems developed to match the nursing load on a ward with resources, in terms of individuals and skill-mix. This sort of function has been performed previously by systems that analysed data collected on a pencil and paper basis. Nursing systems collect such data by direct input to ward-based terminals.

The other function is to collect and maintain information on the nursing care of patients at the time when these events occur. This function is very like that performed by clinical management systems. There is so much common functionality that some health service managers believe that one should not use the term 'nursing systems' but instead adopt some omnibus term such as 'clinical care', thus emphasising the integration of patient care that is the essence of modern hospitals. As it is generally agreed that a ward needs several terminals, a nursing system can be very expensive to install throughout a hospital.

Systems to process and analyse data

The systems described above all support day-to-day functions of a hospital whether they are clinical or administrative. By and large they are not particularly good at analysing the data for managerial, epidemiological or frankly bureaucratic purposes. For this function several different approaches have been tried.

Following the Körner changes, systems were introduced to perform these functions. As they also generate computer tapes to send to the Office of Populations Censuses and Surveys, which provides a national statistical service for the Health Service, these systems are generally located at the Regional Health Authorities. They contain data on in-patients, captured on the in-patient module of district PASs, and aggregated data on a wide range of hospital and community services. Some idea of the extent of such data can be gauged by referring to the reports of the steering group.

Because of the complexity of the databases contained in such a system and because of the desire to provide a flexible inquiry methodology, most are written in a so-called 'fourth-generation language', a '4GL'. Fourth-generation languages enable systems to be constructed from a set of commands that are more akin to everyday language, one does not have to specify the process step by step as one has to do with a high-level language such as BASIC. This simplicity is only apparent, of course. Although it can speed up the process of developing a system, a 4GL has its own subtleties and problems. One of the problems is that it often adds a high 'over-head' to the internal processes of the computer and thus the performance can be substantially degraded.

Information systems for contracting

The most recent round of NHS changes embodied in the National Health Service and Community Care Act 1990 included the innovation of contracting. There are now '*purchasers*' of hospital care; these are mostly the District Health Authority where the patient resides. For certain non-emergency care the purchaser can be the patient's general practice if the members of that practice so choose. As pointed out above, the contracting process sooner or later requires the provider to identify accurately the people whom it treats and what that treatment was. In addition, the information must be timely: a hospital's cash flow depends on the facility and speed with which it gets out its invoices!

The systems described in the previous section have not proved to be suitable for this purpose and software has been devised which has better performance and is easier to use. An example of this is the Nottingham Health Authority's system MEASLES. This extracts the data from the PAS and conducts a number of standard analyses. The system is extremely robust. If the standard output is not sufficient it is possible to produce an output that can be exported to another computer system for more complex analysis. Output from MEASLES can be transferred to the health authority's financial computer systems to generate invoices.

The situation has been made more complicated by a central requirement for an extended data set. Some of these data items are necessary for the contracting process *per se*. Others appear to have been included because they are thought necessary for some vague but, as yet, unspecified purpose connected with the process of determining the health needs of the district. Also included are items that by common consensus have no relation to the contracting process whatsoever.

Whatever view one takes and no matter what strict criteria one adopts, changes in the PAS are inevitable.

Resource management

Another recent innovation in the Health Service is the resource management initiative (RMI).[1,6] The progress of this concept has been rather complex and has been overshadowed by other developments. An exploration of the principles is beyond this chapter. However, a facet of it has been the demand by hospitals participating in this development for *casemix systems*. These are computer systems that take clinical activity and associate it with resource usage such as pathology, radiology, nursing care, etc. The core component of such a system is a record of in-patient stays to which is added the appropriate *diagnosis related group* (DRG). DRG is a system developed in the United States that allocates one of some 470 categories to a hospital stay. Each of the DRG categories has a measure of commonality in that it concerns some specific clinical aspect of medical care and items within each DRG are deemed to use equal amounts of resource. There is a copious literature on DRGs, none of it particularly accessible to the general reader, who is referred to the work edited by Bardsley, Coles and Jenkins.[7]

To this *core* is added, for each hospital stay, data on *resource* utilisation of the services mentioned. These casemix systems have *front ends* that analyse the data and display the results in graphical form if so wished. The consensus is that this service should be made available to clinical managers. However, to provide terminals to the extent implied is an expensive matter as the computing power needed is quite considerable and terminals with graphics capability cost considerably more than the usual text-only terminal. Most installations are in the implementation phase, i.e. the core functionality is in place but the feeder systems are still being added.

Pharmacy systems

One of the resources used by a health service is drugs. Most hospitals have well-developed pharmacy systems. These started out as adjuncts to stock control and financial management. It was soon realised that they could be an important aid to auditing the therapeutic aspect of medical care. Most systems were designed to record 'issues' (of drugs) as being to departments or wards but if the original system design is robust and flexible it is possible to adapt these to function on a individual prescription basis. Such a move, of course, increases the cost and poses a number of organisational problems. There appears to be a consensus that this is desirable and there have been moves in this direction. Such a patient-based approach would have to be integrated with any ward system introduced, as discussed in the section on nursing systems above and in the following section.

Hospital information support systems

It should be apparent from reading the previous sections that hospital systems have been developed piecemeal. Following the publication of the White Paper '*Working for Patients*', doubt was raised on the ability of the information sub-structure of the Health Service to cope. The Government responded by instituting a programme of developing total hospital information systems. This concept, a *Hospital Information Support System* (HISS), was piloted in three sites and subsequently 'rolled out' to other sites in England and Wales.[8,9,10]

At the end of 1990, contracts had been let for two of the pilots. It looks as if the implementations on the roll-out sites will not be so extensive as those for the pilots. One of the problems is that many hospitals will have well-developed systems as outlined above and it is very difficult to specify and procure software and hardware that will tie all this together and make all the information available throughout the hospital.

One of the main components of HISS is the ward orders/reporting system. This enables orders for any hospital service, the exemplar being a pathology investigation, to be ordered using a ward terminal. Upon completion and authorisation the results are available by making an inquiry on a terminal, usually in a ward, but elsewhere if necessary. Similarly, all other data on that patient that is held on any patient-based computer system are available by making an inquiry using the appropriate procedures.

It is quite clear that this is a complicated and expensive undertaking, particularly so if the various 'feeder' systems were not specified and purchased with this sort of integration in mind.

Systems outside hospitals

District Health Authorities have patient-based systems other than those found in hospitals. The original community systems were those designed for scheduling and recording immunisation procedures. These were extended to encompass child-health surveillance. By the time local authority health services were incorporated into the rest of the National Health Service by the changes of 1974, many of these computer systems were very well developed. Data were collected on paper forms, input by data entry staff and subsequently batch processed. The only real disadvantage of this arrangement was that the systems were rather inflexible and the procedure for making *ad hoc* inquiries was cumbersome.

Since then systems have been made more flexible and inquiries are, on the whole, easier. The natural progression appeared to extend this approach to care provided to other age groups. Consequent to the Körner changes systems were developed to capture and analyse the work of district nurses, health visitors and other community-based health service staff.

On the whole these systems have not fulfilled their promise. One of the reasons has been that there is a tendency to overlook them in the queue for resources in contrast to systems designed to support hospital services. Another has been the lack of a centrally driven policy or vision for child-health and other community-based services. The changes in the Health Service have been dominated by managerial priorities that excluded an expansionist view of community-based programmes. What is, perhaps, a more obvious reason was that they were in the second phase of the Körner changes with implementation in 1988 and because of the demands of the first phase, took a back-seat to the developments in hospitals.

The systems in use broadly fall into two groups, those that are based on individuals and the services each individual receives, and those that just record items of service provided, e.g. one just counts the number and type of home visits rather than records who the people were who received these items of care. This second type of system is much easier and cheaper to purchase and implement. It serves the function required for Körner implementation but it will not suffice for contracting and does not enable one to link episodes of community care to individual hospital admissions.

The complexity of possible patterns of care makes it difficult to design and procure a system for community based services that is adequate for present needs and yet has sufficient flexibility and potential for development.

Mental health systems

The same problems arise when one looks at mental health programmes. Such services are amalgams of in-patient and ambulatory care. For many patients the care they receive extends over many years. It is multi-disciplinary and involves different agencies both statutory and voluntary. The record of the care provided is often complicated and to maintain it on computer with the ability to retrieve meaningful information requires careful systems design. At present there is very little software available that fulfils this purpose.

Remedial services

Another set of services that poses difficulties is the remedial services. There are a number of systems in use with a varying degree of success. Again, for the future, these should be patient-based. It should be remembered that these services transcend the hospital–community boundary and their information systems need to be linked by the index to other patient-based systems. Remedial services are an important resource and in the future their cost will have to be included in the equation of balancing services against resource utilisation.

District information support systems

Managerial turbulence created by the introduction of contracting, as pointed out previously, generated a great deal of anxiety about the need for management information. As a result the Government is setting up a project to consider the design and introduction of a computer system to provide the information for districts in their role of purchaser of health services.

The concept was entitled DISS (*District Information Support Systems*)[11] and has four components:

1. Systems to support the contracting process.
2. Resident population register with a record of health events.
3. Planning and needs assessment.
4. Management information.

The view of the authors is that the division implicit in the title is artificial and that systems developed to satisfy the above are equally of interest to provider units. To go further, it could be said that to plan systems otherwise will lead to wasteful duplication and will only enrich the hardware and software providers.

DISS systems are only in prototype at present but it is the declared intention of the Department of Health that districts have such systems fully operational by April 1993.

Health Service information systems and medical audit

It was unavoidable that this chapter should turn out to be a catalogue of systems. There are, nevertheless, some unifying principles to be noted. Although most if not all start out with a limited number of specialised users in mind, sooner or later there comes a time when other staff in the health services wish to access the data or use a system for something extra and beyond what it was originally designed for.

If one accepts this as inevitable and probably desirable, then it has two consequences. Firstly, the strategic development of health services information technology should ensure that this process of growth and adaptation is a relatively easy one. Systems should be designed to a common philosophy so that they can be interlinked at a later date. This often means adopting a common software environment and a common hardware platform.

In the second place, any exercise in gathering and analysing clinical data should include a careful examination of existing systems. What information is already collected? How can it be extracted and analysed?

This principle, it is suggested, applies to medical audit, with the corollary that one should also consider how existing systems can be adapted for this purpose. As pointed out in the introduction, information systems in the Health Service are so expensive to develop that it is often quicker and, thereby, more effective because they are more timely, to look at extending existing installations.

References

1. Ronson, J. (1989). Resource management: The London way. *British Journal of Healthcare Computing*, **6**, 16–17.
2. Steering Group on Health Services Information. *First Report* (1982), *Second Report* (1984), *Third Report* (1984), *Fourth Report* (1984), *Fifth Report* (1985), *Sixth Report* (1984). London: HMSO.
3. Banks, J. A. & Ingram, J. A. (1983). Trent RHA Patient Administration Computer Systems. *Medical Record and Information Journal*, **24**, 150–155.
4. Jones, R. B., Hedley, A. J., Peacock, I., Allison, S. P. & Tattersall, R. B. (1983). A computer-assisted register and information system for diabetes. *Methods in Information Medicine*, **22**, 5–14.
5. Department of Health (1989). *Working for Patients*. London: HMSO.
6. Rea, C. (1989). RM at Guy's: no easy road. *British Journal of Healthcare Computing*, **6**, 24–25.
7. Bardsley, M., Coles, J. & Jenkins, L. (eds) (1989). *DRGs and Health Care. The Management of Case-Mix* (2nd ed). London: King Edward's Hospital Fund for London.

  8. Todd, J. H. (1990). HISS: a hospital's perspective. *British Journal of Healthcare Computing*, **7**, 47–49.
  9. Todd, J. H., Norman, A. J., Thornton, S. V., Rolfe, P., Soady, I. & Cox, E. M. (1990). Developing an integrated information system for a large hospital using information engineering. *Proceedings of MIE90, Glasgow*. London: Springer-Verlag.
 10. Eames, C. (1989). HISS: The Greenwich experience. *British Journal of Healthcare Computing*, **6**, 9–11.
 11. Department of Health (1991). District Information Support Systems (Draft 4 March 1991).

10

Read codes and medical audit

JAMES D. READ

Coding clinical records

In the early days of medical computing it was quite common to see the computer as a way of storing medical records as 'free-text'. That is, clinicians could enter whatever they wanted to record, just as they could with hand-written notes. Nowadays it is generally accepted that the advantages of 'coded' clinical data outweigh the possible disadvantages.

In those early days coded data meant just that; the user would be expected to enter a *code*, such as 'A123', which would represent a medical term. Now, medical data can be encoded 'behind the scenes' without the clinicians needing to be aware of the coding process.

The benefits of encoding clinical data are :

1. It can be much faster than typing in free-text (especially for clinicians, who are not renowned for their typing skills).
2. Once entered, the data are readily searchable and retrievable because of their inherent structure.
3. Also because of the structure of a coding system, it becomes much more feasible to analyse and audit clinical data.

Clinicians have seen the disadvantage of a coding system as being excessive structuring of information – a restriction on what they are able to record about a patient. Whereas it should be recognised that data recording will be constrained, this can also be a powerful advantage. It encourages precision in the use of medical terms, a real benefit when patient data are communicated from one clinician to another, especially when crossing national boundaries.

Clinical coding systems

There are a vast number of coding systems used in medicine and health care. Some are 'home grown' and entirely local to a clinical team or computer system, others are internationally recognised. There are also a number of purposes for which coding systems have been developed. The main ones are:

1. As a rapid and compact way of recording data. (This was the original use of coding systems, and led to a proliferation of parochial systems.)
2. As a research tool, for example for epidemiological studies. (This was the purpose behind ICD-9, the International Classification of Diseases, version 9, which is widely used today for recording data which can be used to assess 'casemix' – the utilisation of health care resources.)
3. As a structured way of making a patient record. (This is the purpose behind the Read clinical classification (Read codes) and one of the subjects of this chapter.)

This chapter is also about the use of coding systems for medical audit. The central thesis of the chapter, and the motivation underlying the Read codes, is that by putting the needs of the clinician first, and developing a coding system primarily to support the clinical process, the best-quality data can be obtained for the purposes of audit or health service management. That is, management data are 'piggy-backed' onto 'clinical data'.

Origins and aims of the Read codes

The Read coding system originated in general practice and has subsequently been adopted for hospital utilisation.

The general practice experience

The Read codes began in 1982 when James Read, as a GP and member of the Abies GP user group, decided to write a simple coding system for recording his practice's clinical data. Initially there were 25 codes! There are now some 100000 codes with 150000 synonyms covering all areas of medicine.

A key step in the development of the Read codes was the endorsement, in 1988, by the Joint Computer Group of the BMA's General Medical Services Committee and the Royal College of General Practitioners. They recommended that the Read codes be adopted as the standard for general practice and that the implications be considered throughout the NHS.

Following this the Read codes were acquired by the Secretary of State for Health, and became Crown copyright in April 1990.[1] The DoH also established the NHS Centre for Coding and Classification (CCC), with James Read as its Director, to maintain and develop the codes for the NHS. The centre has a supervisory board, comprised mainly of representatives of the medical profession and its specialties, to oversee the further development of the codes.

The Secretary of State has licensed Computer Aided Medical Systems Limited (CAMS) to market and make available the Read codes and updates to users inside and outside the NHS. CAMS also provides advice, training, support and regular updates of the codes to major end users and developers of systems in which they are incorporated.

Whereas the aim behind the original 25 Read codes was to produce a brief problem listing for the general practice, the current aim is to support a totally computerised medical record, appropriate to, and communicable between, all health care sectors and all medical specialties.

Underlying this aim, there are three key principles:

1. That data must be easy to enter when making a 'live' clinical record.
2. That once entered, the data can be usefully analysed and audited.
3. That the data can be communicated in a common language between health care professionals.

These were the essential requirements if GPs were to use a computer system for recording medical records during their consultations. Today some 10000 GPs in the UK are routinely using the Read codes in their consultations and the codes are available on most GP systems. It has been concluded by Pringle that by 1992 over 90% of practices will have a computer system and that 'the Read clinical classification is the only coding system to offer full cover for the symptoms, procedures, and events of primary care'.[2]

The hospital experience

Historically, the experience of clinical information systems in NHS hospitals is not an encouraging tale. In stark contrast to the GP experience, which has been clinically led, hospital computing has been administratively led. Although individual clinicians have done some pioneering work in the development of clinical computing, particularly for decision support,[3] the major funding and development has been focused on administrative systems led by IT departments.

One result of this is that, again in contrast to general practice, there has been a distinct dearth of good clinical workstations for use by clinicians.[4] Another factor is that generally the computer-based recording of clinical information has been done for administrative or statistical purposes, for example, the collection of Körner data. Thus, generally the coding of clinical data has been done using ICD-9 (diseases) and OPCS-4 (procedures), neither of which was designed primarily for clinical use.

As a direct consequence, there has been very little involvement or commitment from clinical teams to data collection or use. Thus, for example, in one NHS region an average of 43 % of ordinary and day case admissions went uncoded during the year 1989/90, and the worst District had 80 % admissions uncoded. This says nothing about the accuracy of the coding that was done! We do not wish to suggest that the problem lies with the quality of the work of the coders themselves (who frequently are located in basements, coding far removed in time and place from the point where the information was collected from the patient). The problem lies with the lack of connection between the coding and the clinical process – both in terms of recording the information and also in terms of analysing and feeding it back to the clinical team.

The situation is now changing rapidly as it is recognised that clinical involvement is essential in the information and decision processes. Read codes are playing an important role in these developments.

Read codes in NHS hospitals

In the secondary sector, the Read codes were first implemented at Huddersfield Royal Infirmary where they have now been in use for more than two years. They have enabled the clinical teams, with the support of resource service managers, to produce a wide range of audit and management reports based on clinically valid data.

More recently the Read codes have been implemented in several other major hospitals. In the near future there will be 20 more implementations with another 20 planned, so that all major resource management systems will offer Read. Scotland is about to adopt the codes and all the major medical audit systems either have adopted or are about to adopt the codes.

Changing the culture and the NHS reforms

The advantage of the Read codes is that they are designed *by* clinicians, *for* clinicians. Thus clinical information recording can be primary, with use for management purposes being a secondary application 'piggy backed' onto the clinical information system. This is part of the 'cultural' change that is taking place in the NHS at the moment, primed by the resource management initiative, and carried along by the NHS reforms. However, if it is to succeed it must involve clinicians being responsible at both ends of the information line – as *collectors* of data, and as *users* of that data. In this sense, hospital clinicians are following the same path that GPs have been travelling along for some time now.

Data interchange

Read codes are also vital for data exchange between primary and secondary care. In the not too distant future, GPs will be sending Read coded data to hospitals as part of the referral process. Fund Holding practices will be expecting to be able to cost and assess care based on Read codes recorded by the hospital. For this reason, all sectors of the NHS will need to standardise their clinical language for the electronic communication of data.

We believe the Read codes will become that standard nomenclature for communicating within the NHS, a view shared by Radford and Wallace in a recent review of coding systems:

It seems likely that the Read system will become the standard medical classification system for national use, and as such will become the mainstay of clinical information services both for clinicians and hospital management. The benefits of this should then be seen in terms of better hospital records, better patient care, and better statistics for research, planning, audit and resource management. It is vital that hospital information systems currently under development around the country take account of it.[5]

Read codes and audit

The Read codes were designed for clinical data recording and subsequent audit. However, for that audit to be useful and to lead to an improvement in patient care it is important that:

1. The audit is focused, well managed and the results acted upon.
2. The computer system does not restrict the questions that the clinician or manager may wish to ask.

It is this second aspect of audit – the 'intra-computer' issues – that are focused on in this chapter.

Some general practices are now using the Read codes for a total, computerised medical record. This experience has made it clear that the use

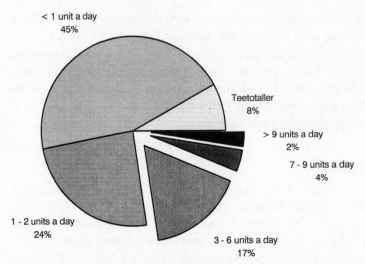

Fig. 10.1. Analysis of alcohol consumption, recorded in the past two years.

of the Read codes, the structure of the medical record and the subsequent analysis of data are all linked and that comprehensive audit needs attention to all three.

The Read codes are a 'gateway' to other classification structures. Because the Read codes are mapped to most of the nationally and internationally accepted classifications, it is possible to translate from a Read code to another system. This gateway facility can be useful for audit, because some coding systems will be more suitable than others for particular types of audit. Thus, for example, by converting from Read code to ICD-9-CM codes it is possible to derive diagnostic related groups (DRGs). Where the DRG is inadequate it is possible to use another method of producing casemix categories, e.g. based on activities.

However, the hierarchical structure of the Read codes aids analysis of clinically related groups. For example, it is easy for a general practice to analyse:

all patients with circulatory disorders;
all patients with ischaemic heart disease for a flu vaccination campaign;
all acute myocardial infarctions in the practice in the past year.

As codes are grouped into clinically useful groups, single searches can often analyse large amounts of data in one step; the results of such searches are illustrated in Figures 10.1 and 10.2.

The Read codes encompass not only diagnoses and procedures, but also social factors, history and symptoms, examination findings, investigations,

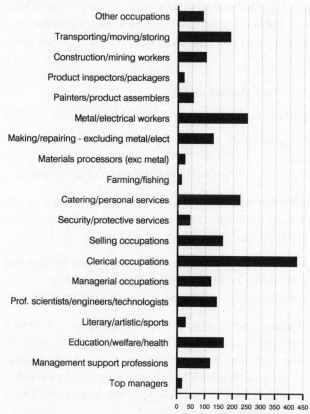

Fig. 10.2. Numbers of patients by occupation (excluding unemployed and retired).

administrative data and drugs. All of these are important aspects of a patient record and may need to be included in a search criterion. The same search logic can act on any Read code and hence complex and multifactorial searches should be easy to set up.

So the same search mechanisms should be able to answer widely different questions such as:

Example 1. Select all of the patients who had a total hip replacement and subsequently developed a chest infection and needed chest physiotherapy and/or an antibiotic – compare the proportion that smoked in that group with the proportion in the original group.

Example 2. Select all of the women due for a smear next month who have not refused, not had a hysterectomy and have so far received only one letter of invitation.

Example 3. Take all of the diabetic patients on diet alone who have been seen in out-patients in the last six months. Analyse what proportion have had fundoscopy in the last year and how many have ever seen the dietician.

The qualities of the software that aid audit

In practice, audit activity on a computer can be divided into two groups:

1. Regular searches and analyses, repeated at predetermined intervals with a well-defined aim.
2. *Ad hoc*, one-off enquiries, often stimulated by intellectual curiosity.

Most clinicians are familiar with the first variety, if only through searches initiated by managers to feedback data from the patient administration system. These well-defined searches are very useful for:

1. Closing the gap between actual and desired performance by showing how we are actually doing rather than how we think we are.
2. Picking up patients who may have slipped through a protocol of care.

Examples 2 and 3 above could well be examples of this type. Example 1 is likely to be a one-off type of search and it is these that will often hold the most interest for the clinician. The information revealed by playful, intellectual, questioning may then lead to the setting up of more regular, formal searches with well-defined aims. It is a great challenge for software designers to be able to provide such a facility.

A clinician needs to be able to interrogate his database quickly and easily in order to be able to audit his own work. This means that the searches and analyses should be:

1. Easy to set up, even for complex searches. These searches should be able to look for the presence or absence of criteria and cope with either/or combinations. Subgroups should be able to be preserved for further refinement.
2. Fast, taking no more than 15 minutes to perform a complex, multifactorial search on thousands of patients.
3. Able to include registration data such as the sex of patient, date of admission, consultant, post-code data, etc.
4. Able to search for the presence of single Read codes, ranges, multiple ranges, from a certain level of the hierarchy downwards and to include other data linked to the code such as the date of entry, a recall date or category of note (current or dormant problem, past history, etc).

5. Able to include 'linkage' between codes, e.g. the reason a drug was prescribed or blood taken for a full blood count. A code may 'qualify' a second code by adding extra detail such as the side of operation, and this needs to be reflected in the searches.
6. Search on the last occurrence of a particular Read code, for example the most recent smoking history or blood sugar.
7. Output the results of searches in a useful way such as an age/sex histogram, pie chart or different format lists. It is also useful to produce data that can be imported into a standard software package such as a spreadsheet or wordprocessor for the production of letters or further statistical analysis.

The requirements of these searches will in turn feed back to the design of the clinical record. It is important that Read codes can be entered in a structured record that establishes links between codes and sets them in context.

Analysis of results and the meaning of terms

Audit should be a circular activity, the results of the audit leading to changes in the way that care is provided. One interesting part of this feedback is that it concentrates the mind on what the data represent, in particular what is meant when we use certain terms. For example in one practice it appeared that a particular GP had many more children under five with asthma than his partner. Further analysis revealed that the prescribing rate for bronchodilators was the same for each partner with each age group. This led to an interesting discussion on the use of the term 'asthma' and a consensus view developed.

New developments in the Read codes

Coding developments and clinical specialties

The new NHS Centre for Coding and Classification has major ongoing work to maintain the Read codes. Each month the drug and appliance codes are updated as are the other code chapters to take into account user feedback.

Some code chapters are undergoing major redevelopment, particularly where the take up in the hospital sector is resulting in new requirements from clinical specialties. The CCC is now working with national groups of most of the specialties. The aim is for each group to make sure that the terms and synonyms they require are defined and included in the Read codes. For many of these specialties a 'specialty flag' is being linked to their terms in the Read code database for use by them as a dictionary, e.g. for audit.

Work is also underway with paramedical groups such as the Chartered Society of Physiotherapists, dieticians and the Disablement Services Agency.

The codes are being developed to incorporate the out-patient grouping number as a cross-reference field in the Read code database. This means that systems using Read codes will have the out-patient grouping number as a by-product of Read code records. Units not using Read codes can still use the out-patient number on its own. The CCC will maintain alterations in the grouping set and relevant mapping changes.

In the longer term, the aim is to work with the profession and other relevant bodies to plan and develop 'Read Six' (Read codes, version six) over the next five years. This will involve a review of the classification structure in close consultation with the specialty groups.

Casemix development and patient management categories

The Read classification system is designed to group terms into clinically meaningful categories. This, of course means that higher levels in the classification do not imply that terms under them are similar in their resource implications. Thus for resource management purposes the Read codes must be linked to resource categories. This could be done in a number of different ways. The simplest is to use the cross-reference tables to convert Read codes into their corresponding ICD-9-CM or OPCS-4 codes (or ICD-9-CM procedures). These can then be fed into a casemix grouper in the normal way.

However, in several specialty areas the groups (based on DRGs) are far too coarse to be useful. Therefore, another way of using the Read codes is to link them directly to clinically appropriate groupings of procedures that are 'iso-resourced'. Thus, for example, the CCC is working with the Resource Management Unit and the Radiotherapy and Oncology DRG Project Working Party to produce *aggregated activity groups* for radiotherapy and chemotherapy groups.

International development

Over the past 18 months there has been considerable international interest in the Read codes.

In Italy a consortium is being put together to establish a national Read code organisation. The setting up of a Norwegian Centre for Coding, with its own Norwegian lexicon and mapping to the Read codes, is being discussed. Plans are under discussion for a national centre for Read codes in Canada, with particular interest coming from the Province of Ontario. In addition negotiations are underway for the use of the Read codes in Finland, Australia and New Zealand.

Technical developments

A key feature of the Read codes is that they are a dynamic system, being updated at frequent intervals. To this end, users can submit requests for new codes or synonyms to CAMS for processing by the NHS CCC. If accepted they are distributed with the next set of release disks.

From early in 1991 the new releases have been available as a file of additions and changes (Read codes are never deleted, they can only become inactive, e.g if a drug is withdrawn). In addition each user licence will have a unique serial number and each Read code update will have a unique code to denote the version.

Early in 1991 a new file structure was also introduced. This contains some important new fields. The medical terms have been offered in three different lengths fields, 30, 60 and 198 characters. A 'specialty flag', to denote a code as a member of a specialty subset, has been included, and a 'language field', to support the automatic translation into other languages, also has been introduced.

The 'key' (usually part of a term or an abbreviation for the term) that is used to search for a term and its Read code will be extended from four to ten characters in length.

A 'term code' field will also be introduced. This will enable the system to store a unique reference to the language with which the user chose to select a term (e.g. a common synonym such as heart attack), so that when the code is output, for example in a discharge letter, the original language of the clinician can be preserved.

Some implementation issues

In general practice, the use of the codes is now well established and there are many experienced users. Most suppliers have now adopted the codes and the conversion from four character to five character Read codes is taking place.

In the hospitals, developments are rapid. CAMS is providing direct training and implementation support backed up by a telephone help-line. The first batch of experienced users is now emerging and different patterns of use are developing.

The most common method of use is for medical secretaries to do the coding as part of the clinical team. In some hospitals coders are still doing the coding, though it appears to be much more effective if the coders do this as part of the clinical team, rather than remaining in the traditionally remote locations.

A particularly important role is emerging, that of the data and coding manager, whose role is to support the clinical team, by assisting with any difficult coding problems, and by ensuring that the team receives regular audit reports generated by the computer system. Former coders can be particularly suitable for this job.

In some teams the clinicians are doing their own data entry, though this is less common than in general practice, most likely because of the lack of sufficient suitable clinical workstations.

In the hospitals the tradition of administratively led requirements is having a marked influence on the current situation. In particular, the 'coding rules' that exist in each region (but not necessarily the same for each region) tend to put administrative expediency before clinical accuracy. Thus when entering clinical data (and therefore choosing a code) a user can be faced with a dilemma between choosing a term that conforms with the local administrative guidelines or one that is meaningful and useful to a clinician. Naturally clinicians tend to choose the latter and coders the former.

We are working, in as many instances as possible, to provide 'compromise solutions' that satisfy both sets of criteria. This is not always possible and we urge that the administrative requirements are reviewed and modified. This may mean, in the longer run, ceasing to require output in ICD-9 or OPCS-4 format. If the principles underlying the NHS reforms and the associated culture change are to be taken seriously, it is important than clinical integrity is taken as primary, and the administrative tail does not wag the clinical dog.

Looking to the future

The Read codes are more and more evolving essentially into a coded nomenclature of medicine, each term having a unique code identifier for transmission purposes, and also providing a 'gateway' for each user to reconstruct the data received or stored into the format of every format to which the nomenclature is cross-referenced. The Read codes are cross-referenced to every other commonly accepted classification system used in the NHS.

The incorporation of ICD-10 and the appropriate mapping will be in place in time for the 1993 release and every system using the Read codes will have no work to do to incorporate the change – they will merely receive and load the new mapping field.

Moreover, by 1993, the Read codes will be in a position to support all medical implementations within the NHS, including all feeder systems. Also by 1993, all primary care (GP and community systems) could be using the Read codes as their key code for electronic transmissions.

It is not unreasonable to expect that by 1995 all feeder systems could have converted to Read as their key code. Thus when an NHS network is introduced it could use Read codes from the start. We would then have a truly common vehicle for communicating clinical information throughout the NHS.

References

1. Chisholm, R. (1990). The Read clinical classification. *British Medical Journal*, **300**, 1092.
2. Pringle, M. (1990). The new agenda for general practice computing. *British Medical Journal*, **301**, 827.
3. de Dombal, F. T. (1979). Computers and the surgeon: a matter of decision. *Surgery Annual*, **11**, 33–57.
4. Rose, C. (1990). Clinical workstations – the Cinderella at the NHS ball. *British Journal of Healthcare Computing*, **7**, 3.
5. Radford, P. & Wallace, W. A. (1990). The code war. *British Journal of Healthcare Computing*, **7**, 22–24.

11
Data capture direct from doctors

DAVID MARSH AND JIM BARRIE

Introduction

In 1987, the Department of Orthopaedic Surgery, Manchester University set out to develop a system for recording and classifying the work passing through the academic clinical unit. Like many others, we were tired of leafing through theatre logbooks to assemble series of patients for study, of depending on patently inaccurate hospital activity analysis (HAA) statistics to tell us what our workload had been, and of relying on rosy memory to retrieve our complications. Moreover, like many others, we had tried paper-based storage systems but found them, in the maelstrom of orthopaedic and trauma work in an understaffed unit, to produce more resentment than usable data.

The rising availability of computers allowed many possible solutions, but all dogged by one question – who keys in the data? We could raise a little money for hardware, though not enough for an extensive network, but salaries for data clerks were always out of the question and our doctors and secretaries were already overworked. In almost all orthopaedic units in the UK, there has for many years been a tradition of typed casenotes, based on dictation by doctors at the time of consultation. So the secretary is already transmitting diagnostic information through a keyboard – why not store the data as a by-product of her/his work?

This has remained the basis of our strategy; it has stood the test of time in several busy orthopaedic units in the last three (at the time of writing) years, with a high level of acceptability from secretaries and doctors alike. As to the quality of the data, that is not a matter for assertion: we have measured it. It is by no means perfect, as will be seen later in this chapter.

Scope of the data

From the outset, we were clear that it was unrealistic to expect to use our system to store all the data needed for actually carrying out clinical research or audit. These require the collection of numerical data describing the severity of presenting conditions, the outcome of treatment and parameters of the process of delivery of health care such as waiting times and so on. Government spokesmen who appear to believe that this sort of data can be collected during routine work, using existing staff, are totally deluded.

We set ourselves the target of storing enough data to achieve two objectives:

- retrieval of series of cases for further study, defined by diagnosis, operation performed, complications encountered, or any combination of these
- summary of admission episodes and all procedures carried out in theatre.

The important thing was that our data were to be of high quality, having been created directly by the doctors looking after the patients and that they would be collected for all the patients being treated by the unit, including those who were never admitted to hospital.

Hardware and software

The system was developed initially on an IBM-compatible 80286 machine, connected to a laser printer and a dot matrix printer, with a tape streamer for backup. Subsequently this configuration was expanded to a network of 80286 machines with an 80386 file server, sharing one laser printer but with a dot matrix or inkjet printer for each workstation. Development is now underway to interface this network to a district network.

The software is based on linked lists of B+ structure, which allows a standard amount of demographic data to be held on each patient, together with an unlimited amount of diagnostic data, without wasting disc space. This chapter will concentrate on the main database program, which stores and retrieves diagnostic and treatment data, plus the maintenance routines essential for this function. Other important elements, such as the waiting list management module, are not described since they are not germane to the issue of doctor-coded data.

Data creation – the doctor's role

Perhaps it will not be too long before we have computers that can automatically analyse a piece of free text, such as a letter from an orthopaedic surgeon to a referring GP, and abstract from it the correct diagnostic codes for the patient to whom it refers. There are two reasons why the sort of computers currently available to the NHS could not do this: they don't know enough English and they don't know enough orthopaedics. These two deficiencies have to be made good by the doctor.

Automatic extraction of codes would require complex analysis of English syntax because not every diagnostic phrase in such text is intended as a true descriptor of the patient being talked about. The author may, for example, be listing diagnoses which should be excluded. It is necessary to help the computer by saying effectively – 'here come the diagnostic terms' – so the doctor has to think about them separately from his thinking about the contents of the letter or note and the secretary has to input them as a distinct step.

Such a separate process is necessary also because the doctor needs to help the computer to know the appropriate depth of detail to code and when a term is a synonym for something else. For example, a letter may contain reference to a patient's 'previous Charnley'. What we want the database to contain as a result of this is the code for a total hip replacement, possibly with 'Charnley' specified as a subtype. We may also want this case to have exactly the same code as other patients who were given the diagnostic label 'low–friction arthroplasty'. The rules for achieving these results are nowhere near being specified completely enough to allow the creation of software that can achieve the task automatically across the breadth of orthopaedics. The only realistic tool available is the intelligence of the doctor, supported or replaced by that of the secretary. This requires knowledge, not only of orthopaedics (which we must assume anyway) but of the aims and structure of the coding system.

Although automatic extraction of codes from free text is not yet possible, it remains true that there can be no better time to access the diagnostic knowledge, held in the mind of a doctor responsible for a particular patient, than when he or she has just dictated the note or letter arising from a clinical consultation or an operation. The doctor is already in communicating mode, striving for perspective, alert to the possibility of some important aspect being overlooked and concentrating on that patient.

Getting the doctor to speak the necessary information onto tape at this critical moment will always primarily be a matter of motivation and discipline. But the task can be made a great deal easier if two conditions are met:

- the doctor should be aware of what data is already held on the database about the patient under consideration, so that only new or missing information needs to be given;
- there should be no, or minimal, need to consult coding books in order to know what to say.

The first condition led to the decision that the contents of the database, for each patient, should be integrated with the clinical record; precisely how this was done is described below. The second condition led to the decision to use a text-based coding system, composed of terms that were as near as possible to the language of ordinary medical conversation. The development of this coding system has been a three-stage process, which is still going on, and to this we now turn.

Data coding

What was needed was a set of orthopaedic terms that would easily be used by the working doctor in the heat of the clinical moment. The model we started with was the well-tutored registrar describing a case over the phone to his consultant. How would he break down the diagnostic picture? What terms and phrases would he use? To this criterion we added some formalisation of syntax, so that similar entities were described by terms of similar structure. With these two rules in mind, a dictionary of keywords was created by simply describing the entire contents of a moderate-sized orthopaedic textbook. This was the first phase of creation of the coding system.

The dictionary of keywords existed in two forms: as a book, which was available in the clinic for doctors to refer to at the time of clinical consultation and as an alphabetically arranged file on the hard disc containing the database. The only way to enter data into the database was to use one of the keywords from the dictionary file. Thus although the keywords are text, they are not free text, and constitute a coding system that can be just as rigorous as a numerical system.

Keywords are of several types: diagnosis, operation, procedure, complication and admission. The difference between operation and procedure keywords is that the latter are reserved for simple activities in theatre,

Table 11.1 *Differences between keyword types*

Keyword type	Meaning of date	Retrieval use
Diagnosis	Presentation to unit or date of accident	Case retrieval
Operation	Date of surgery	Case retrieval Theatre report Log books
Procedure	Date of theatre visit	Theatre report
Complication	Date complication noted	Case retrieval Theatre report In-patient report
Admission	Date admitted and date discharged	In-patient report

which are important for audit of theatre usage, but unimportant for research purposes and should not clutter up the patients' records – e.g. changes of plaster or wound inspections. These are not stored in the patient's keyword record, only in a special file used for theatre audit. Each keyword has a date associated with it; the meaning of the date varies and admission keywords have two. A summary of the differences between keyword types is given in Table 11.1. Examples of keywords are given in Box 11.1.

The second phase of development of the coding system was based in clinical practice. The doctors using the system in the first two installations were asked to use the existing keywords whenever possible, but told that they could invent new keywords if they were sure that they were necessary; this they freely did. Analysis of these spontaneously created keywords, and the very vigorous debate they provoked, led to enormous enhancement of the keyword dictionary in both its breadth and logical consistency.

The facility to create new keywords during routine clinical use of the system obviously carries dangers. A doctor might create a new keyword unnecessarily, being unaware that a similar term already exists; this would then lead to cases with the same diagnosis being split in the database, leading to incomplete retrieval. This danger dictated two features of the program:

● Each entry in the keyword dictionary actually consists of two elements – keyword and masterword. Data entry is by keyword, retrieval is by masterword. When a keyword is initially created, keyword and masterword are identical, but they can be edited. This allows several

---

Box 11.1   *Examples of keywords*

(a)   Typical combinations of diagnosis keywords:

benign tumour – spine – lumbar
osteoid osteoma

osteoarthritis – hip
hallux valgus

multiple injuries
fracture – femur – shaft, open
fracture – tibia – shaft
compartment syndrome, presenting
abdominal injury
head injury

(b)   Common operation keywords

arthroplasty – hip

excision tumour – bone

nerve decompression – median

IM nail – femur

ORIF – tibia

(c)   Complication keywords

deep vein thrombosis

post-operative infection – deep

nonunion

iatrogenic nerve injury – sciatic

implant failure

---

keywords to be synonyms for the same masterword. However, any one keyword always maps onto the same masterword.

- The program was designed to allow a system co-ordinator, who should be medical, to browse the keyword dictionary, looking at newly-created keywords and amending them or their masterwords as necessary. Any change in the keyword dictionary triggers a cleaning process of the whole database, amending all patient records to reflect the new codes. Feedback from the system co-ordinator to individual users was facilitated by a carefully-designed routine that makes full use of the fact that each keyword record includes the identity of the keyword-giver.

We initially intended to close the facility for new keyword creation once the dictionary had reached a certain stage of development. However, it has proved popular with users, who value the ability to make local decisions about the depth of detail to code in areas of special interest, or to create keywords with a local administrative purpose, such as '*interesting case*' or '*July referral*'.

The third phase of development of the coding system is still going on and consists of its fusion with other strands of development into an accepted British lexicon of orthopaedic terms. The philosophy of text-based coding, using terms that are clinically familiar, is universally accepted by the committee. However, for every term developed, a Read code (version 5) is being created, which will in turn map onto ICD-9, OPCS-4 or whatever supersedes them. It is intended that the lexicon of terms will be freely available and we plan to adopt it lock, stock and barrel as a new keyword dictionary. Like everyone else, we will have the headache of mapping the old dictionary onto the new, and users will be responsible for converting their own local terms.

Troublesome though this third phase is bound to be, there is no avoiding it. It is occurring in parallel with the development of a mechanism for linking the orthopaedic departmental network with district networks, such as casemix. This promises the ability for doctor-created diagnostic information to be uploaded directly into district, and thence national, statistics. Such a process demands a universal language of coding.

Data storage: the secretary's role

As with the doctor creating data under the pressure of clinical work, it was important that the business of data storage should not make life more difficult for the medical secretary. This meant that the change from current practice should be minimal and that the computer should save at least as much effort as it required for data storage. The design of our software owes a great deal to the patience with which one of our medical secretaries allowed us to dissect and analyse her style of work. After a few weeks of learning to use the resulting system, she reported that it took her 25% less time to process an audio tape than with her previous typewriter-based system. The hard copy output – letters, notes, theatre lists and so on – was at least as good as previously, *and* we had our data.

In most installations of the system in other units since the original, secretaries have accepted the same method of working, usually because it was very similar to what they themselves were used to, and they have found similar savings in time. However, exporting this precise style of work to other units has not always been straightforward. Potential users have sometimes asked for the software to be modified to reproduce some aspect of their traditional way of doing things. It has been very tempting to agree to this, and of course there is in principle no programming reason why it should not be possible. We have learned however, that it is a great mistake. The existing program logic, which feels smooth and intuitive, only got to be like that by dint of prolonged interaction between secretary, doctor and programmer. Invariably, we have found that requests from new users have turned out to be much more complicated to implement than the users ever suspected, and this necessary close collaboration in developing and debugging new software has been impossible to engender, especially at a distance. We now say, therefore, that the current version of the system is the current version, and people must adapt to it. Any ideas for improvement are welcomed and, if we think they are useful, we will implement them – properly – in the next update.

From the secretary's point of view, the software appears primarily as a simple word processor. When she/he hears a patient's name mentioned on the tape, she/he selects that patient before beginning to type the text; in the case of a letter, the screen is then laid out with name and address of GP and patient in the appropriate places, assuming use of window envelopes. If the patient is new, she/he will have to enter name and address, age and GP before doing this. If the GP is one which has not been encountered before, she/he will have to enter his or her address also; this becomes a progressively rarer event as the system is used. Since the secretaries in the unit are linked via a network and all tied into the same database on the fileserver, the labour of this first-time data entry is shared. In any case it involves no more keystrokes than would have been involved for every letter written about each patient previously. For patients who are already in the database, the saving of keystrokes when a letter is being written is huge: usually around 50% of a reasonably short letter.

Having typed the text, the author of the letter and any recipients of copies are entered, again in a labour-saving way. Just before giving the command to print the letter, the keyword record for that patient is updated according to the instructions the dictating doctor has given on the tape. The existing keywords are displayed in a window on the screen, old keywords can be deleted and new keywords can be added from the keyword dictionary. If a keyword is given that is not in the dictionary, a new entry in the dictionary can be created there and then. Some units decide that this shall not be done without the express approval of the

Table 11.2 *A typical casenote entry*

Current keywords for this patient are:

Type	Masterword	User/ operator	Consultant	Date	Discharge date
D	Osteoarthritis – hip	PK	DRM	16/11/90	
A	Left total hip replacement	JB	DRM	09/02/91	18/02/91
O	Arthroplasty – hip	JB	DRM	10/02/91	
C	Deep vein thrombosis	DRM	DRM	21/02/91	

system co-ordinator. With each keyword is stored a date (Table 11.2) and the identity of the keyword-giver.

When the print command is given, letters and discharge summaries are produced by a laser printer that is shared between all the secretaries. A copy of the output is produced by a dot matrix or inkjet printer that is personal to that secretary and is right by her/his side. It is produced on a continuous roll of paper that is gummed on the back and has frequent perforations. She/he tears this off, sticks it into the notes and can immediately dispose of the latter without waiting for top copies of letters to be dealt with. The updated list of keywords is printed at the bottom of the casenotes copy, looking something like Table 11.2. At future clinical consultations, this will be the last thing in the notes and the doctor will find them a useful summary of events to date. He or she will also be ideally placed to correct any errors or omissions, as well as creating keywords to describe developments that have occurred since the last clinical interaction.

This keyword listing is general for the four formats available on the wordprocessing screen: letter, discharge summary, operation note, and progress note. Only the first two of these produce laser printer output; only the casenotes copies have the keyword listing. Provided the dictating doctors put correct keywords on tape, the task of keyword entry is, for the secretary, extremely easy. The question is how good the doctors are at giving keywords, and evidence about this will be given later in this chapter.

Data retrieval

The original motivation for developing the Manchester orthopaedic database (MOD) was a desire to be able to assemble series of patients for clinical research. Case retrieval is therefore the most developed aspect of the interrogation side of the program. Subsequently, the growing needs of audit led to the development of three methods for quantifying the work of the unit – the admissions report, the operations and procedures report, and the individual surgeon's operating logbook.

Case retrieval

The most basic form of case retrieval is to search for all patients who have a particular keyword in their record. If somebody wants to review all the Klippel-Feil syndromes, or chondrosarcomas, this is all that is needed. The definition of the cases is simple, numbers are small and all that is required are the hospital numbers so that the casenotes can be obtained. However, this simple mechanism needs extending in three respects.

First, it may be anticipated that a researcher may want to know all cases with one of a related group of keywords. Consider, for example, Box 11.2, which encompasses all tibial fractures, a patient group that may well be of interest. It would be tedious to have to search six times, once for each keyword. In a hierarchical coding system, one can often retrieve a broad grouping by only specifying the first few characters of the code and, even with textual keywords, one could achieve the same in this case by searching for 'fracture – tibia – *'.

We deemed it much more flexible, however, to provide a structure called simply a 'keyword group', which could be named, edited and used to search the data. By providing a rapid, string-based routine for creating groups, the above example of tibial fractures could be dealt with almost as quickly as with a hierarchical coding system. But less-convenient combinations, which would defy a hierachical solution, are handled just as easily. For example, one can create a group of all hip operations, including arthroplasties; or a group of all arthroplasties, including those of the hip. This is the sort of flexibility one gets with a modular coding system, but the group concept is yet more flexible, since there need be no common code element at all between group members.

The second refinement required was to be able to define a patient group by a combination of keywords related by logical *and*, *or* and *not*. We decided that this should be done interactively, since one may well start out with a less than perfectly clear idea of the group's desired characteristics. The module that achieves this is called '*building a search file*' and it has proved very effective and easy to use. It works on two screens: 'select', where cases are added by keyword or group of keywords – this provides the *or* relationship; and 'browse', where the cases are displayed with all

---

Box 11.2   *A group of keywords describing tibial fractures*

fracture – tibia – condyle

fracture – tibia – condyle, open

fracture – tibia – shaft

fracture – tibia – shaft, open

fracture – tibia – distal

fracture – tibia – distal, open

---

their keywords and can be eliminated either by possession or non-possession of a particular keyword – this provides the *and* and *not* relationships.

The third requirement was the ability to present the retrieved cases in a variety of ways. The cases can therefore be sorted on three fields: consultant, date and surname, with the priority of these sort fields selected according to the precise question being addressed.

The combination of these features means that there is no serious limitation on the ability to retrieve the names and hospital numbers of patients' groups defined in pretty well any way one can imagine. This greatly simplifies what is often an exasperating first step in any clinical research or in-depth audit project.

Standard reports for audit purposes

It was stated at the beginning of this account that there was never an intention that this system should store the information needed for clinical audit. The strength of the system is that it stores essential qualitative information about all the patients passing through the unit and does so within the compass of routine work by existing staff. It is really a patient tracking system. Nonetheless, as part of this tracking function, information is stored that allows three simple audit functions, of the 'count how many cases' type.*

The first derives from the information stored in admission keywords. These allow a simple report of in-patient work during any given time period. Cases can be listed, with all their diagnostic keywords if required, by consultant and by date of admission. The date of discharge is also

---

* These remarks only apply to the main wordprocessing/database program. The waiting list module is more ambitious in the quantitative tasks it sets out to achieve.

printed but the length of stay is not automatically calculated. As an addendum to the in-patient report, all complications, noted on these patients since the beginning of the time window selected for the report, are listed separately.

The second derives from the operation and procedure keywords, indeed the *raison d'être* for the latter (Table 11.1) is this audit function – a report of theatre activity, again within specified time windows. As well as listing by consultant and time, this report allows grouping and counting of cases by type of operation. Again, the theatre report concludes with a list of complications noted on the patients in the list.

The third standard report is the personal logbook of operations performed. This is possible because every keyword record contains the identity of the keyword-giver and, in the case of operation keywords, this field is used to contain the operator (who would normally be the keyword-giver in any case). Unfortunately, this report does not include operations assisted at, which is a weakness where trainees are concerned; this may be rectified in future.

A study of the quality of data stored

In order to find out how well this sytem works in practice, a retrospective study of the accuracy and completeness of data capture was performed by Jim Barrie. This is one case where a retrospective study is better than a prospective one, since the doctors capturing the data had no idea they were going to be studied at the time! The study was carried out in Ancoats Hospital, Manchester, at a time when the system had been in operation for 18 months. This hospital has four orthopaedic consultants, with five secretaries, each of whom had their own workstation.

The secretaries were pleased with the system but the doctors suspected their data capture was not as complete as it might have been. They had therefore begun a routine of discussing the database at the monthly audit meeting, when the system co-ordinator fed back to the other users examples of inappropriate keyword use and so on. This had been going for about four months at the time of the study.

The study was in two parts. First, 200 random sets of casenotes were pulled, of patients who had passed through the unit (either as in-patients or out-patients) at any time since the inception of the system; the process of keyword ascription throughout their period of care was analysed in detail. Second, the casenotes of 121 inpatients were pulled and the data held on the Manchester orthopaedic database compared with that stored

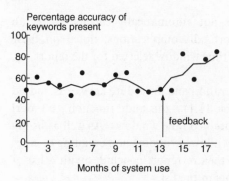

Monthly figures with three-month moving average

Fig. 11.1. Trend of completeness of keyword ascription.

by the NHS coding clerks supporting HAA – the existing source of data to which the MOD might be considered an alternative, or check.

Study 1: Process of keyword ascription

For each case, every occasion on which dictation had been made, when keywords could have been dictated, was examined by an experienced orthopaedic registrar (JLB), noting the keywords in the database just before the dictation (if any) and those present just afterwards. This information was evident from the current keywords lists (Table 11.2). From study of the notes the correct keywords that should have been dictated at that time, given what was already in the database, were determined and compared with what was actually dictated. For each previously uncoded clinical entity (diagnosis, operation or complication), two questions were asked:

- Was an attempt made to describe it in a keyword?
- Was the new keyword accurate?

The aggregated results of these enquiries yielded measures of completeness and accuracy, respectively, in the process of keyword-giving. These were analysed as a function of the time since the installation of the system, the type of keyword and the level of seniority of the dictators concerned. Figures 11.1 and 11.2 depict the cardinal findings of this study. There were unacceptably low levels of completeness which responded dramatically to a modest consciousness-raising exercise in the form of feedback at monthly intervals and extremely high levels of diagnostic accuracy. Figure 11.3 shows that the problem of doctors failing to dictate keywords is most acute in the case of complications. Operative keywords were over 80 % complete

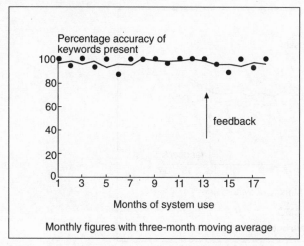

Fig. 11.2. Trend of accuracy of keyword ascription.

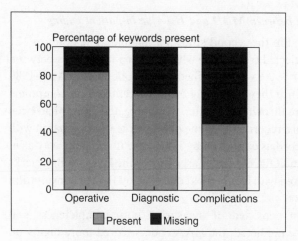

Fig. 11.3. Variation in completeness of keyword ascription.

across the whole period of the study – good news for resource management, bad for clinical audit! It was also found that all grades of doctor were similar in the accuracy of the keywords they entered, but senior registrars were somewhat worse than other grades where completeness was concerned. Completeness was better for in-patients than out-patients. Completeness was lower (only 19%) for creating keywords for long-established diagnoses, in other words dealing with missing keywords, or for correcting wrong keywords (27%), than for responding to the need for a new keyword (71% completeness).

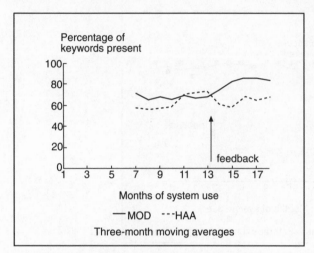

Fig. 11.4. Data quality – doctors versus coding clerks.

Study 2: Comparison between MOD and HAA on in-patient coding

The method employed in the second study was similar. The notes of 121 patients, randomly selected from those who had been in-patients between April 1989 and March 1990, were obtained. HAA codes before April 1989 were not available, since they were only from then entered on computer; prior to that they were thrown away after the aggregated figures had been obtained! The keyword record at the time of discharge was compared with the ideal keyword record as conceived by Jim Barrie in the same way as in study 1. The ICD-9 and OPCS-4 codes ascribed by the HAA coding clerks were similarly compared with ideal codes conceived by JLB, in consultation with the coding books.

The analysis again consisted of measuring both completeness and accuracy. As might be predicted, the HAA coders scored more highly on completeness, and lower on accuracy. Combining the two into a single measure of data quality:

data quality

$$= \frac{\textit{number of correct keywords or codes in the actual record}}{\textit{number of keywords or codes in the ideal record}} \times 100$$

The high accuracy of the MOD codes makes up for their poor completeness and, when completeness begins to improve following feedback, the overall quality of the MOD codes moves significantly ahead of the HAA data (Figure 11.4).

Discussion

In order to serve our research, audit and resource management purposes, what we want is for patients' clinical problems, and our therapeutic response, to end up systematically, accurately and completely described in the information held in a database. Figure 11.5 depicts the steps required to achieve this. The initial step of information creation is when the doctors evaluate and treat the patient; what is held in their minds is the best knowledge there will ever be about that patient – the question is how to change the knowledge into information that can be put in the database with minimal degradation.

The key step is, therefore, the coding; who are the best people to do it? The traditional method has been to employ coding clerks who read the casenotes retrospectively and create coded data. These people have the advantages that they are knowledgable about the structure and aims of the coding system and are dedicated full-time to the task. The doctors do not have these advantages, but they do have the medical knowledge in their heads. By providing a mechanism that eliminates the tedium and impracticality of doctors sitting at keyboards and looking up coding books, we have been able to explore the possibility of doctor-coding, by a group of unselected, ordinary orthopaedic surgeons doing routine work in a busy general unit. Our study produced three significant findings:

- Doctors such as these can produce data on in-patients to a quality as good as that produced by coding clerks, with virtually no special training. They can also create data of similar quality on out-patients, where none currently exists.
- The level of quality is inadequate, mainly because of incompleteness.
- The completeness of data improves significantly with even modest feedback.

Clearly, in the long run, the way to get the best data is to capture them directly from the doctors at the time of clinical action. The question is, how do we combine the talents of doctors and coding clerks to achieve the highest quality and, in particular, how do we tackle the incompleteness problem? Our strategy contains two elements.

The first, short-term, approach is a different way of creating discharge summaries. Previously we believed that GPs liked to receive flowing prose about patients' in-patient episodes and treated discharge summaries like any other letter, with keywords dictated at the end. The incompleteness problem has swept such aesthetic considerations aside. The discharging

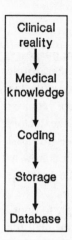

Fig. 11.5. Information flow into a clinical database.

house officer (or above) will now fill out a form with diagnosis, procedure and complications and this will be passed to the medical secretary before being passed to the coding clerks. A semi-automatic discharge summary module will accept these keywords, store them in the database and construct a discharge summary from them. The GPs will at least get accurate information more quickly and we will get our data.

In the longer term, our aim is to team up fully with the coding clerks, whose knowledge and experience is an asset we would not wish to waste. Our new system for generating inpatient episode diagnostic data will run in parallel with their established mechanism of coding to ICD-9 and OPCS-4 codes and inputting to PAS. Quite rightly, they are not going to entrust that statutory duty to medical staff without a great deal of reassurance. However, work is also under way to map our keywords onto Read 5, ICD-9 and OPCS-4 codes, to allow automatic translation of data captured as keywords. Our two parallel systems ought therefore to be producing the same data. Once this situation is achieved, we hope to be able to persuade our coding colleagues to adopt a new role.

The new role is that of supervisors of our system – of the coding aspect of it at least. We would like them to take on both the maintenance of the keyword dictionary, with its mapping onto codes, and the function of quality control. The latter would include monitoring of the quality of keyword ascription by individual users, explaining the mechanism for, and importance of data capture to new doctors and generally educating doctors in the business of converting knowledge into information. Freeing up their time to allow this change demands another quantum leap – episode diagnostic data must be passed directly from our system to a patient administration or casemix system. The technical aspects of this are being tackled now, but the real hurdle is to gain everyone's confidence in the quality of our data, and this cannot happen overnight.

Hopefully, the Manchester orthopaedic database will not be the only system aiming to achieve a complete fusion of the respective strengths of doctors and coders. Unglamorous though their task appears, its importance goes way beyond resource management. In the words of the great nineteenth century statistician, William Farr: 'Classification is another name for generalisation, and successive generalisations constitute the laws of the natural sciences'.

12

Computer systems: practice, limitations and pitfalls

PHILIP J. RADFORD

Introduction

The most difficult thing facing the clinician interested in setting up audit within his/her department must be the means of acquisition, storage and analysis of the data required to support this. Computers are particularly good at storing large amounts of data and at manipulating them, and the enormous advantages of computerisation in aiding these functions have not escaped a large number of clinicians. Many have gone ahead and developed their 'own' computer software to aid their 'audit' activities, and several commercial systems have also been developed. It is important to realise however that there are no 'audit systems', despite the claims of the advocates and salesmen, that will perform all the needs of audit. Rather audit requires the active input of the practising clinician and cannot be done by a computer system alone. The computer can of course be a completely invaluable 'audit assistant' but it is never more than that.

As usual in life whenever one finds a multitude of different approaches to the same thing it usually means that none of them are perfect and that they all have different faults. The perfect solution will be obvious if it arrives. In orthopaedic surgery we see this for example in the 60 or so different operations described for the treatment of bunions (hallux valgus), and in the audit field we see it in the plethora of computer systems aimed at the audit market. To be fair there is no clear 'winner' from all the available systems because they are all trying to encompass multiple tasks, and priorities differ from system to system. For example, some have more emphasis on the medical secretarial role and some on the management of resources.

Many of us must have been in that rather difficult position of thinking that we need some computer assistance, but not knowing how to evaluate systems properly, and feeling rather overwhelmed by the sales 'patter' of the producers. In particular it is difficult to know how to go about evaluation of the multitude of computer systems that all claim to be the answer to all of the problems, ranging from those that are called 'audit systems' to those that claim to 'support' clinical audit functions.

This chapter is hopefully going to be a guide through these troubled and murky waters.

Are computers needed at all?

The answer in theory is no, as all the data required to audit medical practice can be collected manually. However, that is very time consuming, tedious and expensive on staff time, not only for collection of the data but particularly when it comes to analysis, and it soon becomes impractical. Only a very simple audit system can be run exclusively on paper, such as a prospective record of complications occurring on in-patients. In many units including our own, at some stage in the past admissions and out-patient attenders have had their diagnosis recorded by the secretaries on punch cards with holes around the edge. We have filing cabinets full of them, storing a huge amount of diagnostic information stretching back over many years. But try and get the information out, even with a knitting needle that fits through the holes! This is where the computer becomes invaluable as it can store and manipulate huge amounts of information in time spans measured in seconds.

Most authors seem to agree that a modern approach to medical audit will involve some form of computerisation.[1,2]

What types of computer systems are there to support audit?

The systems that are currently available fall into several broad groups the advantages and disadvantages of which we need to consider in turn.

These are:

1. Unit and district based systems.
2. Non-commercial clinically based systems.
3. Commercially available clinically based systems.

Unit and district based systems

These are the standard hospital-based computer systems – called PAS (patient administration system) or similar. These are to be found in every large hospital, health district and regional health authority in the UK.

These systems, one might think at first sight, store a lot of information that could be extremely useful for medical audit. They should also have advantages of scale in terms of hospital-wide coverage, and there are moves in various hospitals to make them into the all-embracing HISS (hospital information support system). For example, all the administrative details about patients are usually stored there – age, sex, place of residence, dates of admission and discharge etc. There is usually a clinical coding module that allows collection of the mandatory statistics on diagnosis and operations developed as part of the Körner NHS data collection process, from which regional and national epidemiological statistics are compiled.

Thus these systems should in theory be able to be used at least for case finding and production of numerical data about length of stay, bed occupancy, readmissions, etc. that could be useful for audit. Unfortunately, practical experience has not borne this out. There are numerous papers in the literature[3,4,5] that show that the information in these systems tends to be wildly inaccurate, in terms of not only the numerical data but also the clinical details stored. Not only are the numerical data often inaccurate but the level of clinical detail is usually insufficient to be of much use to the clinician.

In addition to the quoted papers, as a further example we have performed a study in our own unit to look at the accuracy of computer recording of diagnoses and operations performed on the same patients independently by our medical staff/secretaries and by the clinical coding section of the medical records department. Before we even got to the accuracy of the actual coding the first finding was that 30 % of the patients recorded by the clinical system did not appear in the hospital system at all for the consultant episode in question, revealing a major deficit in the process by which the data are captured. In fact, as in many hospitals coding relies on the patient's notes reaching the coding office and many sets never do, for example because patients have been transferred to another hospital taking their notes with them, or because they have outpatient visits scheduled for soon after discharge for which the notes are needed. In our study the accuracy of the actual coding done on the patients was very good by both coding staff and secretaries, there being over 95 % correspondence when ICD-9 and OPCS-4 codes were compared. This is not as good as it seems however because a further and major problem for supporting clinical audit is the level of clinical usefulness of the codes themselves. We had great difficulty translating the clinical terms used in our computer system and in everyday practice into ICD-9 and OPCS-4 codes so that we could compare them with the codes used by the coding staff. Indeed for patients where I had actually performed the relevant operation I found it difficult to decide which OPCS-4 code should be used.

To be fair, ICD-9 and OPCS-4, the standard NHS coding systems, were never designed for clinical use. They were designed for administrative use and in particular for epidemiological use. As a result the ways in which diagnoses and operations are grouped do not necessarily reflect clinical practice and the terminology used is often very cumbersome albeit factually correct.

The clinical shortcomings of these systems were one of the main pressures that brought about the production and development of the Read clinical classification. It is very revealing to survey the commercially available clinical information systems with regard to the way in which they capture and record clinical data. None of these uses ICD-9 and OPCS-4 codes as the primary method of data capture, which is interesting when one considers that in its wisdom that is what the Körner committee has committed the NHS medical records departments to doing.

In addition to the accuracy and coding problems, the actual hospital computer systems themselves suffer from several other drawbacks when looked at from the point of view of clinical audit. These problems all stem from the fact that these systems were designed for administrative use within the health service and not to satisfy the information requirements of clinicians, and no matter how many 'add-ons' are added to them this fundamental problem remains. Thus whilst it may be quite straightforward to request a clinic appointment for a patient, or find out what clinics they have been to before, you will not find any details of what they were there for or what happened to them as a result. Even within the in-patient clinical coding module, it is easy to code a patient in the system but try and get information out again! In our own region to do a search of the regional PIS (patient information system) where unit data are aggregated is a major task that has to be done by the computer staff and typically takes several days to come up with a printout, of what we have already said are data of questionable accuracy and completeness. So in addition to the data quality problems already outlined there are major difficulties with rapid access to the data when required.

Is there any light at the end of this tunnel? The answer is yes, mainly because with the advent of a greater financial emphasis to the NHS it is becoming very important that hospitals have accurate patient-based information, because of course the hospital that is undervaluing the work that it does will be getting paid less than it should. This has led to the development of the 'casemix' systems, which are large hospital-wide computer systems that are intended to keep track of patients' clinical details so that the correct resource implications are documented. These systems rely on good-quality clinical information and as a result the clinical coding function of the medical records department is being brought out of the basement into a more prominent position. Some of the developers of these systems have finally realised what many clinicians have known for some time, and that is that the only way to get the best-quality clinical data is to get them directly from the doctors, rather than the standard NHS way which for years has been for staff unconnected with the clinical staff trying to divine the information from often badly written casenotes. Several casemix systems have rather attractive modules that clinicians can use for storing their 'own' data in addition to the basic diagnostic and operative information that both they and the management require. Whilst most large hospitals are going to have to invest in such a system, most are a long way away from providing it for every clinician to use as desired.

Non-commercial clinically based systems

The unmet needs of clinicians within the NHS have led many to set up their own clinical computer systems and many of these have led on to commercial developments later.[6,7] With the recent and continuing rapid advances in computer technology, the power and data storage facilities of the average desktop personal computer (PC) are more than adequate to run such a system. The most attractive feature of these systems is that they, and the data within, belong to the medical staff themselves. Not only are the data there to be looked at whenever desired, but also the format of the data and indeed what data are stored are determined by the clinician themselves. Equally, as is often the case, if after a few weeks it becomes clear that some facet of the data storage needs to be changed then it can be done, without recourse to anyone else.

How does the average system of this type work? Almost universally these are PC based systems, running on computers sitting on the desk in the clinical office. They use a piece of software known as a database, which is basically a program that allows information to be recorded in a structured way for ease of retrieval. Data are usually recorded in a series of parcels or boxes known as 'fields', which are organised into a series of forms or 'records'. One field might be Surname, or Date of birth or Diagnosis, and a record would be like a whole printed form with various boxes for individual pieces of information. Database software comes in varying levels of sophistication, the latest types being 'relational' allowing different records to be related by common fields. For example, a patient's hospital number can be the link between several different records about the same patient.

Some databases either have their own wordprocessing software attached, or can be linked to a wordprocessor, and this allows the possibility of generation of secretarial documents from the stored data. The commonest example in practice is the automatic generation of a discharge summary from data entered into various fields.

When one looks at the organisation of these systems, most indeed revolve around the collection of data during a hospital in-patient stay and the production of an automatic discharge summary as a by-product. There is often a printed proforma that is completed during the admission, onto which data are recorded in a structured way – structured because the form has spaces for certain pieces of information that act as a prompt reminding the doctor completing the form that an answer is required. The recorded data then have to be entered into the computer, either by the doctor or the medical secretary. This is where the carrot of the automatic discharge summary comes in, because as a general rule of course all NHS medical and secretarial staff have more than enough work to do already, and the addition of an extra task without immediately obvious benefit is not a winning strategy. Most systems have additional secretarial facilities aiding their implementation into the clinical office.

There is a certain attraction in doing away with paper recording of data completely and several systems allow data entry directly into the computer by the doctor. This is a rather different strategy because it requires adoption of a new task by these doctors, whereas secretarial staff are already used to keyboards, typing and increasingly to computers. There is a danger that direct medical data entry will be viewed as rather a chore and hence delegated to those most junior in the unit. The most junior staff are usually the most transitory with the least to gain from these data, and hence their level of motivation to enter accurate and complete data may not be high.

Setting up standard commercial database and wordprocessing software to do these tasks is a time-consuming but not unduly complicated task, and many clinicians have done this for their departments. The main problem with this approach is that such systems are highly individual and although they work well with their originator they may not elsewhere where their foibles are not understood. The data stored in such systems are usually not easily comparable with those in other systems, even within the same hospital, rendering the increasingly important concept of comparable audit difficult. Furthermore, these systems are usually for technical and financial reasons independent from the central hospital PAS system and so require their own entry of patients' demographic data, duplicating what is already in the PAS system.

Commercially available clinically based systems

The unmet needs of clinicians have not escaped the commercial computer world. Several systems on the market have had their beginnings in the enthusiasm of a clinician developing his/her own system and then expanding this with commercial help. Equally, computer firms have produced software of their own to subserve these functions.

The method of organisation of these systems is usually very similar to those of the non-commercial systems from which they gain their impetus. Again, the input method is usually a structured form, either on paper or on screen requiring certain pieces of data to be entered. There are various output 'carrots' such as office automation features with wordprocessing and automatic discharge summaries.

The commercial systems are inevitably much more polished than the non-commercial in terms of ease of use. They usually have more features, such as waiting list modules, graphics and statistics for reports, etc.

In the commercial arena the major problem however is cost. Compared to standard PC database and wordprocessing software this type of customised software is usually an order of magnitude more expensive, being measured in thousands of pounds per user for the software rather than hundreds. There are also usually significant ongoing costs amounting to around 10–15% of the original cost for maintenance and upgrading of the software. It can be extremely foolish to buy such software without taking up the ongoing costs as these cover any breakdowns of the software. These, the users will not usually be able to sort out themselves, because the technical workings of these programs are designed to be inaccessible to the user in order to protect the copyright of the developer. Equally, such software will probably be upgraded from time to time to take advantage of new developments, and not to have these upgrades means that a local system may quickly become outdated.

The other more fundamental problem with these clinically based systems is that they are essentially designed as independent systems from the central hospital PAS systems that already exist. Electronic links can often be made so that demographic patient data already stored in PAS can be used by the system, but this requires extra work and funds.

On the other hand, there can be great advantages to purchasing a commercial system 'off the shelf'. Firstly it already exists and development work by the clinician should be minimal, indeed it should be possible to get a 'plug in and go' system, given what specific features are required in advance. On entering into a commercial contract with a supplier specific requirements can be written into the contract together with follow-up facilities such as guaranteed call-out times in the event of failure. This can be a slightly two-edged sword, however, as it does require the supplier to be still in business in order to honour the contract!

Of greater importance, one can purchase a system that other units around the country are using already, so ensuring that firstly the system is tried and tested, but also that data can be compared between units. In the surgical field there are several 'user groups' for particular software programs, meeting regularly, and as a result in general surgery and more recently orthopaedic surgery the concept of *'confidential comparative audit'* has appeared.[8] Here, initially, the same data have been collected from clinicians using the same computer software and comparative complication rates, workload figures, etc. produced in a non-identifiable way. This has great promise as a method of inter-unit audit, but it does rely on the involved clinicians collecting the same data in the same format, which is easiest to ensure if they are using the same computer system.

What is the ideal system?

Clearly the answer is a fully PAS integrated, user-friendly, system allowing for secretarial office automation features, clinician designed data storage facilities and unlimited on demand reporting facilities for the stored data in any format desired. Data storage methods should be undemanding on clinical and secretarial time with high accuracy and reproducibility.

Such a system does not exist, and there has been a remarkable lack of central vision in the NHS in terms of developing such systems. The potential cost savings to the NHS if such a system had been produced centrally and then provided free of charge to those that wanted it, could have been huge. However, in practical terms this may be an unrealistic goal, for the NHS as an organisation seems to have great difficulty in standardising anything nationally, whether it is the cost and supplier of toilet-paper or computer software.

What would be ideal for most hospitals would probably be the development of an in-house clinically based information system integrated with the central hospital PAS, that could use technology based around the friendly PC on the clinician's desk rather than around the complicated mainframe-type central hospital computers. Such a system could then be spread around the whole hospital rather than each department having its own independent and probably incompatible systems. With certain notable exceptions[9] these systems have been very slow in arriving, one suspects because systems aimed at financial administration have been given a higher priority than those aimed at clinical audit. However, times are changing largely because the importance of timely and accurate clinical data is being realised, and this can be best obtained direct from clinicians or their computer systems.

How should you set about looking at systems?

This largely rests on planning and research before launching into getting a computer system[10,11] and the two referenced publications can be strongly recommended. None of us would embark upon a completely new method of treatment for our patients without a great deal of planning and research of the literature, especially of any negative reports. It is surprising how many clinicians have embarked on a completely new method of working for their department, and secretaries in particular, without much more than seeing system demonstrations by those selling them. Of much greater importance than a demonstration is researching the current users of a system to see what they think of it.

This process can be divided into several steps which I will discuss in more detail, as a practical guide.

1. Draft out a plan on paper without thinking about any particular system.
2. Discuss this with all interested parties – secretaries, doctors, your local unit computer services department and managers for their comments.
3. Evaluate systems that you see by means of a checklist for particular features.
4. Ask for formal written quotations from potential suppliers covering in detail your written requirements.

Planning and consultation

It is extremely helpful to produce a written outline of what you want. Not only does this crystallise your plans, but if you cannot produce a written outline of your system you cannot hope to get one that will do what you want it to do. This outline, when revised in more detail, can hopefully become a specification for suppliers to work from. This applies both to the software program and to the hardware on which it is to be run.

Data organisation

Firstly decide on the following points

(a) What data do you want to record (and later analyse) in your system?

For example, how much demographic data on patients do you want? – will date of birth and sex do, or do you want marital status, ethnic origin, etc.? These requirements will differ from specialty to specialty so it is no use copying someone else's list. It is necessary to make a list on paper of each individual piece of data, together with their level of priority to you. Some will be essential, others advisable and others optional.

(b) In what form do you want the data recorded?

This is especially important for clinical data, in terms of diagnostic data. Do you want to use any of the standard coding systems? Are they good for your specialty? Will you have to produce your own list of diagnoses, etc. and if so can you keep them compatible with other systems?

(c) On which patients are you going to record these data?

Are you going to start off the whole of your department in one go or will there be a phased introduction? Are you going to record data on all patients or a subset? Are you going to deal with just in-patients, out-patients or both?

(d) Where, and more particularly who, are you going to get these data from?

This needs some analysis of the processing of data in your department. If for example the house staff in hospital complete all the in-patient records, summaries, etc. you may wish to aim your system at them. If you have good dictation facilities you may be able to specify data yourself on ward rounds, in clinics, etc.

(e) How are the data going to be recorded?

Are you going for a paper/proforma based system with later entry into the computer or a system using the computer as the primary medical staff recording medium. The former may be easier to implement as the latter requires a completely new task to be introduced to the medical staff. It will be more cumbersome, however.

(f) Who is going to enter the data into the computer?

This requires careful thought, as whoever it is must regard this as an important task and not as yet another chore without any obvious benefit. Is there any chance of you getting a specific new member of staff for this? If not how can you motivate your junior staff or secretarial staff to do this? Will it save them any other work in compensation? – e.g. by producing automatic letters, summaries or helping with research projects.

(g) What other computer systems exist locally that you need to take account of?

There are two areas to consider here. Firstly, if other departments have already obtained a particular clinical audit system there may be compelling reasons for you to consider the same one. Such systems are usually cheaper the more that is bought on one site and maintenance etc. is usually easier the more that there is in one place. Secondly, will your system need to interface with existing systems such as PAS, laboratory systems, etc.? This does need to go into your written specification before evaluating systems, although it will usually need detailed discussions with the district IT department.

Hardware organisation
What sort of computer hardware do you want?

Whether you have a system that runs on personal desktop type computers or on a large central hospital computer with terminals, depends to a certain extent on what other tasks you want to do with the hardware. For example, if in addition to the audit system you want to supply your secretarial staff with wordprocessing facilities, the local availability and their preferences for software will be important. Few large hospital systems have such office automation features, whereas they are plentiful for PCs. The use that you wish to make of your data is also important. If you wish to make colour graphics, 35 mm slides, overhead projector sheets etc. for presentation of data, these are tasks that at the moment are basically PC based.

Where do you want your data to be physically stored and what are the security and backup implications?

If all your data reside in one PC in an office, there are potential dangers of access by unauthorised users and of loss of it all if, for example, the PC were to be stolen. Despite claims to the contrary the PC is a very insecure device as those with a reasonably knowledge of such computers can usually 'hack' into the data around security features such as passwords. Thus both the security of the data on the machine and also the physical security of access to it must be considered. Equally, whilst data stored in a large central hospital computer system may seem at first sight more secure, who in fact will have access to it? Remember that the responsibility for unauthorised access to potentially sensitive clinical information rests with the clinician recording it, who must make sure that it is secure.

The related topic of data backup must be considered. Computers, whilst usually reliable, do go wrong and if there is only one copy of your data in a machine that goes wrong, is destroyed in a fire, or is stolen then that is a disaster. Regular copies, preferably daily, must be made of the entire database, and this requires both hardware, software and a mechanism and person identified to do it.

Discussions

There are important groups of staff who should be involved from the start in plans to implement an audit computer system. These are not only the actual users, who will often not be clinicians, but those who have to pick up the financial costs of supporting the system, which can be considerable. These are covered by the headings below.

(a) What do your secretarial and/or medical staff think of your plan?

All too often those staff who are going to be using the system day in and day out are not adequately consulted in advance. Do your secretaries and medical staff like the idea and will they use it? What are the implications for alterations in their current workload?

(b) What does your management think of the idea?

Without support from your managers things will be very difficult. In particular, the ongoing costs of the system in staff time and contracts for hardware and software maintenance may not be supported leaving you in a difficult position when things go wrong.

(c) What is the opinion of your unit/district information and computing department?

There may be major advantages in getting your local computing department involved with your system. In particular, they usually control access to the local PAS system and so if you want your system to have access to patients' demographic data they will have to be involved. There may also be advantages to their taking over responsibility for your hardware and/or software maintenance. On the other hand there may be a danger of you losing control of your system if you relinquish it to such a department, where a departmental clinical audit system may carry rather low priority compared to the PAS, appointments, financial, telecommunications and other large systems that these departments run.

(d) What is the opinion of the coding staff in your hospital ?

Coding of diagnostic and operative data is a difficult and time-consuming task performed by often undervalued staff in every hospital in the UK by statutory requirement. If you are recording such data yourself in your audit system there may well be common ground in which the coding staff can gain benefit from your data, and may be able in return to assist you, for example by input of data.

Evaluations

It is only too easy when looking at a computer system to be carried away by what it appears to do, and not notice what it doesn't do. Such systems need a proper evaluation in a structured way, like a new medical treatment, and not just a superficial inspection. The main areas to consider are as follows.

(a) How does this system cover your written requirements ?

The only way to decide this properly is to write down, with reference to your previously written requirements, which features this system has, which features it can be made to have and which it will not have. This needs to be considered in two sections – the software program and the hardware on which it is to be run.

(b) If modifications are needed to the system before installation, will the supplier provide a written commitment to do these ?

Beware the salesman! Suppliers of such systems are only too willing to promise that certain features that you want incorporated are easy to do. Only a written agreement, with exact costings, can be relied on. This is especially important when it comes to things like interfacing with PAS, which can be a difficult and expensive task. Therefore, the fact that something can be done with a computer system (and in theory virtually anything can be done) does not mean that it will be done.

(c) Arrange a demonstration of the system to all interested parties in your department.

This is extremely important as different members have different viewpoints. For example, you, as a clinician, cannot possibly assess the secretarial aspects of a system whereas your secretaries can. This demonstration is not a sufficient evaluation on its own as it will invariably be given by the supplier or an enthusiastic user who will therefore gloss over any deficiencies. You need to know what the 'warts' of the system are now, and not after you have bought it.

(d) Ask the supplier for a list of departments already using this system and arrange a visit.

It is better to ask for a list like this rather than asking the supplier to arrange a visit for you, as they will inevitably arrange for you to visit an enthusiastic user. If you have a list of users then you can telephone a few and visit one of your own choosing which may be more informative. It is always much more enlightening to talk to a user who has had problems than to one who has not. Ask such users about the quality of follow-up by the suppliers as well as the quality of the actual system. Interestingly, of the eight quoted departmental users of a particular commercial system who I contacted personally as part of our departmental evaluations, the only two that were happy with the system were the department of the original clinical developer and the department that it was suggested that one visited. I learned much more from my conversations with the other six departments some of whom were not using the system at all, despite having bought it, because of various problems.

(e) Ask the supplier for a commitment-free trial of the system.

Unfortunately, this is often not possible, but also often not actually asked for. A supplier secure in their system should have no particular reason for not leaving you a trial version for a week or so to look at yourself in more detail and to try out.

(f) Ask the supplier for details of their company.

If purchasing a system from a commercial source, what will happen if that source ceases to exist. If the company ceases trading you may get into a very difficult situation in which you have a system that nobody else can deal with. The trading record and viability of the company is therefore important and you may need independent advice on this.

Quotations

It is vital to get down on paper exact details of the software and hardware with prices before making any commitment. Such quotations need to cover certain specific areas as follows.

(a) Obtain a written detailed quotation for the system covering both hardware and software.

There may be merit in getting your hardware and software from different sources, but the same principle applies to both. A written quotation can form the basis of a written contract with the supplier and this is the only way to be sure to get what you have asked for. Clinicians have poor business training in general and it is only too easy to rely on verbal assurances that are never brought about. Every aspect of your system to be supplied should be on paper in all the categories already discussed, including a detailed specification of what the software will do.

(b) Obtain written details of installation costs.

There are a number of 'hidden' costs to installing such a computer system. Actual installation of the hardware must be considered together with any cabling costs, etc. Similarly, installation of the software on the hardware requires time and may be charged for. Written manuals will be needed for the software, and lastly and most importantly the staff using the system will need to be trained in its use. Written costs for all these aspects are vital in advance of installation.

(c) Obtain written details of follow-up and maintenance agreements.

Written commitments to maintenance are vital. These should include specific guaranteed call-out times in case of a system failure, of either hardware or software. Details of upgrading of software with future developments should be made clear, and the cost of these agreements for the foreseeable future made clear. It is not sensible to install either hardware or software without getting these aspects sorted out in advance, as computer systems inevitably do go wrong from time to time and need specialist repair.

(d) Obtain written details of the procedure if the supplier ceases to exist.

Computer software often cannot be modified without access to what is known as the 'source code' which is the original writing of the program. Understandably, suppliers are often not willing to let you have this as it is their main protection against piracy of their programs. If they cease to exist, however, you will need the source code if anyone else is to modify your system for you or to sort out any problems with it. It is preferable to insist on a written agreement to be supplied with such access in that event, as no matter how secure the company they may not be here in a year's time.

Conclusions

The whole process of acquiring a computer system to support clinical audit may seem a daunting procedure. However, the pitfalls that I have outlined in this chapter are only too real and it is only too easy to find clinicians who have fallen into them. Indeed, we have done so ourselves in the past. This should not diminish the incalculable benefits that can be gained from such systems, properly installed. All members of staff involved can become very enthusiastic about the system, from the secretarial staff who may feel that their worth has been recognised by the introduction of technological help in their day-to-day work, to the medical staff who are at last able to get hold of data for meaningful audit and to support research projects. These computer systems are relatively new and this is still an area of continuing development and so it may be unrealistic to expect to get a system now that will last. However, I firmly believe that any lasting and comprehensive system of medical audit cannot be run without access to computerisation of some sort.

Happy hunting, but remember the old adage – 'to err is human but to really foul things up requires a computer' !

References

1. Pollock, A. & Evans, M. (1989). *Surgical Audit*. London: Butterworths.
2. Shaw, C. (1989). *Medical Audit: A Hospital Handbook*. London: The King's Fund Centre.
3. Sunderland, R. (1985). Inaccurate coding corrupts medical information. *Archives of Disease in Childhood*, **60**, 593–594.
4. Whates, P. D., Birgzalis, A. R. & Irvine, M. (1982). Accuracy of hospital activity analysis operation codes. *British Medical Journal*, **284**, 1857–1858.
5. Knight, L., Yardley, M. & Jones A (1991). The dangers resulting from inaccurate computer-based operative records. *British Journal of Clinical Practice*, **45**, 41–42.
6. Ellis, B. W., Michie, H. R., Esufali, S. T., Pyper, R. J. D. & Dudley, H. A. F. (1986). Development of a microcomputer system for surgical audit and patient administration: a review. *Journal of the Royal Society of Medicine*, **80**, 157–161.
7. Dunn, D. C. (1988). Audit of a surgical firm by microcomputer: five years' experience. *British Medical Journal*, **296**, 687–691.
8. Emberton, M., Rivett, R. & Ellis, B. W. (1991). Comparative Audit: A new method of delivering audit. *Annals of the Royal College of Surgeons of England* (Supplement), **73**, 117–120.
9. Purser, H., Secker-Walker, J. & Curzon, S. (1989). Exploring Medical Audit in Bloomsbury. *British Journal of Healthcare Computing*, **6**, 11–15.
10. West Midlands Regional Health Authority and Anderson Consulting. Royal Society of Medicine Services Ltd. (1990). *Computers in Medical Audit*.
11. Joint Commission on Accreditation of Healthcare Organisations, USA (1990). *How to buy QA/RM Software*.

13

Paediatric audit

PHILIP C. HOLLAND

Introduction

As in other medical specialties the increasing emphasis on medical audit should be welcomed by the paediatricians. The need to review critically specific aspects of paediatric care is of particular importance. What is implemented by paediatricians may have long-term consequences, potentially into adult life. These consequences may on occasions not be appreciated if they subsequently present only to the adult physician or if adequate follow up is not achieved. It may be difficult to measure every aspect of paediatrics and child health, although a wide spectrum of paediatric care can be covered from child health surveillance, neonatology, paediatric surgery and general paediatrics. It should begin with perinatal care and the developing foetus and thus by definition cross into obstetrics. Although audit in the form of, for example, perinatal meetings have taken place in the past, the recent impetus in initiating more formal audit should remind us that previously some new procedures, drugs and techniques have been accepted with enthusiasm without critical review. Intrapartum foetal monitoring of the full-term baby is so accepted by some that it is thought negligent not to monitor during labour, although a recent study now questions this.[1] Before accepting specific audit procedures as a measure of quality of care then we have to be certain that our guidelines are reliable, as shown in the preceding example. Establishment of reliable audit of patient care is accepted by all involved in the care of children; however, there are immediate problems. Death, one hopes, is an uncommon outcome and, therefore, quality of care becomes as important but more elusive to measurement and comparison. Audit must look at the total work of a clinical team as well as compare the management of individual conditions.

To enable evaluation and comparison of care to be achieved within paediatrics then 'predetermined objectives' must be established by an acceptable body of paediatricians. In conjunction with this, paediatricians must be prepared to evaluate their work critically and be prepared to change if necessary. These predetermined objectives must include 'quality of life' as a variable. Attempts to define quality of life have been used in assessment of handicap subsequent to neonatal intensive care and may also include attempts at estimating total financial costs. *Quality adjusted life years* (QALY) are calculated based on a number of parameters including physical disability, social and emotional function and health problems. The relative value of these health states (utility scores) are scored from 0 (death) to 1 (normal health). These utility scores are then used to adjust life years for quality, the greater the handicap the lower the number of quality adjusted life years.[2] It is sobering to note that some parents rated certain chronic handicaps as worse than death, and thus scored below nought. Questions about perceived quality of life, patient (parent) satisfaction and physical health should be constructed to enable outcome to be assessed. In its broadest sense 'quality of life' to a child may include number of days off school, exercise tolerance or side effects of drugs, for example. All paediatricians know that even with severely debilitating conditions and terminal diseases, the help provided by the paediatric unit can be invaluable support to the family. Ultimately, the paediatrician is judged not only by his/her management of specific conditions but also by his/her relationship with individual children and parents.

Outcome measures in child health were addressed in a report published by the British Paediatric Association and included suggestions on how these may be applied.[3] The report published in February 1990 demonstrates that audit within paediatrics is still in its infancy. Highlighted in the report is the difficulty in determining 'outcome measures' and this will be discussed under the relevant section later in the text. In an attempt to produce a set standard in the management of common conditions, individual 'expert' groups have produced or are about to produce 'consensus statements' on the management of conditions such as asthma[4] and epilepsy. The British Paediatric Association working party has published a report on paediatric audit which briefly outlines the role of audit and includes specific audit report forms in relation to general paediatrics, community paediatrics and neonatology.[5]

Working parties involved in the establishment of medical audit use the framework of *structure* or *resource, process* and *outcome*. This will have been discussed in detail elsewhere but specific examples of its application to paediatric audit will be given within the context of these headings, although overlap occurs. Audit should not only compare one's own management against a recognised standard but also look at ways paediatric care is given in each unit and constantly reappraise this.

Data collection and coding

The British Paediatric Association has been instrumental in the drawing up of paediatric codes based on the ICD-9 coding system; this is likely to be superseded by the Read coding system. The problem of data collection is paramount if successful audit is to be achieved. In paediatrics, with the wide variation in admission rates along with the relative short admission time, it is obviously important that accurate and reliable data collection is achieved. Incomplete data collection may obviously lead to erroneous conclusions when the audit is complete. The difficulty in obtaining data on routine admissions such as length of stay and diagnostic categories is unfortunately still a problem here, as in many hospitals. This problem is highlighted not to show the deficits of this hospital but to stress the need for good-quality data collection. The average length of stay on a children's ward is two days. Eighty per cent of admissions are acute via general practitioners or casualty. To enable accurate data collection with reliable discharge diagnosis there must be some way of reviewing diagnosis and coding at discharge. An approach taken in this hospital is to combine the discharge summary and coding under the responsibility of a ward secretary. Summaries are dictated at discharge as per standard protocol. This protocol will ultimately be adapted to enable specific data collection. We have elected to code for certain procedures such as lumbar punctures as well as for diagnoses. Summaries are typed and dispatched after review at the weekly ward audit meeting. Random checks are made to insure that no discharge has occurred without a summary. An immediate benefit of such a system is to reduce the average time to the GP receiving a summary from six weeks to ten days.

Medical care of the newborn

Audit of the medical and nursing care of newborn babies is important not only because they are more likely to die on the first day of life than on any other, but because the well-being of babies in the first few weeks of life has a bearing on their health throughout childhood and adolescence and into adult life. Of approximately 650 000 births in England and Wales annually about 3500 are born dead and a similar number die within a month. Some

5–7% of births are preterm and 1% of total births are very immature requiring intensive care. The Royal College of Physicians' report published in 1988[6] lays down guidelines for medical staffing of neonatal units thus giving a base line for resource audit. Financial limitations make these recommendations unlikely to be achieved. Traditional perinatal audit includes perinatal mortality meetings with comparison of annual perinatal and neonatal mortality rates. (Perinatal mortality being the number of babies who die from 24 weeks of gestation to one week of age per 1000 total births. Neonatal mortality is the number of babies who die within 28 days of birth per 1000 live births.)

Mortality rates, although important, are relatively crude and the fall in mortality rates makes it more important to assess outcome, particularly in relation to handicap as well as incidence of specific neonatal problems during intensive care. Neonatal units should be able to extract with ease the figures for standard neonatal problems. Comparison between units can only occur however, if the condition is clearly defined and the data are collected uniformly. Comparison between studies is often confused as some collect data in groups based on gestational age, others on birthweight, and yet others do not distinguish between inborn and outborn babies. The report on outcome measures mentioned earlier only refers to the minimum data collection such as death rates in weight categories < 1000 g, 1000 to < 1500 g, for example. Neonatology is an area where there is a relatively finite number of common problems (Box 13.1) and, therefore, comparison between units could occur with ease. Long-term outcome with follow up till at least five years of age is imperative if reliable neurological outcome measures are to be achieved.

Ultimately, the benefits of audit will only be seen if there is accurate data collection enabling not only comparisons annually within a unit but between units. Specific audit projects may then allow further analysis of other aspects of neonatal care. The potential scope is wide and should include parental involvement in areas such as the recognition and management of handicap, the management of the dying neonate and assessment of how parents are informed of the neonatal problems that have occurred or may occur. Minimal audit requirements must include the analysis of the annual perinatal mortality rates within the different age brackets but there is the need and potential to move beyond this. The British Paediatric Association or the Perinatal Society could take the lead in promoting audit between neonatal units. Consensus guidelines are needed on 'acceptable' levels of the complications of neonatal care as seen in Box 13.1. This is becoming increasingly important in association with

Box 13.1   *Common neonatal problems*

- Hyaline membrane disease
- Pneumothorax
- Aspiration syndromes
- Persistent foetal circulation
- Bronchopulmonary dysplasia
- Patent ductus arteriosus
- Necrotising enterocolitis
- Intraventricular haemorrhage and grade
- Periventricular leukomalacia
- Metabolic bone disease
- Retinopathy of prematurity
- Congenital abnormalities

the government White Paper and perhaps the move for more intensive neonatology to be done in the local unit and a possible reluctance for transfer to regional neonatal units.

Paediatric pathology

The clinical importance of reliable autopsy data is not always appreciated. In the neonate or aborted foetus, diagnoses made at autopsy may have clinical and genetic relevance for future pregnancies. Porter and Keeling, in a survey of 150 stillbirths and 150 neonatal deaths, showed that in 36 % of stillbirths and 44 % of neonatal deaths important clinical information was obtained at autopsy.[7] The perinatal autopsy is an important method of audit for the obstetrician, paediatrician and radiologist. The commonest cause of death from one month of age to a year is the sudden infant death syndrome. Accurate pathology may diagnose inborn errors of metabolism (e.g. fatty acid oxidation defects), which have genetic implications, and rarely non-accidental injury, which has important social ramifications.

The Yorkshire region recently completed a survey of perinatal and foetal autopsies performed in 1986.[8] The perinatal autopsy rate for the region was 62 %, lower than the recommended rate of 75 %. Important problems were highlighted, in particular the lack of facilities to weigh foetuses, perform whole-body X-rays and photograph pathological findings. In the region as a whole 37 % of the autopsied deaths were of macerated but normally formed foetuses, 14 % had congenital abnormalities, 17 % had conditions associated with immaturity and 27 % conditions associated with pregnancy or labour. The last three groups in particular may have important clinical implications. Of the aborted foetuses 21% were associated with congenital malformations and 7% with an infective process although the majority were normal. The relatively few perinatal autopsies performed in some districts, fewer than seven per year, may be important concerning the training of future pathologists.

This report demonstrates the importance of regionally based audit projects. It highlights deficits in the specialty and compares them with the recommended standard. The project was financed by the region and a doctor was employed full time to visit each hospital and collect the data. It was published at the beginning of 1991 and it is obviously too early to assess whether the lessons learnt in the audit will be acted on.

Paediatric surgery

The *National Confidential Enquiry into Perioperative Deaths* (NCEPOD) was established to enquire into clinical practice and to identify remedial factors in the practice of anaesthesia and surgery[9]. It was estimated that one in five of all deaths occurs within 30 days of a surgical or gynaecological procedure. In the first year a smaller easier defined group was chosen, namely children ten years of age and under. It is not possible to highlight all features of this report but it is taken as an example of national paediatric audit. A specific target group has been defined, i.e. children under ten requiring surgery. This group, particularly towards the younger age, and especially in the neonatal period, generate specific problems both preoperatively and during surgery. These may include not only the ability to recognise how sick a child actually is (not always easy), but also complex fluid management problems and maintenance of body temperature. A total of 417 deaths were investigated. The study looked at surgical and anaesthetic management, particularly reviewing the paediatric experience of those responsible for care. The collection of information on perioperative deaths was highly successful with only 0.2% of consultants refusing to participate. The general conclusions are worth highlighting. Overall surgical and anaesthetic management were good with consultants being involved in care. Problems were more likely to arise when locum staff were involved or when the staff at all grades did not recognise their lack of paediatric expertise. The needs of children in sub-specialist surgical units such as neurosurgery and burns were not always met. The natural dominance of surgical requirements are paramount but could have been supplemented by the skills offered by paediatricians and paediatric anaesthetists. As already highlighted, data collection systems were inadequate making the routine review of specific events, e.g. postoperative complications, time consuming and difficult. The study was made possible by the availability of national funding and the involvement of the Royal Colleges in promoting professional led audit. Its benefits will only be seen if it is read, acted upon and repeated.

Surgeons have led the field in relation to audit of postoperative complications and it would be considered poor surgical care if a system was not functioning in all surgical units. In relation to the NCEPOD report, specific attention to complications in children should, therefore, be considered by general surgeons and audited independently.

Medical care of children

Recommended levels of medical and nurse staffing of paediatric wards have not been clearly established, although guidelines have been issued by appropriate authorities. This needs to take into consideration not only the age range but also type of paediatric care required. Occupancy levels cannot be too high or children will then have to be nursed on adult wards, although no real figures exist for ideal occupancy rates in children's wards. Due to wide fluctuations in admissions rates, an average of 75% occupancy will minimise the risk of the ward closing or children being nursed on adult wards. Cubicle space to allow isolation and/or a parent to sleep next to the baby needs to be available. A DHSS building note refers to the need for 0.9 to 1.1 children's beds per 1000 population under 16, excluding mentally handicapped children and special care cots. Advice was also given that eight out of 20 beds should be as single cubicles.[10]

Under the auspices of general paediatrics the opportunity exists for audit of not only acute admissions and out-patients but also of select populations. Diabetes, asthma and cystic fibrosis are areas already highlighted for regular medical audit. The collection of children in such clinics allows specific targets to be set. Comparisons may be made between clinics, or in the same clinic over different periods of time.

The British Paediatric Association working party recommendations on diabetic services list the minimal criteria for each district.[11] This includes the establishment of a diabetic clinic with a consultant paediatrician taking a specific interest in diabetes, and a health visitor and dietician with expertise in diabetic care. Resource audit should establish that such a clinic exists and that appropriate staff are available. Audit should go beyond this and involve the children and parents in looking at the deficiencies of the clinic and correcting them. This may include access to adult diabetic services, British Diabetic Association camps, psychiatric help, educational literature and diabetic evenings. Diabetic complications are rare in childhood with the subsequent appearance of retinopathy or nephropathy in particular not necessarily being known to the paediatrician. Satisfactory transfer of care to adult clinics as well as successful follow up can both be achieved with the development of joint liaison with adult diabetologists. Biochemical audit may rely on regular monitoring of glycosylated haemoglobin. The British Paediatric Association's report on outcome measures has suggested an average glycosylated haemoglobin of 1.5 times the mean of the normal range of the laboratory as an acceptable level. We are initiating audit meetings between paediatric diabetic groups to enable us to compare facilities and standards of care between districts, enabling the sharing of individual ideas amongst other clinics.

Asthma affects 10 % of the childhood population and is one of the major causes of admission to paediatric wards. A recent review of 35 asthma deaths in the Northern region shows that 80 % had some preventable factor.[12] The major factors in their deaths included chronic undertreatment in 51 % and suboptimal management of the final attack with delay in seeking medical advice in 57 %. At present we are establishing audit of both our acute asthma management as well as the asthma clinic. A major component of this audit assesses the parents understanding of asthma and the use of score cards and peak flow meters by the parent and child in the management of their asthma. Guidelines for asthma management have been published by a consensus group of paediatricians from Europe and North America; this acts as a useful comparison to ones own management both of the acute admission as well as chronic asthma care.[4]

Minimal audit of childhood asthma should include looking at asthma deaths, asthmatics requiring ventilation, frequency of readmission to hospital and parent's/child's understanding of asthma, in particular knowing when to seek medical advice. Quality of life variables could include exercise tolerance, sleep pattern and time off school. Audit of such clinics is hampered by the problem of defining what are good outcome measures in the management of asthma. We are tackling this by initially trying to establish what the parents and child feel are the benefits of the clinic and what is lacking in the clinic. Score cards are completed by the parents or child and those children over five years of age are assessed for peak flow monitoring. These cards are scored in an attempt to define more accurately whether better control is achieved. Having established the deficits in the clinic, we can attempt to correct them and repeat the audit a year later. Data are collected straight on to a lap top computer so that the information can be collated and analysed with ease.

The publication by Phelan and Hey in 1984 comparing the mortality statistics in cystic fibrosis between the UK and Australia serves as an important introduction to audit in this disease.[13] The authors (rightly or wrongly) attributed the improved survival in Australia to the fact that these children all attended specialist centres. Comparison of median survival in different clinics here shows wide variation but also demonstrates the problem of regional comparisons. Social class may well affect outcome, those less well off and less able to travel may attend the local clinic, but may also be less compliant with therapy. Poor mortality may reflect poor compliance and social circumstances rather than a poor clinic.[14] Similarly, well-established supraregional centres may include more highly motivated parents – those wanting the 'best for their child'. The median age of death from cystic fibrosis has risen from 6 months in 1957 to 17 years in 1986; this must act as the gold standard to clinics. Audit cannot simply include death as the outcome measure; access to genetic counselling, to heart lung transplant, state of nutrition with dietetic services being available are all important. Audit meetings between such clinics with comparison of nutritional support and antibiotic policy, for example, would help highlight such differences.

A major problem in paediatrics is to establish process audit of the general paediatric workload. Attempts should be made by looking at access to paediatric services. Measures of this can include out-patient waiting lists, delays in acute admissions via casualty or directly from the general practitioner and delays in diagnosis. The commonest reasons for admission to paediatric wards are listed (Table 13.1); this may act as a guide to audit of specific categories of children such as those with abdominal pain, febrile convulsions and infections. We recently reviewed here the management and investigation of all cases of abdominal pain in children under 14 years referred in 1990 (Table 13.2). Specific cases from this audit were highlighted, in particular the three cases of peritonitis in relation to appendicitis of which two occurred in the paediatric medical wards. All investigations with respect to abdominal pain were also audited and the role of such investigations assessed. Ultrasound was performed in 8/53 surgical cases as opposed to 13/32 medical in-patient cases as an example. To complete the audit loop we need to define defects in our management of such a symptom, change our policy and re-evaluate later. Perhaps we should have similarly audited the 67% of medical cases and 40% of surgical cases where no diagnosis was made.

Little help is given in all the reports on audit as regards the setting up of audit in paediatric departments whether in district general hospitals or

Table 13.1 *Some of the commonest reasons for admission to a paediatric ward*

Diagnosis	%
Wheeze	18
Infections	12
Convulsions (febrile)	10
Convulsions (epileptic)	8
Vomiting/Diarrhoea	10
Stridor	4
Crying	—
Headache	—
Abdominal pain	—
Accidental ingestion	—
Deliberate ingestion	—
Relief care	—
Oncology treatment	—
Routine for investigation	—
Non-accidental injury	—

Table 13.2 *Audit of acute abdominal pain*

	Medical admissions	Surgical admissions
	21 in-patients	53 in-patients
	1.5% total admissions	3.9% total admissions
	33% diagnoses confirmed	60% diagnoses confirmed
In-patient diagnoses		
Appendicitis	2 (peritonitis)	13 (inflamed)
		6 (normal)
		2 (1 primary peritonitis)
Intussusception	1	1
Mesenteric adenitis	0	5
Urinary infection	3	0
Chest infection	1	0
Constipation	0	4
Miscellaneous	1 infective diarrhoea	1 ovarian cyst
Out-patient diagnoses		
(medical cases only)		
Constipation	4	
Irritable bowel syndrome	3	
Helicobacter pylori gastritis	2	
Gastro-oesophageal reflux	1	
Migraine	1	
Abdominal wall pain	2	
Mesenteric adenitis	1	
Total number of diagnoses	54	

specialist referral centres. The minimum data which needs to be readily available is a breakdown of admissions by diagnosis, age and length of stay, as well as the readmission rate over a given period. Statistics produced by many departments have little meaning and are in danger of being misinterpreted. Work-load on a paediatric ward is generated by the number of acute admissions and their severity and age distribution. Statistics of average occupancy mean little as it may not include the number of new admissions but simply reflect bed occupancy. In our ward, paediatric referrals by GPs are sent directly to the assessment area of the paediatric ward. Day attenders account for half our acute referral work load but will not appear on standard statistics unless collected separately.

Community paediatrics

As part of the recent changes in health care in this country we have seen the adoption of certain screening policies by the general practitioner as part of their new contract. This coincides with a rationalisation of screening programmes by community paediatricians, after recommendations on child health surveillance made following the report in 1989 on '*Health for All Children*'.[15] These recommendations act as very sound guidelines to screening procedures, which should be adopted throughout different health regions. They have succeeded in reducing a number of screening tests which have in general been of no proven value. Audit is not just part of assessing whether a specific screening programme is justified. It should examine, in the wider context, whether such a programme is working effectively. Audit is generally lacking in such cases, although recommendations have been made in the report referred to earlier from the British Paediatric Association.[3] An example given in the report is the assessment of the number of children diagnosed with congenitally dislocated hips after six months of age; this figure should be low. The increasing trend of early discharge may result in an increased incidence of late diagnosis, as it is known that a single examination at birth may well miss dislocation. Audit should also include false positive diagnosis, reflecting poor examination technique.

Audit of preschool checks must include failures to attend, perhaps those most in need of follow up. Selective medical examinations of school entrants have been proposed in an attempt to eliminate unnecessary medical examination, an area open to audit.[16] In *Health for All Children* ideas for establishing audit are briefly listed. These include the age at which serious defects are diagnosed, although this must be related to the age at which they are likely to present. Ventricular septal defects are rarely diagnosed at birth, for example, as the murmur is not present until right ventricular pressure falls. Further suggestions include examining the efficiency of the community service in relationship to special needs and education, maintenance of a register of the number of special needs children in the district and facilities available for them. Few places are able to produce a comprehensive list of children with special needs.

The publicity given to child abuse over the last few years highlights the major problems in auditing this area. Accurate and reliable data collection is essential and can only be achieved by recording the relevant data at the time of either examination or via the secretaries at the time of writing the report. Data that need to be available includes the age distribution of specific forms of abuse, the incidence of types of abuse and possible ways of detecting clustering of types of abuse in certain areas. Basic audit can include looking at missed cases of abuse, whether under paediatrician, casualty or orthopaedic departments and with more difficulty looking at incorrectly diagnosed cases of abuse.

Establishment of paediatric audit

As suggested in an editorial on medical audit a lot of thinking, talking and writing about audit is ill-focused and vague.[17] Due to the potential value of audit it is essential that paediatricians do take a lead in establishing audit correctly, ultimately leading to benefit in the care of children. It must be the responsibility of each paediatrician to set standards in his/her own field, where possible using 'consensus statements' as their guidelines. Paediatric guidelines on audit give little concrete advice on its initiation. By defining the minimum acceptable level of audit that should be achieved, we can then establish the resource implication. A major problem found here, as in all busy clinical departments with a large turnover, is not only collecting the data but finding the time for analysis of the data.

Casenote audit based on the British Paediatric Association checklist[5] is easy to establish. It is limited in what it can achieve and allows for a more formal check of the quality of the notes. Paediatric casenote review obviously takes more account of obstetric history, the child's developmental progress, growth, social circumstances and immunisations. Casenote audit is liable to become monotonous and is best done (in my mind) when new housemen start and less frequently once they are well established.

Auditing the paediatric ward service requires adequate and reliable information. The system here involves defining certain steps in the admission procedure and then logging these data. At all times we need to collect the basic demographic information. We need to know the age distribution of each diagnosis and the length of stay. Children seen and not admitted and day cases need to be quantified. More detailed data may best be collected as a series of regular audit programs. For example, this could be collected over a two-week period every six months, with a specific aim in mind. This might include such aspects as looking at the time from arrival in hospital to examination, being admitted to the ward, having investigations performed and the diagnosis finally made. Investigations and procedures performed acutely may be collated and the information gained from these investigations examined.

Due to the difficulty in defining outcome each paediatric unit must initially look at the service it provides and define problems in that service. Parent questionnaires as in the asthma study may bring these deficits to light. Having defined these deficiencies then attempts can be made to correct them and the audit repeated a year later. An out-patient audit, recently performed here, relied on a patient questionnaire to assess the deficits of the out-patient service. The aims of the study are listed (Box 13.2) and the questions were designed to assess whether these aims were being achieved. The most promising aspect was that 92% of parents felt that they had spent enough time with the doctor and good explanations were given. The major complaint was lack of car parking space; this may have the added effect of delaying out-patients because of late arrivals.

Future developments in audit require more sophisticated data collection as well as specific national audit projects, as seen in the NCEPOD study. Areas we are exploring, especially on the neonatal unit, are ways of collecting data on ward rounds. For this to be successful it must ultimately save time and remove some of the administrative workload from the junior medical staff. Neonatal units are ideal for this due to relatively low numbers, long stay and a limited number of diagnostic categories. The data are collected on hand held or lap top computers during each ward round and if tests are requested these can be printed out automatically. Very accurate data could be collected without extra staff and the annual neonatal unit statistics would be available immediately. Checks could be written into the program such that if a specific diagnosis is made then appropriate investigations are listed; this may be particularly useful if research projects are in progress in particular areas. Collection of data like this enables more accurate yearly comparisons which may highlight early any increase or decrease in incidence of specific conditions. Establishment of a full paediatric classification on the Read coding system allowing not

Box 13.2 *Paediatric out-patient questionnaire – this was constructed with the aim of answering the following questions:*

- Age distribution of out-patients
- Mode of transport to hospital
- Ease of directions within hospital
- Welcome provided by staff
- Arrival in relation to appointment time
- Time seen by doctor in relation to appointment time
- Whether enough time was spent with the doctor
- Whether adequate explanation of diagnosis was given
- What tests were done and when
- Time of leaving the department
- Quality of facilities, toys, etc

only for disease classification but drug, procedure and severity classification, will in the end allow for accurate annual comparisons as well as comparison between units and quality control.

National or regional audit projects looking at paediatric management of common childhood problems as well as specific conditions such as epilepsy, cystic fibrosis, diabetes, growth disorders and child abuse need considering. Reported examples of paediatric audit projects are few. The lead needs to be taken by the British Paediatric Association and individual societies within paediatrics to promote such audit and to move away from the rather limited approach taken at present.

References
1. MacDonald, D., Grant, A., Sheridan-Pereira, M., Boylan, P. & Chalmers, I. (1985). Dublin randomized controlled trial of intrapartum fetal heart rate monitoring. *American Journal of Obstetrics and Gynecology*, **152**, 524–539.
2. Boyle, M. H., Torrance, G. W., Sinclair, J. C. & Horwood, S. P. (1983). Economic evaluation of neonatal intensive care of very low birthweight infants. *New England Journal of Medicine*, **308**, 1330–1337.
3. *Outcome measurements for Child Health* (1990). Report of the Outcome Measures Working Group of the BPA Health Services Committee.
4. Warner, J. O., Gotz, M., Landau, L. I., Levison, H., Milner, A. D., Pedersen, S. & Silverman, M. (1989). Management of asthma – a consensus statement. *Archives of Diseases of Children*, **64**, 1065–1079.
5. British Paediatric Association (1990). *Paediatric Audit*. Report of a BPA Working Group. London: BPA.
6. Royal College of Physicians (1988). *Medical Care of the Newborn in England and Wales*. London: RCP.

7. Porter, H. J. & Keeling, J. W. (1987). Value of perinatal necropsy examination. *Journal of Clinical Pathology*, **40**, 180–184.
8. Batcup, G., Boddy, J. E. & Allibone, E. B. (1987). *A Survey of Perinatal and Fetal Autopsies Performed in the Yorkshire Region During* 1986. A report prepared by the Yorkshire Regional Health Authority.
9. Campling, E. A., Devlin, H. B. & Lunn, J. N. (1990). *National Confidential Enquiry into Perioperative Deaths*. London: Kings' Fund.
10. *Hospital Accommodation for Children* (1984). DHSS Health Building Note 23.
11. The British Paediatric Association (1989). *The Organisation of Services for Children with Diabetes in the United Kingdom*. Report of a BPA Working Party.
12. Fletcher, H. J., Ibrahim, S. A. & Speight, N. (1990). Survey of asthma deaths in the Northern region. *Archives of Diseases of Children*, **65**, 163–167.
13. Phelan, P. & Hey, E. (1984). Cystic fibrosis mortality in England and Wales and in Victoria, Australia 1976–1980. *Archives of Diseases of Children*, **59**, 71–83.
14. Britton, J. R. (1989). Effects of social class, sex and region of residence on age at death from cystic fibrosis. *British Medical Journal*, **298**, 483–487.
15. Hall, D. M. B. (1989). *Health for All Children. A Programme for Child Health Surveillance*. Oxford: Oxford Medical Publications.
16. Richman, S. & Miles, M. (1990). Selective medical examinations for school entrants: the way forward. *Archives of Diseases of Children*, **65**, 1177–1181.
17. Smith, T. (1990). Medical audit. *British Medical Journal*, **300**, 65.

14

Audit in obstetrics and gynaecology

HELEN K. GORDON AND NAREN B. PATEL

Introduction

The basic ideas of '*Health for All by the Year 2000*' were outlined in 1978 at the Alma Ata Conference organised by the World Health Organisation (WHO) and the United Nations Children's Fund (UNICEF). Subsequently, the WHO Regional Office for Europe devised criteria to monitor some practical ways of implementing the basic ideas and in their document they suggest 'By 1990, all members states should have built effective mechanisms for ensuring the quality of care within their health care systems'.[1] Medical audit is one way of monitoring the mechanisms implemented to ensure the quality of care and indeed, medical audit is a key part of the UK's White Paper that proposed reconstruction of the National Health Service.[2,3]

Maternal mortality audit

Maternal mortality audit is not a new phenomenon in the specialty of obstetrics and gynaecology. In Scotland, for example, the first special enquiry into maternal deaths was instituted in 1930 by agreement between the Scottish Board of Health, the local authorities and the medical professional organisations. The perinatal mortality rate was first recorded in Scotland in 1939, when it was 68 per 1000 total births. The information elicited by the first enquiry led directly to the *Maternity Services (Scotland) Act* of 1937 and laid the foundation for the immeasurably improved hospital services of today. Since then the perinatal mortality rate has fallen steadily, and was reported as 9.8 per thousand live births in 1985.[4] Although the enquiry continued subsequently, a different system of collecting data was introduced in 1965, in line with the method started in

1952 in England and Wales. Medical audit for maternal deaths takes the form of the Confidential Enquiry into Maternal Mortality and, indeed, is the most successful and longest running audit of practices in the UK. The audit is conducted by the Royal College of Obstetricians and Gynaecologists (RCOG) and the Department of Health. It is a voluntary and not a statutory duty. The audit itself depends entirely on peer review. Data on obstetric mortalities are collected, then reviewed by experienced obstetricians, pathologists, anaesthetists and GPs who assess the avoidable factors that may have played a part in the ensuing death. When appropriate, specialist advice from other specialties is always sought. The intent of this exercise is to indicate situations where the level of care falls short of commonly accepted practice. It is considered that the careful assessment by both the doctors concerned and the regional assessors has made a considerable contribution to the reduction in maternal mortality; and it provides an opportunity to consider possible errors of management, or faults in the organisation of maternity services. In this particular method, confidentiality is of paramount importance, and is protected by the Secretary of State for Health, acting in the public interest.[5] Only one copy of a report on a maternal death is made. This is passed from the district medical officer to the regional adviser in obstetrics (or anaesthesia) and thereafter, to a central committee. All patient identification is removed; the report is seen by only a small staff of doctors and their assistants; and once each three-yearly enquiry is completed, all documents are destroyed. No copies of any confidential enquiry document should be retained in the patient's hospital case notes as these could be made available to lawyers; they should be in the possession only of the chief medical officer or his representative.[6] Reviewing the triennial reports for England and Wales up to 1984, an HMSO document comments that the data covers a period of more than 30 years during which 24 million births have been registered in England and Wales.[5] Over the period covered by the eleven triennial reports the maternal mortality rate fell from 69.1 to 8.6 per 100 000 total births roughly halving between each given triennium. In comparison, the general fertility rate in 1982–84 (60.1 births per 1000 women aged 15–44) was only slightly lower than the rate in 1955–57 (78.4). For the period covered by these data – more than three decades – a maternal death has been defined as: one occurring during pregnancy or during labour or as a consequence of pregnancy within one year of delivery or abortion. From January 1985, in line with the *International Classifications of Disease, Injuries and Causes of Death* (ninth version), and as adopted by the International Federation of Gynaecologists and Obstetricians, only deaths of women while pregnant or within 42 weeks of termination of the pregnancy are included.

Perinatal mortality

As well as maternal mortality rates, perinatal mortality rates are indicative of the effectiveness of the maternity services. In Scotland, maternal mortality and perinatal mortality statistics are published together.[4] It is thought that by publishing the results in one report, the findings of the two groups of clinicians who have separately been investigating maternal and perinatal death should increase the value of each and assist in identifying aspects of the service where there is scope for further improvements. Initially perinatal surveys were carried out on a research basis – the Scottish Perinatal Mortality Survey of 1977[7]; and in England, the Mersey Region 1982[8] and the Northern Region 1984.[9] Like the review of maternal mortality, the casenotes for all these deaths are reviewed by a peer group and likewise, an important procedural detail is that the assessor does not know where the death occurred, the name of the deceased, the hospital, or the identities of the consultants concerned. As has been recognised regarding maternal mortality, the purpose of medical audit is to improve patient care not to attribute blame to an individual neonatal team. In Scotland since 1983 the surveys of perinatal deaths have been dealt with by the information and statistics division of the Common Services Agency and have been published annually. Due to the larger numbers involved, an epidemiological approach is used as distinct from the more detailed analysis carried out on the individual maternal deaths. In order to cover perinatal deaths as fully as possible, late abortions (20–24 weeks) are included and it is intended to move towards the eventual inclusion of deaths up to one year after delivery as they may be the result of perinatal causes. A particular problem is the low birthweight group, which is the subject of the ongoing Scottish low birthweight study. During 1981–85, the downward trend continued in the stillbirth and first week death rates which together comprise the perinatal mortality rate. In 1981 this rate was 11.6 per 1000 total births, less than half the rate of 1971. By 1985 the rate had decreased further to 9.8 per 1000. The steady improvement was probably due to a variety of influences – social factors, continued developments in neonatal care and improvements in maternal care. The surveys of perinatal mortality in Scotland and the Northern Regional Health Authority in England[4,9] regularly analyse the obstetric factors that lie behind each death using the modified classification first used in Aberdeen by Sir Dugald Baird and his colleagues.[10] However, discussion between the clinicians and epidemiologists responsible for the two surveys showed that differences had developed in the way the classification was being used and interpreted in these two areas. Differences had also developed in Scotland between the way the classification had first been used by the original authors and in the way the classification was now used in Scotland,[11] and as it is important to be able to compare like with like, important guidelines had to be drawn up to prevent discrepancies.[12] Different assessors can classify a series of deaths with considerable unanimity, provided close attention is paid to the published definitions and 'working rules'. Cole[11] found that when a group of clinicians were asked to classify the same cases after an interval, 99 % of the cases were classified in the same way, while differing groups reached similar conclusions in 97% of cases submitted for assessment provided they have a copy of the 'ground rules' before them. It has been found that good clinical records are essential, and an autopsy report helpful, although the classification can work even when these are incomplete. The classification can also be used on babies born dead between 22–27 weeks gestation.[13] The 'rules' only take into account the maternal factors involved with the death and, as yet, no account of the various diseases or conditions in the foetus or infant. However, since 1986, revised stillbirth and neonatal certificates have come into use in England and Wales in line with WHO recommendations,[14] which take into account foetal clinico-pathological reasons. Already, several regions in England and Wales have on-line computerised systems with perinatal data, which permit them to contribute to inter-regional comparisons[15] and these will be used to re-examine the pattern of perinatal mortality across and within the whole of the United Kingdom.[16]

Screening audit

Audit can be useful in assessing screening methods. Of course before setting up a screening service, it is important to know whether or not a selected screening programme is of sufficient practical benefit. From a theoretical point of view screening may be an efficient preventative measure but, except in a few instances, firm evidence of this is still lacking. There is often a public demand for screening, e.g. cervical screening, and whether these demands should be satisfied is still an open question, as scientific considerations need to be weighed against the desire for 'doing something'. Any programme which is implemented should be continuously monitored in relation to effects and costs. To quote an example, a recent report on audit of laboratory workload and rates of referral for colposcopy in a cervical screening programme in three districts[17] demonstrates that with increasing referral for minor abnormalities in line with Department of Health Guidance[18], and an Intercollegiate Working Party[19], the increased workload on the department devoted to follow up might jeopardise the maintenance of even five-yearly call, recall and quality control. It was also concluded that in their screening programme, the audit disclosed a steady increase in the proportion of women with minor abnormalities being referred for colposcopy. This has implications not only for financial and manpower resources but may also result in investigation of up to 40 times the number of women likely to benefit. Audit used in these cases can help the Department of Health and Social Security (DHSS) and RCOG to realise the implications of their stated policies and may help health authorities to target resources more effectively. Quite apart from targeting resources to 'popular' causes, the costs of recognised practices can be assessed by means of medical audit.

Resource implications

Caesarean section is a commonly used procedure in obstetrics and an impressive study shows the savings obtained when providing antibiotic prophylaxis prior to caesarean section.[20] In 58 controlled clinical trials involving the use of antibiotics prior to caesarean section, covering some 7777 women, the probability of wound infection was reduced by between 50 and 70 per cent. For 41 women recorded as suffering from infection, the average extra cost of hospital care was estimated at £716 per case. It was concluded that routine antibiotic prophylaxis would reduce the average cost of post-natal care (at 1988 prices) by between £1300 and £3900 per 100 cases, depending on the cost of the antibiotic used and its effectiveness. No attempt was made in this study to compare the effectiveness of different antibiotics. The authors simply concluded that 'as well as reducing serious post-operative infection and the associated unpleasant symptoms, such a policy results in reduced hospital costs'. Similar studies in anaesthetic agents have similar implications for obstetric and gynaecological services. A study from the United States compared the reduced demands on recovery-room resources when the anaesthetic propofol was used, as compared to anaesthesia using more conventional thiopentone-isoflurane; the study covered a total of one hundred patients. At each of the sites used for the study, patients were randomly allocated between the two anaesthetics. The estimated mean, direct patient care required was reduced in the propofol group by 18.8 % and by 6.5 % in two different series of cases – 40 female patients undergoing laparotomy in Illinois and 60 mixed patients receiving a variety of procedures in Chicago[21]. Length of patient stay is also an important resource implication, measurable by audit. The length of time that patients are kept in hospital, usually confined to bed, has important connotations not only for the efficient use of resources but also for the effective clinical management of the individual patient. Both of these aspects of medical care have been promoted by investigations examining traditional assumptions about desirability of prolonged bed-rest for most hospital diseases and particularly after operative surgery. An analysis of hospital in-patient statistics in Scotland showed that even within one country, the median stay of patients varied greatly by individual consultant for similar types of condition or operation. For example, the median postoperative stay for hysterectomy ranged from three to 18 days, the variation between consultants being greater in non-teaching hospitals.[22] More clinically orientated investigation had shown that prolonged bed rest was not wholly desirable or even necessary. Early postoperative ambulation with consequent early discharge might not merely be safer and make more economical use of resources, but may also reduce the incidence of complications such as chest infections and deep venous thrombosis. Quite apart from surgery, the obstetric unit at St. Mary's Hospital, London, reporting on a scheme of early post-natal discharge, showed that over two thirds of patients could be sent home at 48 hours after delivery, and the scheme was shown to be safe and desirable.[23]

Computerised systems in obstetrics

It is all very well to collect data, but there must be a manageable system for handling them. Obviously, improved computerised systems will allow easier comparison and analysis of data in the future; manual systems involve time-consuming sorting of data that may often be inaccurate. In the early 1980s, several units began utilising on-line data collection related to maternity information, for immediate production of reports and audit.[24] In 1981–85, the *Steering Group on Health Services Information* (*The Körner Committee*) drafted their maternity proposals made in collaboration with representatives from the Royal College of Obstetricians and Gynaecologists and the British Paediatric Association.[25,26] These provide a minimum data set, which is designed to provide enough information for clinical audit and effective service planning. Regional Health Authorities in England and Wales agreed to implement these final recommendations by 1988. Six units were used initially to pilot the Körner committee proposals and the findings of these were published by the computer policy committee.[27] The major objective of these systems, for example the 'Mary's System',[28] is to improve the care of the mother and the baby by using a computer system for collecting accurate computer data for dissemination to the primary health care team and planners. The system meets the Körner requirements by collecting a recommended 'data-set'. By using modern computer technology without an increase in staff, it also meets further requirements by linking into the regional mainframe computer and the child health system, assisting in operational tasks such as production of forms and avoiding duplication of data entry and outputs. The system relies heavily on midwives and medical staff for data collection but, for the first time, it provides them with readily available information on all women booked for delivery. This is invaluable should notes be lost, and when dealing with telephone enquiries. Better communications with general practitioners, community midwives and health visitors are likely to improve the shared ante-natal care system and encourage an early visit to the mother and baby on return home from hospital. Summaries are sent more quickly to general practitioners and hospital staff are freed from the drudgery of dictating routine letters and discharge summaries. The care of the women too has been improved because of the ease of highlighting risk factors, often overlooked by busy clinicians in routine ante-natal clinics, and by the use of clinical prompts, as in the case of rubella-susceptible women needing vaccination in the puerperium. The Mary's group report a high degree of accuracy between the computer and clinical records.[28] Data are now collected on babies admitted to the neonatal intensive care unit, which allows audit of current practices to take place locally within the neonatal unit and also regionally; and eventually it will be possible internationally. Up until recently the DHSS performance indicators were of limited value in obstetrics because so few data were available but with the introduction of these computer systems in England and Wales, the auditing of ante-natal, intrapartum, puerperal and neonatal care is now possible, allowing for inter-hospital and regional comparisons in terms of outcome for mother and baby and for comparison of resource and manpower utilisation. While health authorities in England and Wales have grappled with the implementation of the recommendations of the Körner Committee, Scotland has already achieved a national system for recording the outcome of every pregnancy with a viable outcome. Using such contemporary records, up-to-date reports on perinatal mortality, with geographical analysis, have been used to improve obstetric management.

The Scottish Health Service has the advantage of utilising an information service appropriate to a central government with a close-knit maternity service; by contrast there are 14 English regions, each with a population of 3–5 million.[29] It is proposed that when similar patterns of data collection and classification are established throughout the UK, NHS regions can, as well as auditing their own practice, make valid comparisons between foetal and neonatal mortality rates in their own and other regions.[16]

Doctor–patient relationship

There are many uses for medical audit in obstetric practice. The overriding objective, of course, is to improve practice, so that the patient (currently, perhaps 'consumer' is a better concept) receives not just minimal care but an excellent standard of care. In this connection, quite apart from the physical expertise used in a clinical procedure, the patient–staff relationship is of paramount importance, including concern for the mother and child as people, and part of a family. Audit should not deal solely with outcome measures or use of resources but also with the access to and process of clinical care, which involve the doctor–patient relationship and communication skills. The doctor–patient relationship and the ability to communicate are particularly important in the specialty of obstetrics and gynaecology as compared with, for example, pathology. In the past, these topics have been given more attention by general practitioners, for example, by video recordings of a doctor's approach to a patient.[30] Analysis of the approach as indicated on the video has been shown to alter practice and to alter the stated objective measurements of the quality of care in patients who have chronic disease. This method should be considered as a potential tool for obstetrical audit probably using techniques usually employed by social scientists. More recently, patients have been 'auditing' care as a consumer.[31,32] Several studies have assessed the opinions of the mothers towards for example ultrasound, home confinement and artificial induction.[33,34,35] The real challenge is determining the quality of care, adapting yesterday's standards to tomorrow's science and balancing science with the patients' expectations. Standards of care that were used yesterday inevitably will change by tomorrow. How much they will change is not known with any certainty, but what is known is that today's definitions of good-quality care will not fit future practices and expectations. Society seems to assume that scientific discoveries and technological innovations will solve all problems. Unfortunately, too often the pitfalls that are not necessarily well presented with the reports of new discoveries are overlooked. Well-conceived clinical trials need to be encouraged. New technologies have to be evaluated on a scientific basis but when they are more expensive and provide no better care than the old ones, they should be discarded. With the explosion in medical technology has come an explosion in costs. In the United States, employers and unions, who bear the brunt of financing health, are beginning to ask questions about the cost as well as the quality of care received by employees. These are just a few of the problems faced by the medical community today.

Education

Medical audit can also be used as an educational tool. Even prior to the publication of the Government White Paper that advocated the use of medical audit[36], the RCOG had instituted some methods of audit within the college. The introduction of the 'LOGIC' system of self-assessment, multiple choice questions for furthering postgraduate education was a revolutionary idea at the time.[37] The professional examinations in obstetrics and gynaecology for the Membership of the Royal College of Obstetrics and Gynaecology (MRCOG) also involve a form of professional audit. They include an assessment of clinical standards, as well as knowledge, and have been supplemented by log books that require the documentation of clinical and surgical experience gained under supervision. As an educational tool, too, audit can be utilised in the undergraduate programme. When discussing with students the nature of peer review as a form of audit (e.g. as used in the collection of data for maternal and perinatal mortality), it is possible to pass on to these potential practitioners the value of listening to the opinions of colleagues, and the usefulness of evaluating professional responsibility and accountability to the profession (RCOG); to the licensing body (General Medical Council); to the public; to the individual patient; and not least, accountability to oneself.

Guidelines in audit systems

As has already been said, obstetricians and gynaecologists in the United Kingdom are more used than other branches of the profession to the concept of audit. The Royal College of Obstetricians and Gynaecologists has been involved in the longest running medical audit, namely the Confidential Enquiry into Maternal Deaths. More recently the Royal College of Obstetricians and Gynaecologists has established initial guidelines on audit for their own specialty.[38] This idea has already been in use in the USA. The American College of Obstetricians and Gynaecologists (ACOG), published as early as 1972, *Indices for Use in Peer Review of Obstetric and Gynecologic Practice*, followed by *Indices for Outcome Audit* in 1977, by *Quality Assurance in Obstetrics and Gynaecology* in 1981 and by *Standards for Obstetric–Gynecologic Services*, 7th edition.[39] The American College has in progress an active quality assurance programme. It is a two-pronged process. In the first part – the voluntary review of the quality care programme – trained teams of ACOG fellows and members of the nurses association of ACOG serve as peer reviewers for hospital obstetric and gynaecology departments if they request a voluntary evaluation of their departments. The team provides a comprehensive report to the hospital. It sums up the inquiry data and makes specific recommendations based on the group review of the data, interviews with key hospital staff, and summaries of the observations obtained from the evaluation of the facility. The report becomes the hospital's property. What they do with it is their responsibility. Of the first 14 programmes evaluated, three issues were seen as problems in all the institutions – protocols, quality assurance activities and provision of education. Half of the institutions had problems with forms and documentation, department function, staff relationships, 24 hour coverage, hospital relationships, staffing and credentials and privileges. The second part of ACOG's process to ensure quality of care is a *task force on quality assurance*. This involves the use of a manual for peer review within a hospital practice setting. These involve 'clinical indications' used by the abstractors who flag patient records when they contain material indicating that a physician should again review and evaluate some aspect of that patient's care. 'Clinical criteria' are used to help review the decision making process of physicians to determine when a particular procedure is indicated. It was designed to represent a base level of acceptable care below which no facility or practitioner should fall. The manual is to provide ongoing review and change where appropriate. It is proposed that as the data are accumulated, the use of the manual in developing physician profiles, department profiles and practice trends, and in identifying educational needs, will become increasingly evident. ACOG have set out to provide a quality assurance programme that changes appropriately and continuously with proven advances in science and technology.

Measurements in health care

Any audit method used for health care evaluation is concerned with evaluating the extent to which a health care programme, or a medical intervention, or an organisation has achieved its objectives. These goals can be defined by changes in the health of individuals and/or populations by patient or community, or by professional satisfaction. In any enterprise, it is logical to have in mind goals or objectives or outcomes, and to plan a process to achieve these goals. The only way of knowing whether or not goals are achieved is to evaluate the end product, if possible against pre-set measurable criteria. This is the general rationale for medical audit – in effect a variation on the scientific method – and although the scientific method can be discussed in different ways, these variations can be summarised as a process using assessing, planning, implementing and evaluating. To take a selected obstetric activity as an example, one would require to assess whether or not the activity occurs sufficiently commonly to merit audit, define it, and then set goals, plan what must be done to meet these goals using realistic criteria and mindful of available resources, implement the plan, and evaluate the end product against the criteria. Of course goals may be too idealistic, or may be unrealistically expensive, or complications may occur that make them unachievable, or the planned process may be faulty. This is why obstetric audit must be considered as an 'open' system with frequent feedback so that adjustments can be made to the plan. Once an obstetric practice has been shown to be desirable, and it is approved by the profession, to the extent of being included in guidelines, audit must be continued to evaluate whether or not the guidelines continue to be useful in practice. Guidelines for medical practice can contribute to improved care only if they succeed in moving practice closer to the behaviours the guidelines recommend. In one survey carried out in Ontario, Canada[40] on assessment of guidelines, recommendations were widely distributed, and nationally endorsed consensus statements recommending decreases in the use of caesarean section were widely circulated. Hospitals and obstetricians were surveyed before and after circulation. These surveys along with discharge data from hospitals reflecting actual practice revealed that most obstetricians (87–94 %) were aware of the guidelines and most (82.5–85 %) agreed with them. Attitudes towards the use of caesarean section were consistent with the recommendations even before their release. One third of the hospitals and obstetricians reported changing their practice as a consequence of the guidelines, and obstetricians reported that rates of caesarean section in

women with a previous caesarean section were significantly reduced, from
72.2 to 61.1%, in keeping with the recommendations.

Conclusion

Generally speaking, in the UK, most audit evaluation studies carried out
so far in the field of obstetrics have shown important advances, especially
concerning mortality (stillbirths, perinatal mortality, maternal deaths).
However, there have also been some reported improvements in pre-natal
care, changes in economic and social conditions, and demographic factors.
When attempting to evaluate the true effect of an intervention technique in
a population, one is confronted with many methodological problems
related to the fact that it is generally far removed from an experimental
situation in which the population can be randomised. As a consequence,
the inevitably conflicting results give rise to dispute about the evaluation of
one intervention over another.[41] Another difficulty in the evaluation of
obstetric interventions is that the risk level measured by the usual indicator,
mortality, is quite low (less than 10%) and the interventions are many.
Incidence of morbidity is higher but it can take longer to show since it may
only become apparent several years after birth. This means that even if the
intervention is effective, the impact on the population as a whole is limited
and can only be shown on very large populations. However, such
difficulties are, in effect, challenges. As Yudkin and Redman conclude[42]:
'Routinely collected computerised data enable ongoing clinical audit, but
it becomes a reality only when clinicians agree on standards of practice,
and have a flexible attitude towards change...'. Obstetricians and
gynaecologists will have to be convinced of the value of audit, and be
helped to use it effectively.

   To quote an old Chinese proverb,

   A journey of a thousand miles begins with a single step!

References

1. World Health Organisation (1985). *Targets for Health for All.*
   Copenhagen: WHO.
2. Department of Health (1989). *Working for Patients.* London: HMSO.
3. Department of Health (1989). *Working for Patients: Medical Audit:
   Working Paper No. 7.* London: HMSO.
4. *Report on Maternal and Perinatal Deaths in Scotland 1981–1985* (1989).
   Edinburgh: HMSO.
5. *DHSS Report on Confidential Enquiries into Maternal Deaths in England and
   Wales 1982–1984* (1989). London: HMSO.
6. Chamberlain, G. (1983). Ninth report of the confidential enquiries into

maternal deaths in England and Wales 1979–1981. *British Journal of Obstetrics and Gynaecology*, **90**, 689–690.

7. McIlwaine, G. M., Howat, R. C. G., Dunn, F. & MacNaughton, M. C. (1979). *Scotland 1977 – The Scottish Perinatal Survey*. University of Glasgow.

8. Mersey Region Confidential Enquiry into perinatal deaths in the Mersey region (1982). *The Lancet*, **i**, 491–494.

9. Northern Regional Health Authority perinatal mortality (1982). *British Medical Journal*, **288**, 1717–1720.

10. McIlwaine, G. M., Dunn, F., Howat, R. C., Small, M., Wylie, M. M. & MacNaughton, M. C. (1985). A routine system for monitoring perinatal deaths in Scotland. *British Journal of Obstetrics and Gynaecology*, **92**, 9–13.

11. Cole, S. K., Hey, E. N. & Thomson, A. M. (1986). Classifying perinatal death: an obstetric approach. *British Journal of Obstetrics and Gynaecology*, **93**, 1204–1212.

12. Chiswick, M. L. (1986). Commentary on current WHO definitions used in perinatal statistics. *British Journal of Obstetrics and Gynaecology*, **93**, 1236–1238.

13. Whitfield, C. R., Smith, N. C., Cockburn, F. & Gibson, A. A. M. (1986). Perinatally related wastage – a proposed classification of primary obstetric factors. *British Journal of Obstetrics and Gynaecology*, **93**, 694–703.

14. WHO (World Health Organisation) (1977). *Manual of the International Statistical Classification of Diseases, Injuries and Causes of Death*, 9th edn. Geneva: WHO.

15. Mutch, L. M. M. (1986). *Archive of Locally Based Perinatal Surveys*. Oxford: NPEW.

16. Barron, S. L. (1986) Commentary. How can we improve perinatal surveillance. *British Journal of Obstetrics and Gynaecology*, **93**, 1201–1203.

17. Raffle, A. E., Aiden, B. & MacKenzie, E. F. D. (1990). Six years 'audit' of laboratory workload and rates of referral in a cervical screening programme in three districts. *British Medical Journal*, **301**, 907–911.

18. Department of Health and Social Security Health Services Management Cervical Cancer Screening (1988). DHSS HC 88 (1): London.

19. Sharp, I., Duncan, I. D., Evans, D. M. H. *et al.* (1987). *Report on Intercollegiate Working Party on Cervical Cytology Screening*. London: Royal College of Obstetricians and Gynaecologists.

20. Mugford, M., Kingson, J. & Chalmers, I. (1989). Reducing the incidence of infection after Caesarean section: implications of prophylaxis with antibiotics for hospital resources. *British Medical Journal*, **299**, 1003–1006.

21. Mavais, M. L., Maher, M. W., Wetchler, B. U., *et al.* (1989). Reducing demands on recovery room resources with propofol (dipriven) compared to thiopental-sofluarare. *Anaesthetics Review*, **XVI**, 29–40.

22. Heasman, M. A. & Carstair, V. (1971). Inpatient management: Variations in some aspects of practice in Scotland. *British Medical Journal*, **1**, 495.

23. Pinker, G. D. & Fraser, A. C. (1964). Early discharge of maternity patients. *British Medical Journal*, **ii**, 99.

24. Maresh, M., Beard, R. W., Coombe, D., Gilmer, M. D. G., Smith, G. & Steer, P. J. (1982). Computerisation of obstetric information using a microcomputer. *Acta Obstetrica Gynaecologica Scandinavica (Suppl)*, **109**, 42–44.

25. Steering Group on Health Services Information (1981). *Report of the Working Group A*. The Körner Committee, vol. 39. London: DHSS.

26. Steering Group on Health Services Information (1985). *Suppl. to the First and Fourth Reports to the Secretary of State*. London: DHSS.
27. Computer Policy Committee (1985). *Evaluation of Maternity Pilot Trials NHS*. Birmingham.
28. Maresh, M., Dawson, A. M. & Beard, R. W. (1986). Assessment of an on-line computerised perinatal data collection and information system. *British Journal of Obstetrics and Gynaecology*, **93**, 1239–1245.
29. Scottish Health Service (1985). *Perinatal Mortality Survey Scotland* 1984. Edinburgh: Information Services Division.
30. Batsome, G. F. (1990). Educational aspects of medical audit. *British Medical Journal*, **301**, 326–328.
31. Garcia, J. (1989). *Getting Consumers Views on Maternity Care*. London: HMSO.
32. Mason, V. (1989). *Women's Experience of Maternity Care. A Survey Manual*. London: HMSO.
33. Garel, M. & Franc, M. (1980). Reaction des femmes a l'echographic obstetricale. *Journal of Gynaecology, Obstetrics and Biological Reproduction*, **9**, 347.
34. Kitzinger, S. & Davis, J. A. (1978). *The Place of Birth*. Oxford: Oxford University Press.
35. Cartwright, A. (1975). Mothers' experience of induction. *British Medical Journal*, **2**, 745.
36. The Health Service (1989). *Working for Patients*. Medical Audit Working Paper 6. London: HMSO.
37. Royal College of Obstetricians and Gynaecologists (1986). LOGIC.
38. Royal College of Obstetrics and Gynaecologists (1990). *Interim Royal College of Obstetricians and Gynaecologists Guidelines on Medical Audit*. London: RCOG.
39. Malkasian, G.D, (1990). The conscience and the specialty. *Obstetrics and Gynecology*, **75**, 1–4.
40. Lomas, J., Anderson, G. M., Pomnick-Pierre, K. D., Vayda, E., Enkin, M. W. & Hannah, W. J. (1989). Special article. Do practice guidelines guide practice? The effect of a consensus statement on the practice of physicians. *New England Journal of Medicine*, 321, 1306–1311.
41. Chalmers, I. (1976). British debate on obstetric practices. *Paediatrics*, **58**, 308.
42. Yudkin, P. L. & Redman, C. W. G. (1990). Obstetric audit using routinely selected computerised data. *British Medical Journal*, **301**, 1371–1373.

15

Audit in general surgery

J. R. W. GUMPERT

Introduction

Each surgeon treats his own patients as he thinks best. The time honoured concept of clinical freedom must today be balanced by contemporary demands for accountability and value for money.

The argument that critical assessment of our work is part of the surgical ethic and anyway built into our professional lives, is powerful but no longer good enough. All of us want to make the best use of our time, and the vast majority would honestly wish for accurate information about the appropriateness of our surgical endeavours. The aims of abolishing the unnecessary, while treating the patients with the minimum morbidity and maximum satisfaction are right and proper. Audit is the cornerstone of these endeavours. It should, therefore, become an integral part of surgical practice, just as much as ward rounds, out-patient clinics and operating lists.[1]

It is fashionable to divide audit into three components: *structure*, *process* and *outcome*. This may be helpful administratively but less so clinically, since undue emphasis is placed on the audit of structure and process and outcome is neglected.

Since doctors are responsible for nearly all spending on health care, they need to ensure that resources are used wisely by administrators and politicians as well as by themselves. However, the audit of structure, the facilities available, and the audit of process, the delivery of those facilities, are not the primary concern of the surgeon. The clinician is rightly far more concerned with outcome – how things worked out for his/her patient. Surgical audit is predominantly about the outcome. One of the reasons why audit has been welcomed by the profession with less than open arms, is an undue emphasis on the audit of structure and process. They are so much easier to audit than outcome, particularly by administrators and nurses.

Concern that audit is a euphemism for cost cutting remains. Worse still, audit is perceived by some as unwarranted prying into the professional domain, and that it is synonymous with 'big brother'.[2] However, those familiar with surgical audit will appreciate that it is a 'state of mind'. To find fault is *not* the object. The aim is to enhance quality.

Definition

Clinical audit is the process by which medical staff collectively evaluate and improve their practice.[3]

The Shorter Oxford English Dictionary defines:

Audit – Official examination of accounts with verification by reference to witness and vouchers.
Review – The art of looking over something (again) with a view to correction or improvement.

By definition this chapter should really be called 'clinical review in general surgery'.

Rationale

Why should surgeons audit?

Quite apart from the compelling ethical reasons mentioned above, the 1989 Government White Paper states that we are now obliged by law to audit our work, whether we like it or not. 'Every doctor should participate in systematic medical audit'. At the same time it recognises that 'The quality of medical work can only be reviewed by a doctor's peers'.[4] The Royal College of Surgeons response to the White Paper is: 'It has for some time been official college policy to make regular audit a condition of recognition of hospitals for surgical training'.[5] Audit is a form of education and merges into research. The process is educational for both senior and junior surgeons. It is probable that in the future evidence of surgical audit may become necessary for the accreditation of a hospital's surgical services.

Evidence of adequate audit will also become a defence against medical litigation, which is increasing exponentially. The chairman of the GMC recently said 'I am convinced that the introduction of performance review procedures for doctors ... will serve to demonstrate how the profession can regulate itself effectively for the mutual benefit of both the public and the profession'.[6]

In the brave new world of the provider and purchaser of health care, whether or not hospitals opt to become trusts, it seems likely that the purchasing authorities will require evidence that the provider audits a surgical procedure (e.g. herniorrhaphy or laparoscopic cholecystectomy) prior to entering into a contract for that procedure. They are already showing signs of opting for the safest and not necessarily the cheapest contract.

The policy makers within the Department of Health and Regional Health Authorities are continually seeking surgical economy. The drive to increase day case surgery[7] or to lessen the postoperative length of stay are just two examples. Although it seems likely that an ever-increasing number of surgical procedures can be safely and effectively performed on a day or short stay basis, surgeons must beware of allowing this trend to go too far. Accurate audit of complications and the readmissions that result is essential in case the brakes need to be applied.

Only through accurate audit data can the wisdom or otherwise of wholesale bed or even hospital closure be assessed. Without such information surgeons will be even more powerless to modify those political decisions, which are made more for financial expediency than the good of the patients. Rationalisation is all very well, provided the patient does not suffer as a result. If we assert that they have suffered without objective evidence of deteriorating outcomes, we will certainly be ignored. If we have hard data the politicians might just listen.

Very few surgeons fall below the accepted standards of surgical competence, but all of us know one or two who would benefit the community by referring certain patients to colleagues with specific specialist interests. No one wishes to pillory them, but a system that demonstrates as unaggressively as possible the error of their ways should be encouraged.

Audit can be boring and repetitive, but the honest discussion of surgical complications can also be cathartic. It is reassuring to be reminded that every general surgeon who performs major surgery particularly in elderly or frail patients will have complications. Furthermore, these discussions are an invaluable method of teaching.

Any service that swallows up as much of the public purse as does the NHS, must be not only accountable but seen to be accountable. George Bernard Shaw felt 'all the professions to be a conspiracy against the laity'. Contemporary demands for accountability will ensure that if we do not audit ourselves, it will be imposed upon us. Sanctions for the poor performers will result[8]. Those familiar with surgical audit will appreciate that to find fault is not the object. The process aims to encourage doctors to think constantly *why* they are doings things. It should be facultative rather than regulatory.

Audit is no longer the 'flavour of the month' – it is here to stay.

What information should surgical audit provide?

In order to satisfy those who hold the purse strings, the politicians and managers, data concerned with management resources will be needed, including the total number of patients, the diagnoses, casemix, length of stay, emergencies, length on waiting list, numbers and categories of operation and delays in hospital for medical or non-medical reasons.

Data concerned with teaching and learning will be needed by the Royal College of Surgeons. This should include total numbers of operations undertaken by surgeons in training, and the type, complexity and degree of consultant help. Similar data will be needed for the consultants themselves. At the end of his/her stay each surgeon in training should be given a list of operations performed by him/her, with and without assistance.

Data concerned with the quality of care are what most surgeons really want. These will include mortality (expected and unexpected), complications, (avoidable and unavoidable), prolonged in-patient stay and the reason for it, unexpected return to the operating theatre, and transfer to the intensive therapy unit. Even more important is assessment of the severity of illness on admission and the casemix, or the patient's strength to withstand surgical intervention.

In summary, surgical audit must provide data about the volume of work, the casemix, unit management, teaching and quality of care.

Types of surgical audit

Surgical audit has many dimensions:

1. *Individual* – the best example of this is private practice. The variables are less than in any other system. The surgeon is the same. There are few emergencies and really ill patients. The morbidity should, therefore, be very low. Such audit would be useful in setting standards. Inexperienced surgeons or patients with more severe disease could be compared with those standards.
2. *Firm* – consultant (one or two) and juniors. This is the basic firm. The exact manpower should be defined because firms vary.
3. *Departmental* – all the general surgeons and junior staff in one hospital.

4. *District wide* – all the general surgeons and juniors throughout the district. This audit would be co-ordinated by the district medical audit committee.
5. *Inter-departmental* – where responsibility for the patients care is shared by more than one discipline, e.g. ITU, trauma, gastro-intestinal bleeding, diabetic vascular disease.
6. *Regional* – specific conditions treated in several districts and compared within the region, e.g. transurethral prostatectomy or ruptured aortic aneurysm. This audit would be co-ordinated by the Regional Audit Committee as is audit in small specialities such as maxillofacial surgery.
7. *National* – CEPOD (Confidential Enquiry into Perioperative Deaths[9]) and now NCEPOD (National CEPOD[8]) or the Royal College of Surgeons Confidential Comparative Audit Service.[10]

Besides variation in the width of surgical audit there are many different methods of surgical audit:

(a) *Hospital patient record analysis.*[11] This can be performed by non-medical staff who pick out deficiencies in standards predetermined by peers. This sort of audit produces consensus views on the ideal investigations and treatments of specific conditions, as well as setting standards for the quality of the patients' surgical notes. However, it is time consuming, potentially boring, retrospective and of limited value. Even in the USA where it originated, its usefulness is being questioned and it is falling from favour. However, it is a good starting point.

(b) *Criterion based audit.*[12] Measurable criteria of good practice are agreed and local practice compared with these standards. This can be prospective, but is usually retrospective. Such audit also produces consensus views on the optimum investigation and treatment of specific conditions, an invaluable exercise in itself and one that is by no means easy. An example of such audit might be the time taken for patients with gastro-intestinal bleeding to come to endoscopy.

(c) *Adverse occurrence screening.*[13] This is also a transatlantic development. It involves the identification and analysis of events or occurrences in a patient's treatment that might indicate some lapse in the standard of care. Again the notes are screened, usually by a trained nurse, and any detected occurrence is then reviewed by a clinician. A judgement is made, and if appropriate a change is implemented. For example, unplanned return to the operating theatre might be chosen as the adverse occurrence. This form of audit is worthwhile and undoubtedly improves teaching, but it is time consuming. This method of audit can be threatening, and instead of recognising that the vast majority of patients are successfully treated without problems, its punitive approach is in danger of being counter-productive.

(d) *Routine prospective unit* (departmental audit). This is described in detail later in the chapter.

(e) *Specific detailed audit projects.* This is the detailed study of a small specified group of patients.

Practicalities (nuts and bolts) of surgical audit

What data to collect and how to collect them

Data collection whether standard or detailed should be considered under the following headings:

1. Patient details
2. Admission details
3. Diagnosis details
4. Operation details
5. Outcome details
    (a) Complications
    (b) Histology
    (c) Discharge
    (d) Non-surgical treatment
    (e) Discharge details
    (f) Severity of illness
6. Additional information
7. Optional extras

(Based on *Guidelines for Surgical Audit by Computer* – May 1991 – RCS of England.)

Good audit precedes the computer age. Indeed there is a potent argument that the computer muddies the water by making it too easy to collect excessive amounts of unnecessary data without due thought.[14]

However, there is no doubt that surgical audit in particular is enhanced by the use of a computer. Comprehensive surgical audit requires collection and analysis of the same data on every in-patient (and ultimately every out-patient). Comprehensive surgical audit is impossible without a computer.

The pro forma is the linchpin of surgical audit data collection.

There are two types:

(a) A routine short pro forma – to be collected on all in-patients.

Most widely used is the Micromed pro forma.[15] This small card was devised to fit into the houseman's pocket. The card is filled in by him/her for each patient on arrival, and it stays with the houseman until discharge, when at a weekly firm meeting, its accuracy is checked, any complications discussed, and the data entered into the computer. The advantage of this system is that the houseman has an *aide memoire* of all his/her patients immediately available in his/her pocket. It should, therefore, be to his/her advantage to keep it up to date. In practice however, it is difficult to persuade housemen to do this. Furthermore, effective audit must be consultant led and the responsibility for accurate coding, should be the consultant's. A more practical system is a pro forma (see Fig. 15.1) that occupies a prominent position in the patient's notes. This pro forma is then filled in at various stages of the patient's admission. The responsibility for filling in the pro forma falls on different members of the surgical team.

The ward or admission clerks are responsible for making sure the pro forma is in the patient's notes. This is no problem with elective cases, but there is a major problem with out of hours emergencies and ward transfers.

The senior operating surgeon is responsible for ensuring that patient, admission, diagnosis and operation details are filled in. This is the cornerstone of meaningful surgical audit, and is absolutely crucial. At the end of the operation, after writing or dictating the operation note the audit pro forma must be filled in. Surgeons accept that the operation note is their responsibility – the pro forma must be an extension of that responsibility.

The outcome details should be filled in by the house staff, prior to discharge. Ideally the patient should not be allowed to leave the hospital until the pro forma is complete. In practice this is extremely difficult to achieve. A doctor's handbook explaining the computer system, the coding and the generation of discharge summaries is given to all house staff when they start work on the firm. The house staff are far more likely to fill in outcome details dispassionately than are the surgeons who performed the operation. With the best will in the world, surgeons tend to minimise their complications.

A weekly verification meeting is essential. For about half an hour each week, the firm together with the firm secretary must go through the week's pro formas, to ensure their accuracy prior to entry on to the computer. At the same time, as part of the educational process, the patients and any complications are briefly discussed. Indeed, it is possible to tell how accurately and seriously surgical audit is taken by studying the minor complication rate. Superficial audit does not detect minor complications.

GENERAL SURGERY AUDIT PRO FORMA

Patient   Hospital Identity No.   Admitting Hospital ....   **Details**
Surname.

     1st Name
     DoB
     Address & Post Code   Male/Female

     Telephone No. Work............... Home..................

     GP Name, Initials
     Address

Admission   Date of Admission ../../..   Time (24 hours)...........
Details   Admission type: Emergency/Waiting list   (urgent)/waiting list (soon)/waiting list (routine)/Booked/Internal transfer

     Date put on waiting list or booked ../../..   Consultant (name) ....
     Clinical presentation (free text) ....
     Initial Diagnosis (free text) ....
     Main investigations (free text) ....

Diagnosis   Diagnostic category (see explanation) ....
Details

     Main Diagnosis .... ICD 9 Code..........Lt/Rt/Bilat.
     2nd Diagnosis .... ICD 9 Code...........Lt/Rt/Bilat.

     3rd Diagnosis .... ICD 9 Code..........Lt/Rt/Bilat.

Operation   Date ../../..   Time (24 hours)
Details   Operation Priority: Emergency/Urgent/Scheduled/Elective (see explanation)

     Main surgeon.. Grade .... (state if locum)

     Assistant Surgeon .... Grade ....

     Consultant in Attendance Yes/No

     Main Procedure .... OPCS Code............Lt/Rt/Bilat.

     2nd Procedure .... OPCS Code .... Lt/Rt/Bilat.

     3rd Procedure .... OPCS Code .... Lt/Rt/Bilat.

     Procedure Complexity: Minor/Intermediate/Major/ > Major (see explanation)

     Anaesthetic Type: General/Local/Regional/Other   Consultant Anaesthetist Present. Yes/No

     Procedure details (Free text) ....
Details

     Complication 1 .... Code No ....

     Complication 2 .... Code No ....

     Complication 3 .... Code No ....

     Complication due to surgery: Yes/No/In part.   Complication due to underlying cause: Yes/No/In part.

     Nursed in ITU: Yes/No   If yes no of days...   Ventilated: Yes/No
     Return to theatre: Yes/No. If yes fill in 2nd proforma.

Histology: Yes/No. If yes result...................................... Code

Non-operative treatment (free Text) ....

Discharge   Date of Discharge   ../../..   Discharging Hospital ....
Details

    Mode of Discharge: Home/Nursing Home/Other speciality/ Died (if so P.M. Yes/No)

    Future Plans: Follow up Yes/No   In .... weeks

                            at ....(specify)

                  Refer to other speciality...(specify)

    Information given: Patient told diagnosis Yes/No

                  Relative told diagnosis Yes/No

    Furtherinformationgiventopatient&relatives (free text) ....

    Drugs on discharge ....

    Other comments (free text) ....

    Severity of Illness score. ASA clarification: 1....... 2....... 3....... 4....... 5.......

Additional   Special Interest Case: Yes/No
Information

    Expected length of stay (to compare with actual length of stay) .... days

    Discharge delayed for non medical problems: Yes/No If yes specify ....

    Other field for specific projects eg Smoking, Time of decision to operate

    Other field for amplification of summary and comments (free text) ....

CONFIDENTIALITY STATEMENT

THE INFORMATION CONTAINED IN THIS DOCUMENT IS PROTECTED BY THE RULES OF CONFIDENTIALITY IMPOSED ON ALL HOSPITAL PERSONNEL BY (Insert relevant) HEALTH AUTHORITY. UNAUTHORISED DISCLOSURE OF THIS INFORMATION IS FORBIDDEN AND MAY BE SUBJECT TO LEGAL ACTION WITHIN THE DATA PROTECTION ACT (1984)

Form completed by ....

Form verified by ....

Form entered in to computer ....

Fig. 15.1. General surgery audit pro forma. (Modified from the Brighton General Surgical pro forma.)

A modification of the Brighton General Surgical pro forma for routine use in all patients is shown in Figure 15.1. It is designed to fit on both sides of a single sheet of A4 paper and is included in the front of the notes.

Explanation of the short pro forma. Those sections of free text in brackets amplify the basic data that are computerised. The free text is not retained by the computer but is used partly for generation of the discharge summary and partly for teaching purposes at the verification meetings.

Debate about the computer-generated discharge summary continues. The vast majority of surgical admissions do not require a detailed personalised discharge summary. Indeed, general practitioners do not have time to read them. More details, either for the general practitioner or more likely for a comprehensive synopsis of an admission may be required. If so, the free text and extra fields for discharge summary and comments can be used. Most GPs are happy with the stilted computer-generated discharge summary because it is short and should reach them within a few days of discharge.

Diagnostic category. A long list of unstructured diagnoses and operations presented at an audit meeting can be very tedious. It is helpful to subdivide general surgery into groups as follows:

Mouth, pharynx and neck
Thyroid, parathyroid and adrenal
Skin, connective tissue, bone
Breast
Hernia
Oesophagus
Stomach, duodenum, upper GI tract
Small bowel, omentum, peritoneum, abdominal cavity
Appendix, gynaecology
Colon, rectum
Anal, perineal
Liver, gallbladder, bile duct
Pancreas
Amputation
Venous, lymphatic
Arteries
Spleen, haemopoiesis
Urology

Box 15.1   *Procedure complexity and IE (Intermediate Equivalent)*

Minor: e.g. Skin lesion excision (IE = 0.5)
Intermediate: e.g. Herniorrhaphy (IE = 1.0)
Major: e.g. Cholecystectomy (IE = 1.75)
Major plus: e.g. Cholecystectomy and exploration of Common Bile
Duct (IE=2.2)
Complex Major: e.g. Oesophagectomy (IE = 4.0)

Ultimately, such groups should be standardised throughout the country, particularly with the advent of comparative audit.

Operation priority. NCEPOD has classified operations in terms of their urgency as follows:

Emergency: Immediate operation, resuscitation simultaneous with surgical treatment. Usually within a hour, e.g. major trauma – ruptured aneurysm.
Urgent: Operation as soon as possible after resuscitation. Usually within 24 hours, e.g. intestinal obstruction; irreducible hernia.
Scheduled: Early operation, but not immediately life threatening. Usually within three weeks, e.g. malignancy.
Elective: At a time to suit both patient and surgeon, e.g. herniorrhaphy, varicose vein surgery.[16]

Procedure complexity. This is based on the British United Provident Association (BUPA) reimbursement scale[17] and is divided into minor, intermediate, major, major plus and complex major.

Operative work load must be distinguished from caseload. Caseload, the number of cases operated upon, is extensively used by management in assessing workloads and service requirements. Much more relevant is operative workload which takes into account the complexity of the operation. All operations should be classified in terms of their intermediate equivalent (IE) (Box 15.1).[18,19] For example, a typical operating list might be equivalent to four IE's. If audit data is to be compared nationally, then all surgical procedures should be given an intermediate equivalent value.

Severity of illness score. The most important determinant of the outcome of an operation is the patient's ability to withstand the illness that made the operation necessary.

This depends on:

1. the severity of that illness;
2. his/her state of health.

Both are extremely difficult to measure.

This I believe to be the main challenge to the ultimate success or failure of surgical audit. All other determinants pale into insignificance when compared with these two variables. Prolonged faecal peritonitis is incomparably more serious than an early perforated diverticular disease with a localised abscess but both might be classified as perforated diverticular disease. A 'hot' aneurysm with early or localised rupture is so different from a massive rupture with profound shock, yet both are 'ruptured aortic aneurysms'. In the same way a straightforward cholecystectomy in a patient with advance pulmonary insufficiency may have a much more uncertain outcome than a technically formidable cholecystectomy in a young otherwise fit patient.

These problems have not yet been seriously addressed, but attempts are now being made to categorise the so-called casemix. The American Society of Anaesthesiology has devised a classification:[20]

Class 1: No organic, physiological, biochemical or psychiatric disturbance.
Class 2: Mild/moderate systemic disturbance caused either by the condition to be treated or other diseases, e.g. mild diabetes, anaemia, slightly limiting heart disease, obesity, chronic bronchitis.
Class 3: Severe systemic disturbance, e.g. severely limiting organic heart disease, severe diabetes with vascular complications, angina, previous myocardial infarction.
Class 4: Severe, already life-threatening systemic disorders, e.g. organic heart disease with cardiac insufficiency, advanced pulmonary, hepatic, renal or endocrine insufficiency.
Class 5: Moribund patient with little chance of survival, e.g. ruptured abdominal aortic aneurysm with profound shock.

(b) A more detailed longer pro forma for use on specific audit projects

Examples of this are pro formas prepared for all anterior resections, all screen detected breast carcinomas, all patients undergoing a specific operation – anterior resection, thyroidectomy or whatever.

Figure 15.2 is an example of an audit of an individual consultant's

PATIENT IDENTIFICATION

Name _____

Sex   M   F   Date of Birth ___ / ___ / _____   Age _____

G.P _____

PRESENTING SYMPTOMS

Routine Admission [ ]   Emergency Admission [ ]

Rectal Bleeding [ ]   Change in Bowel Habit [ ]   Constipation [ ]

Diarrhoea [ ]   Abdominal Pain [ ]   Obstruction [ ]

Perforation [ ]   Anaemia [ ]   Others [ ]

Duration of Symptoms   1mth   2mth   3mth   6mth   12mths

Saw G.P. Prior to Admission   Yes   No   Family History of Cancer   Yes   No

ASA Classification Class   1   2   3   4   5

PREOPERATIVE ASSESSMENT

Site:

Caecum [ ]   Ascending Colon [ ]   Transverse [ ]

Decending Colon [ ]   Sigmoid [ ]   Rectum [ ]

Palpable mass [ ]   No palpable mass [ ]

Fixity:

Mobile [ ]   Tethered [ ]   Fixed [ ]

Distance of lower edge of tumour from Anal verge by rigid sigmoidoscopy _____ cm

If Rectal:

Quadrants: Anterior [ ]   Posterior [ ]   Right [ ]   Left [ ]

Biopsy:

Primary Adenocarcinoma [ ]   Other [ ]

Differentiation [ ]   Poor [ ]   Other [ ]

Metastases present [ ]   No Metastases [ ]

Liver scan: US.   CT.

Metastases   [ ]   [ ]

Number: solitary Multiple   _____   _____

Location: Right/ Left   _____   _____

Fig. 15.2. For caption, see p. 215.

special interests, in this case colorectal cancer.[21] These may be long-term projects, or perhaps pulsed audit, collecting such data for a few months every few years. Help may well be needed from a computer professional working for the clinicians rather than for the district department of

OPERATIVE ASSESMENT

Surgery

Elective ☐   Emergency ☐   State procedure _____

Number of Tumours _____

Site:

Caecum ☐   Ascending Colon ☐   Transverse ☐

Descending ☐   Sigmoid ☐

Rectum: Above peritoneum ☐   Below peritonium ☐

Fixation:

Mobile ☐   Tethered ☐   Fixed ☐

Complications:

Obstruction ☐   Spontaneous perforation ☐   Local abscess ☐   Operative perforation ☐

Metastases present   Peritoneal ☐   Mesentric ☐   Para aortic ☐

Number of Liver Secondaries _____   Left ☐   Right ☐

Excision of Local Tumour

Complete ☐   Incomplete ☐   Unsure ☐

Lateral quadrant biopsies   Yes   No

Bowel preparation:

Picolax ☐   X prep ☐   Others ☐   Clean ☐

Fluid ☐   Faeces ☐   Loaded ☐

Antibiotics

Pre-op ☐   Cefuroxime ☐   Flagyl ☐   Gentamicin ☐

Anastamosis

Yes   No   Stapled   26   28   30   31   33

Hand Suture ☐   Suture Used _____

Anastamosis Air Tight   Yes   No

Height of Anastomosis on Sigmoidoscopy _____cm

Arterial Blood Supply of Proximal Bowel 0-10 _____

Mucosal Blood Supply of Proximal Bowel 0-10 _____

PaO$_2$ Proximal Bowel _____

Complete Doughnuts   Yes   No

Tension of Anastamosis   Nil   Some

Pre-op DXT _____   Previous Excision _____

Intra-op Chemotherapy   Yes   No

Fig. 15.2. *Cont.*

information. The audit co-ordinator or facilitator is therefore an essential member of the team. Although modern software is becoming increasingly flexible, most consultants are not computer literate and need help with their individual projects.

OUTCOME

Early: (30 days)

Patient Died ☐   Patient Survived ☐

Anastomotic Leak: Radiological ☐   Clinical ☐

Wound Infection ☐   Perineal Infection ☐   Colostomy Problem ☐   Chest Infection ☐

DVT ☐   PE ☐   MI ☐   Others ☐

Late: (+30 days)

Patient Alive in Months: 3mth   6mth   9mth   12mth   18mth   2yr   3yr   4yr   5yr   6+yr

If Dead: Cause of Death _____

If Alive: Recurrence: Yes   No

If Recurrence

Bowel ☐   Pelvis ☐   Abdo ☐   Liver ☐

CEA.

Pre-op ☐   Post-op ☐

3mth   6mth   12mth   2yr   3yr   4yr

COLONSCOPY FOLLOW UP

Post-Operative _____   Time from Resection _____

3mth   6mth   12mth   2yr   5yr

Findings: _____

Defunctioning Stoma Performed   Yes   No

Caecostomy ☐   Transverse Colon ☐   Small Bowel ☐

Blood Transfusion Performed   Yes   No

Blood Group _____   Nos Units _____

PATHOLOGICAL REPORT

Date ___/___/___

Length of Specimen _____ cm   Length of Tumour _____ cm

Bowel circumference at Tumour _____ cm   Width of Tumour _____ cm

Appearance: Ulcerating ☐   Protuberant ☐   Stenosing ☐   Others ☐

Local Spread:

Cannot be assessed ☐   No invasive cancer (dysplasia) ☐   Submucosa ☐   Muscularis Propria ☐

Beyond Muscularis P ☐   Penetrates peritoneum ☐   Invades adjacent organs ☐

If beyond Muscularis Propria: distance beyond bowel wall _____

Lateral excision margins free of tumour _____

Margin of normal colon distal to tumour _____ cm   Complete excision ☐

Cytology of lateral pelvic walls,   Tumour ☐   No Tumour ☐

Lymphatic spread:

Number of nodes identified ☐   Number of nodes +ve ☐   Peri-colonic nodes ☐

Meso-colic ☐   Para-aortic ☐   Invasion of Extramural Veins ☐

Distant Spread   Liver ☐   Peritoneum ☐   Others ☐

Histology: Adenocarcinoma ☐   Mucinous ☐   Signet ring ☐   Others ☐

Differentiation: Poor ☐   Others ☐

Invasive margin: Expanding ☐   Infiltrating ☐   Lymphocytes at Tumour ☐

Adenomas present in remainder of specimen ☐   Synchronous Tumour Present ☐

UC. present ☐   Fam. Polyposis present ☐

Fig. 15.2. Colorectal cancer follow-up.

How to ensure its accuracy

Unless the data are accurate one is not auditing, merely sampling. Comprehensive, accurate data, depend on:

1. Weekly verification meetings of the whole firm. This must be part of the firm members' weekly programme. It must be within office hours and be as important a part of firm activity as, e.g., an out-patient clinic.
2. Intermittent checks with data collected elsewhere, e.g.:
   (a) A & E admissions or A & E computer.
   (b) Theatre operating books or theatre computer.
   (c) The district patient information system, e.g. PAS – patient administration system. (This is well known to be far from accurate.)
   (d) Other comprehensive data collection systems, e.g. individual research projects.
3. Manual checks:
   (a) Housestaff should keep a note of every patient admitted to their unit. The patient's name, registration number and date of admission should suffice.
   (b) The unit secretary should keep a similar list. This must include details of those patients most likely to be missed; patients referred from other specialties and wards not used to audit data collection. In particular, patients in medical wards and patients treated conservatively, tend to escape.
4. Audit data 'back up': At the end of every week, all in-put data have to be transferred to a floppy disk in case the hard disk fails at any time.

How to store data (once collected)

In the long term and the ideal world, all surgical beds will be adjacent to the unit secretarial office. In practice, units operate in different theatres, and different hospitals. Multi-user computer systems can solve these problems, so that data can be recorded on several sites. As information systems improve there will be terminals on every ward and audit data will be recorded by the nurse or house staff or even the consultant in the ward at the workstation. Such information systems are so expensive that in the short and medium term, each surgical team or even surgical department will have to be content with one terminal, which should be kept in the surgical office.

In several centres, it is the consultant who physically inputs the data.

However, consultants are often absent, and their time is more purposefully spent elsewhere. Similarly, there are limits to the housestaff's time and their commitment to audit. I sympathise with the opinion they often express, that they should be by the bedside whenever possible.

Some centres employ audit assistants whose main job is to input data, but the surgical secretary is best placed to do this. A good surgical secretary is essential for accurate surgical audit. However, this requires considerable expertise and dedication and must be rewarded with an adequate salary. 'The loyalty and enthusiasm of the National Health Service workforce is legendary.'[8] If we require decent audit, we must be prepared to employ and remunerate good office staff. The dedicated secretary makes sure that the pro forma are assembled in the office, correctly filled in, and entered expeditiously. Feeding data into the computer, day in, day out (as done by an audit assistant) is as dull as typing out-patient letters and dictated discharge summaries day in, day out, and should be done frequently and briefly. The secretary who keeps her/his fingers on the 'audit pulse' knows all about the firm and the patients and, besides being an invaluable member of the team, has enhanced job satisfaction.

How to process data for audit meetings

Getting audit data out of the computer is the forgotten step. Some of the software companies boast of the ease of inputting, only to fall down because it proves difficult to retrieve and process the data. To present one consultant or firm's annual data in an interesting and meaningful form may take several hours, and considerable expertise. It is not just a matter of a few minutes work prior to the audit meeting. The firm secretary may well be able to manage but often the audit facilitator needs to be involved.

The forum for the presentation and discussion of surgical audit is the audit meeting which should take place once a week.[22] Some departments meet at the same time each week (e.g. Friday 1 pm – 2 pm), but others feel that there is less service disruption if the meeting is on every eighth working day. Since the Royal Colleges as well as the politicians have decided that audit is mandatory, it should therefore take place between 9 am and 5 pm. If it is eventually decided that the benefits of audit do not justify the time taken, then audit will cease. Until that time audit must take the place of some clinical care.

Above all, surgical audit is an educational process. Outside the teaching hospitals we have traditionally 'worshipped at the altar of patient care' and anything that distracts us, including teaching, has been viewed with suspicion. At last we have the opportunity, indeed we are being encouraged, to include audit and teaching in our weekly programmes. We must grasp the opportunity. Formal audit and teaching should take up one session per week. Elective surgery for that session should cease. Two hours every week should be 'ring fenced'. The verification meetings and other routine weekly meetings, such as X-ray meetings and teaching, should take up the rest of the weekly session set aside for audit.

All the surgical staff except those unavoidably detained by emergencies must attend the weekly audit meeting, consultants included. There should be a senior nurse representative from each surgical ward and ITU, as well as the audit facilitator and particularly the ward secretaries involved in audit.

The district general manager, or his/her representative (usually a member of the Department of Community Medicine), should be invited to attend every so often. This is contentious and horrifies many clinicians. However, his/her department holds the purse strings, and most of the deficiencies unearthed by audit have financial consequences.

Audit is a three part cycle; defining standards, comparing them with observed practice and effecting the necessary improvements in clinical practice.[23] District finance is usually necessary for implementing these improvements. Minutes of the meeting should be taken. A record of each meeting should be kept. This should include attendance,[24] subjects discussed, proposals arising at the discussion and in particular action required to implement these proposals. Confidentiality is of the utmost importance. As far as possible material identifying particular patients and particular members of staff should be kept to a minimum and destroyed at the end of each meeting. Confidentiality at audit meetings is discussed in detail by Walshe and Bennett.[25]

The problems of surgical audit

Audit is beset with problems. *Data collection* is not easy, particularly in multiple sites and wards unfamiliar with the concept of audit. Problems also arise when regular staff are on leave. Patients admitted straight to the operating theatre from the accident and emergency department are often missed. The more complicated the problems the more likely it is that they by-pass surgical audit, especially if they ultimately die. This is because of the delay in the notes being returned to the secretary in the surgical department. These complex problems in seriously ill patients are the very ones most needing to be audited. The problem should become soluble as audit becomes routine in all departments, particularly when audit data generation is automatic and an integral part of patient treatment. In the short term most problems will be solved if the patient's discharge is dependent on completion of the audit pro forma.

More of a problem is *data accuracy*, especially if data are to be compared. Verification of the data is spasmodic and complications can be missed, usually by a mistake but sometimes on purpose. Wholesale publication of audit data, as reputedly occurs in parts of the USA, will ensure that audit data are not accurate. Surgeons and institutions could either audit what they know they are good at or worse 'cook the books' because they feel threatened. Once threatened there is a danger that surgery will become defensive and surgeons will be unwilling to take risks because the stakes have become too high.

Audit has the potential to be inordinately *boring*, particularly if the same complications are discussed repeatedly. Worse still, if audit fails to demonstrate an improvement with the passage of time, enthusiasm evaporates and disillusionment sets in. However, audit has to make the same point again and again, otherwise changes and improvements resulting from audit are forgotten and standards slip.

Confidentiality has already been mentioned. Audit is a peer review activity, performed by doctors for doctors. How much audit data the purchasers of health care will require is uncertain and worrying. How surgeons should respond to this remains to be seen.

Meaningful *interpretation* of surgical audit can be extremely difficult. Superficial interpretation, particularly by nurses and administrators, is all too common. The number of variables that influence structure and process, but especially outcome, are so great that it is seldom possible to conclude that one unit is better or more industrious than another. Such claims, however, are frequently made. The usual explanation is to be found in the casemix. Indeed, the greater the expertise the higher the complication rate and the lower the throughput is likely to be because experts are referred the most difficult problems. If data are to be compared, like must be compared with like, and audit must be standardised.

Coding is a major problem. The more comprehensive the coding the less likely the data are to be accurate, because coding takes time.[26] Most computerised audit systems try to balance simplicity with comprehensiveness and accept that if the coding is too complicated it will not be done properly. This is satisfactory until data from different systems are compared. Such comparisons are not valid. The coding of diagnoses, operations and complications must be standardised. Assessment of the severity of the illness and the patient's general state of health, facetiously but accurately called the 'crumble factor', must also be standardised if meaningful comparisons are to be made. The Colleges of Surgeons are beginning to address these problems as comparative audit gains momentum. Ultimately, national standards may be developed that predict the chances of success or failure of a specific procedure, in a patient with a particular severity of illness and a particular general state of health. Enormous volumes of audit data will have to be collected before this can be achieved, although as the volume of comparative audit data increases so do their accuracy.

The interpretation of *complications* is particularly difficult. Many result from the underlying poor general state of health, and are not directly related to surgical treatment. Some are operation related. Others are related to the severity of the illness rather than the surgical treatment. It will, therefore, be extremely difficult to standardise complications, and in particular to decide whether they are avoidable or unavoidable.

The greatest problems of all are the measurement of *outcome* and the *appropriateness* of the treatment. Even death, surely the most untoward complication of all, can at times be the most appropriate outcome. We need more indicators of outcome, but for the time being audit should concentrate on the review of the untoward events, such as unexpected transfer to the ITU, out of hours surgery, sepsis rate, chest infection, pulmonary embolism and prolonged in-patient stay.

The future

We must strive towards automatically generated audit information, as an integral part of a surgeon's daily work, collected and stored only once. Coding of diagnoses, operations, complications, and of the severity of illness and the underlying frailty of the patient will be standardised. All surgeons will participate. They will collect standard information about all their activity (a little about everything) and much more detailed information about their own special interest (a lot about a little) perhaps intermittently for a few months every few years.

The Colleges of Surgeons will have well-defined consensus views on the desirability of particular treatments. These 'indicator' sets will be organised and updated by college working parties. Comparative audit meetings will be organised and run at the colleges. Truly accurate information, for *all* clinicians to see will modify our practice so that we 'whittle' away at the complications. Perhaps really accurate information will even allow us to turn off the tap of excessive treatment as it becomes more clear that the outcome does not justify it.

The process of audit will thus become an integral part of teaching and clinical research and will be seen to be facultative rather than regulatory.

Conclusions

No longer can we shrug off routine data collection as not being our concern.[8] If we do not participate voluntarily, public scrutiny will be imposed upon us.

The success or failure of surgical audit ultimately depends on four factors:

Time – in the working week to collect, verify, prepare and present audit data.

Co-operation – of all surgeons, led by enthusiastic and respected practising clinicians.

Accuracy – of prospective, comprehensive, comparable data. and above all *Proof that it works*.

If the deficiencies unearthed by audit really are corrected and clinical practice is modified and improves as a result then surgical audit will flourish.

References

1. Pollock, A. & Evans, M. (1989). *Surgical Audit*, p. 12. London: Butterworths.
2. Kettlewell, M. G. W. (1990). Surgical audit. *Annals of the Royal College of Surgeons of England*, **72** (Supplement), 70.
3. The Royal College of Surgeons of England (1991). Brochure – page 6.
4. Secretaries of State for Health, Wales, Northern Ireland and Scotland (1989). *Medical Audit Working Paper* 6, pp. 3–6. London: HMSO.
5. Royal College of Surgeons of England (1989). *Response to the White Paper – Working for Patients*, pp. 4–5. London: RCS.
6. Sir Robert Kilpatrick (1990). President's foreword, *G. M. C. Annual Report*.
7. Audit Commission Review (1990). *A Short Cut to Better Services – Day Surgery in England and Wales*.
8. Devlin, H. B. (1990). Audit and the quality of clinical care. *Annals of the Royal College of Surgeons of England*, **72**, (Supplement), 3–14.
9. Buck, N., Devlin, H. B. & Lunn, J. N. (1987). *The Report of Confidential Enquiry into Peri-operative Deaths*. London: Nuffield Provincial Hospitals Trust and the Kings Fund.
10. The Royal College of Surgeons Comparative Audit Service. Meeting 5 June 1991 at the Royal College of Surgeons of England.

11. Williams, J. G., Kingham, M. J., Morgan, J. M. & Davies, A. B. (1990). Retrospective review of hospital patient records. *British Medical Journal*, **300**, 991–993.
12. Shaw, C. D. (1990). Criterion based audit. *British Medical Journal*, **300**, 649–651.
13. Bennett, J. & Walshe, K. (1990). Occurrence screening as a method of audit. *British Medical Journal*, **300**, 1248–1251.
14. Crombie, I. K. & Davies, H. T. O. (1991). Computers in audit: servants or sirens. *British Medical Journal*, **303**, 403–404.
15. Ellis, B. J., Michie, H. R., Esufali, S. T., Pyper, R. J. D. & Dudley, H. A. F. (1987). Development of a microcomputer-based system for surgical audit and patient administration: A review. *Journal of the Royal Society of Medicine*, **80**, 157–161.
16. *The Report of National Confidential Enquiry into Peri-operative Deaths in* 1989 (1990). London: Royal College Surgeons of England.
17. British United Provident Association (1989). *BUPA Scheme of Procedures*.
18. Collins, C. D. (1990). Model workload agreement for DGH general surgeon: discussion paper. *Annals of the Royal College of Surgeons of England* (suppl), **72**, 48–50.
19. Emberton, M. (1990). Audit and quality assurance: Micromed user group meeting. *Annals of the Royal College of Surgeons of England* (suppl), **72**, 27–29.
20. Owens, W. D., Felts, J. A. & Spitznagel, E. L. (1978). *Anaesthesiology*, **49**, 239–243.
21. Farrands, P. A. (1991). Personal communication.
22. Gumpert, J. R. W. (1988). Why on earth do surgeons need quality assurance? *Annals of the Royal College of Surgeons of England*, **70**, 85–92.
23. Shaw, C. (1989). *Medical Audit. A Hospital handbook*. London: Kings Fund Centre.
24. Bowden, D. & Gumpert, J. R. W. (1988). Quality versus quantity in medicine. *RSA Journal*, **136**, 333–346
25. Walshe, K. & Bennett, J. (1991). *Guidelines on Medical Audit and Confidentiality*. South East Thames RHA.
26. Nixon, S. J.(1990). Defining essential hospital data. *British Medical Journal*, **300**, 380–381.

16

Orthopaedic audit: guidelines and hints

SIMON P. FROSTICK

Introduction

As with all other specialties, orthopaedic and trauma surgeons have been undertaking 'audit' in its broadest sense for decades. However, in terms of formalised, structured audit orthopaedics is well behind other specialties. It is self-evident that for any specialty to develop some form of systematic review has to be undertaken. Orthopaedic surgery differs from many specialties in that the true effect of any treatment/management regime and any complications that may arise may not be apparent for many years. Audit in orthopaedics must, therefore, be looked at in two levels – (i) short-term effects and (ii) the eventual outcome whenever that occurs. Any guidelines to implement audit in the specialty have to include review at both levels. Further, in order to be realistic about audit in orthopaedics resource management cannot be ignored. Many orthopaedic operations involve the use of expensive implants. There is a tendency to use the 'flavour of the month', which may also be the most costly available at the time. Orthopaedic surgeons must, therefore, act responsibly in using new implants and be able, and willing, to justify their use when challenged.

Like many other specialties orthopaedics has undergone dramatic and irreversible changes in the last 20 years or so. Historically, orthopaedics grew up as a result of the high incidence of skeletal tuberculosis and other major diseases such as polio. The advent of chemotherapy and effective vaccination successfully and rapidly eliminated these diseases as a major source of musculoskeletal patients. It was then possible for orthopaedic surgeons to turn their attention to other areas such as osteoarthritis.

Orthopaedic trauma grew up alongside elective orthopaedics but has usually remained the poor relation, frequently run by inexperienced juniors with little consultant input. Recently, however, trauma has started to receive appropriate attention and interest and is now developing as a primary major interest alongside the other orthopaedic specialties.

Both elective orthopaedic surgery and trauma surgery have rapidly developed into technically demanding specialties where minor defects of technique can have major effects on outcome. Further, some skills that orthopaedic surgeons who trained in the 1940s and 1950s developed have been gradually lost to more recently trained individuals but still have their place in routine practice. Audit, therefore, serves an important educational role in orthopaedics as it does in other specialties.

Problems in orthopaedics and trauma

At the present time orthopaedics is receiving a great deal of media attention because of long and increasing waiting lists. Compared with most other Western nations the United Kingdom has a significantly lower ratio of consultant orthopaedic surgeons to population. The estimated ratio in the United Kingdom is one consultant per 63000 population, whereas in the United States the figures are one per 20000 and in most other European countries one per 30–40000 head of population. These figures suggest that there should be a need to increase the size of the consultant ranks. However, a number of problems exist in determining the true level of consultant staffing in the specialty. Due to differences in work practices between the United Kingdom and other countries there is little point in making direct manpower comparisons. In order to determine the true level of the consultant establishment a considerable amount of information concerning work patterns, workloads and patient demography needs to be acquired, otherwise, at best, the suggested levels would be a poor estimate. There is now an obvious need for a much more rigorous acquisition, storage and interpretation of workload and staffing data.

The management of resources cannot be separated from clinical audit activity in orthopaedics. The operation of total hip replacement illustrates some of the problems that orthopaedics faces in the 1990s. Total hip replacements started to appear in the early 1970s and over the last 20 years increasing numbers of operations have been successfully performed. Parallel with this is the fact that during the same period the general public have become more aware of health care in general and aspects such as total hip replacement in particular. Further, there has been a large rise in the population requiring joint replacement surgery. Therefore, the general public are familiar with the fact that orthopaedic surgeons can successfully replace not only hips but now other joints and will expect the service to be readily available. The success of the surgery has bred a demand that is difficult to keep pace with and would appear to be increasing. Thorngren (Chapter 23) details the rate of total hip replacement in Sweden based upon a national survey. Comparable figures are not available for the United Kingdom at present, so that it is impossible to plan for the likely demands on the orthopaedic services for total joint replacement over the next 10, 15 or 20 years. The Department of Health have suggested that an acceptable rate of hip replacements should be 1050 per million population per year. The problem with this figure is that the Department of Health have failed to realise that they have included hemiarthroplasties for fracture. A rate of 1050 per million population is significantly lower than that described by Thorngren in Sweden where the rate is 1200 per million population *excluding hip fractures*. In the USA the rate is 2500–2700 per million population.[1] The problems outlined here may seem to be simply the perennial grouse for increased resources. However, more importantly it demonstrates the lack of accurate information that is available for planning orthopaedic and trauma services. At the other end of the scale orthopaedic surgeons have been very poor at introducing measures of outcome and quality assurance making it difficult to judge the worth of the treatments provided.

Therefore, in orthopaedic and trauma audit we will need to discuss two areas which are both fundamental to the audit activity. The first area is the traditional audit including peer review of small groups of patients. As with audit in other specialties this type of audit is extremely important and must effect a change in working practice. The second area of orthopaedic audit is much broader and comes into the realm of what the editors of this book have called patient care audit, i.e. the acquisition and interpretation of clinical data in order to plan future clinical activity in the light of changes in demand for resources.

Clinical research versus audit in orthopaedics and trauma

Many orthopaedic surgeons have misunderstood the fundamental difference between clinical research and audit. The main effect has been to the detriment of clinical research, as few comparisons of treatment have been studied using prospective randomised controlled trials based upon a scientific hypothesis. Statistical methods have often been inappropriately applied and bias has been introduced making comparisons invalid. The contribution of retrospective review and anecdotal reporting (i.e. the audit of personal experience often over a long career) must not be ignored. These studies have frequently led to further discovery and stimulated others to pursue lines of research.

Audit is concerned with quality of care including patient satisfaction. Audit requires that data are acquired and recorded in a systematic and accurate way but 'control' data are not required for audit purposes. The purpose of clinical research is usually to demonstrate that one treatment regime is better than another. The control group will probably be an established method of treatment. A clinical trial must be performed in a prospective, randomised fashion. Ideally, the only variable that is not controlled is the specific treatment regimes that are going to be undertaken. Otherwise age, sex, surgeon, etc. should be as closely similar in both groups as possible.

Methods of audit in Orthopaedics and Trauma

At present few orthopaedic units have the capacity to acquire, store and process large volumes of data. Adequate computer hardware is still not available and very little software is commercially available specifically for use in orthopaedics. A number of enthusiasts have written their own computer databases and others have influenced or are trying to influence the hospital information technology departments to adapt hospital based systems to orthopaedics. Therefore, at present most orthopaedic audit needs to be undertaken as a paper based exercise. The advantages of this type of audit are that it is relatively simple. The disadvantage of paper based audit is the often inadequate sources from which to obtain case records and to extract the appropriate data. If similar audit techniques are used all the time then the process is also in danger of becoming very boring even for the enthusiasts. It is, therefore, necessary to organise audit activities using a variety of different methods.

Provision must be made for recording relevant information even for a paper based audit. Complications should be properly and thoroughly recorded. If necessary, pro forma can be designed and distributed to Senior House Officers to record specific pieces of data.

Possible audit methods in orthopaedics and trauma
Notes review

A random sample of case records from patients under the care of one consultant should be assessed by another consultant. There are several aims for this very simple method of peer review:

1. The content and adequacy of documentation can be assessed. Table

Table 16.1 *A scoring system for case record assessment*

Legibility	
All notes legible	3
Not fully legible but comprehensible	2
Not fully comprehensible	1
Signature	
All signed, dated and identifiable	3
All signed, some identifiable	2
Not all signed	1
Regularity of entries	
Daily	4
Alternate days	3
Two entries per week	2
< two entries per week	1
Diagnosis	
Definite diagnosis within 24 hours of admission or pre-admission	4
Definite diagnosis during admission (after 24 hours)	3
No diagnosis before surgery	2
No stated diagnosis	0
Investigations	
All ordered and acted upon	3
Some not ordered or not acted upon (treatment not affected)	1
Some not ordered or not acted upon	0

16.1 shows a very simple method of scoring in-patient case records. This scoring system has not been fully validated as yet but some form of semi-quantitative analysis is useful in order to compare with future sets of notes to ensure an improvement in case record keeping.

2. The diagnoses and treatment regimes can be discussed. This will be educative for all individuals attending the meeting. As with all specialties there is often more than one way to treat patients; the decision making, the appropriateness and alternative means of treatment can be discussed. With these points for discussion in mind it might be reasonable to suggest that at the initial consultation or at the time of admission a care plan is formulated and stated in the case records. The accuracy of the diagnosis and how closely the treatment regime has adhered to the initial care plan can be assessed. Once again this can be very useful in developing decision making skills as well as diagnostic skills.

This type of audit method, if used as the sole means, will rapidly become boring. Further, there is the possibility of public embarrassment and the possibility of litigation if confidentiality of both clinicians and patients is not maintained.

Topic based audit

In this type of audit a particular topic is given to an individual (often a junior) to review all the cases passing through the unit in a given time. The topic can be chosen for any reason – simplicity, complexity, rarity, etc. An attempt should be made to locate and review all the case records and radiographs relating to the topic. A brief literature review can also be undertaken. A full discussion can take place; any major problems, complications, etc. can be highlighted and decisions taken in order to alter the structure and/or process in order to improve outcome.

Occurrence screening[2]

This type of audit is often seen as very threatening. It reviews problems that may have occurred. The problems can be related to any aspect of patient care including hotel services, delays in operating, etc. In the USA occurrence screening is often used as the major type of audit method. Some units in the UK are also introducing it for regular audit purposes. As it is seen as a threat it would probably be most reasonable to use occurrence screening intermittently during randomly selected periods. For example, there is a universal problem of fulfilling the Royal College of Physicians' recommendations to operate on patients with fractures of the neck of the femur within 24 hours after admission.[3] Occurrence screening could be used for a two or three month period to gather baseline data on the problem. This could be reported to the unit, probably in conjunction with the anaesthetists and geriatricians and recommendations used to improve the provision of the service. At some later date a second group of data are collected and the improvement (or lack thereof) assessed.

Occurrence screening may be useful to assess para-medical and nursing processes intermittently but must be undertaken by the group concerned themselves and not imposed by the clinicians. Given that at present, detailed data about many aspects of patient care cannot be easily acquired, stored and most importantly, analysed, intermittent occurrence screening may be helpful to the Clinical Director in order to obtain data to formulate contracts. Variations from the recognised 'norm' can be examined in detail, reasons determined and if found acceptable it may be necessary to consider specific inclusions in the business plan for the following year. Further, occurrence screening could be used to record details of all complications occurring in a given period. Once again this is important for the overall day-to-day functioning of a unit and the hospital managers require information about the incidence of complications when formulating contracts. However, caution must be exercised about all aspects of occurrence screening as bias can be introduced due to rogue months.

Morbidity and mortality reports

These reports have been the cornerstone of audit meetings for decades. Complications will be considered in more detail later but the recording of morbidity and mortality data on a pro forma such as shown in Figure 16.1 is very valuable and can form the basis for useful discussion. However, witch hunts must be avoided.

Comparative audit

The Royal College of Surgeons of England have recently instigated confidential comparative audit meetings in a number of specialties including orthopaedics. The purpose of these meetings is for consultants to enter data onto a pro forma about workload, types of work and specific enquiries and for these data to be compared in a completely confidential fashion with all other data submitted. The main problem with this at present is the low number of consultants who are willing to provide data and the poor quality of that data. If the initiative is successful then eventually national standards for comparison could be created. It is intended that these meetings are held annually. Data concerning the previous year's activities are submitted for analysis. Absolute confidentiality is fundamental to this activity.

Outcome measures

In order to perform audit and clinical research an adequate, workable and comprehensible set of outcome measures is required. The measures may differ in some ways depending upon whether the measures are for audit or research purposes. In audit, measures of patient satisfaction are very important; these will be entirely subjective. Quantitative measures are also required for audit but are fundamental to clinical research. Differences between a study group and a control group must be tested statistically for research.

A large number of scores for assessing various conditions and operations have been described, e.g. the Harris hip score,[4] the Constant shoulder score[5], etc. These have been developed by interested individuals who wish to assess the effectiveness of, say, a particular total hip replacement. Pain

MORBIDITY AND MORTALITY REPORT
DEPARTMENT:

DOB: CONSULTANT: WARD: SEX:

PMH:

ADMISSION DATE: DRUGS:

DIAGNOSIS/OPERATION (INCLUDING TIME/DATE):

MORTALITY:

RESULT PRE-EXISTING DISEASE	
RESULT OPERATION/TREATMENT	

MORBIDITY: Major morbidity is a complication resulting in a prolongation of hospital stay, results in a further treatment or which is life threatening.

Major	
Minor	

SPECIFIC COMPLICATIONS:

	Pre-operative	Peroperative	Post-operative
Wound problems (specify) Use ASEPSIS scale			
Thromboembolism (specify)			
Fixation/implant failure			
Anaesthetic			
Pressure area problems			
Urinary retention			
Cardiovascular			
Respiratory			
Neurovascular			
Haemorrhage			
Unplanned hypotension			
Transfusion reaction			
Allergic reactions			
Fracture blisters			
Secondary fracture			
ARDS/Fat embolism			
Compartment syndrome			
Other infection (specify)			
Problems of # Union			
Other			

Fig. 16.1. Morbidity and mortality report.

assessment is often an important component of these scores, which is reasonable as many of the operations are performed for the relief of pain. However, none of the scores attempt to assess patient satisfaction and quality of care. Further, the assessment of pain is notoriously difficult. A combination of the McGill Pain Questionnaire (short form),[6] used at the beginning and end of each treatment episode, together with a visual analogue pain scale at more frequent intervals, is probably an appropriate way to assess pain.

A comprehensive review of all the scoring systems that are in usage at present needs to be undertaken and new measures that take into account patient satisfaction developed. This is a potentially massive task and will take a long time to complete adequately.

Complications

Complications are frequently used as outcome measures especially by managers as part of contracts. Purchasers of health care expect that complications are kept to a minimum and demand that such 'quality' measures are stated in contracts. A complication is defined as an adverse event arising as a consequence of a pre-existing disease or as a result of an intervention. The term co-morbiditor is increasingly used in the North American literature as an alternative to the term complication.[7] This author uses the term co-morbiditor only in reference to diseases that are co-existent with the orthopaedic or trauma condition and may modify the outcome. The term complication is still used as a generic term referring to any medical adverse event.

It is obvious that an accurate record of complications is fundamental to all clinicians. A change in expected complications may be the first indicator of a problem. Inexperienced surgeons will often have a higher complication rate compared with more experienced surgeons. This may reflect lack of skill (Is counselling needed?), poor general education (Does the teaching programme need to be improved?) or poor supervision (Should supervision increase?). Complications may also be an important outcome measure when introducing a new method of treatment. Figure 16.1 is a morbidity and mortality report that can be carried by the senior house officer. The report is filled in for each complication at the time that it is diagnosed. The accumulated reports can then be reviewed at the audit meetings.

Complications, however, are notoriously difficult to diagnose; especially those of particular interest to orthopaedics and trauma – thrombo-embolism, wound infection and implant failure.

The clinical diagnosis of deep vein thrombosis (DVT) is of very limited use.[8] Venography is regarded as the gold standard for the investigation of the complication. Other methods are available such as venous occlusion plethysmography[9] but the methods are not entirely proven to be specific

Table 16.2 *ASEPSIS scoring for wound infections*

Wound characteristic		Percentage of wound				
	0	< 20	20–39	40–59	60–79	> 80
Serous exudate	0	1	2	3	4	5
Erythema	0	1	2	3	4	5
Purulent exudate	0	2	4	6	8	10
Separation of deep tissues	0	2	4	6	8	10

Criterion	Points
Additional treatments	
Antibiotics	10
Drainage of pus (LA)	5
Debridement of wound (GA)	10
*Serous discharge**	
Erythema*	Daily 0–5
Purulent exudate*	Daily 0–5
Separation of deep tissues*	Daily 0–10
Isolation of bacteria	Daily 0–10
In-patient stay > 14 days	10
	5

* Given score only on 5 of first 7 postoperative days
Total score: 0–10 Satisfactory healing;
              11–20 Disturbance of healing;
              21–30 Minor wound infection;
              31–40 Moderate wound infection;
              > 40 Severe wound infection.
From Wilson *et al.*, *The Lancet*, 1986.

and sensitive. Until a thoroughly reliable method of diagnosis is found, underreporting of DVT, especially the potentially lethal thromboses, will continue.

Wound infection is probably one of the greatest hazards orthopaedic and trauma patients are exposed to. Infection around an implant may result in death, multiple operations (including amputation) or chronic ill health. Somewhat spuriously, wound infection has traditionally been divided into deep and superficial, early and late. As far as orthopaedics is concerned all wound infection will involve the deep tissues until proven otherwise. The term late infection is probably a misnomer in most cases as most infections are probably introduced at the time of the surgery.[10] There is a need for orthopaedists to accurately assess wound problems. The *Surgical Infection Study Group*, an interdisciplinary committee, has recommended the use of ASEPSIS[11] to assess wound infections in all

Table 16.3 *American Society of Anesthesiologists classification of physical status*

Class 1	No systemic disturbance
Class 2	Mild to moderate systemic disturbance
Class 3	Severe systemic disturbance
Class 4	Life threatening systemic disturbance
Class 5	Moribund, little chance of survival
	+ E for emergency

Table 16.4 *CEPOD classification for operation priority*

1.	Emergency	Within 1 hour
2.	Urgent	Usually within 24 hours
3.	Scheduled	One to three weeks
4.	Elective	No specified time

patients including orthopaedic patients. Table 16.2 details the ASEPSIS scoring system.[12] The scoring system has not been validated in orthopaedics and trauma.

A further problem in diagnosing and recording complications is that an event recognised as a complication by one consultant may not be regarded as a complication by another. Simply recording an event as a complication is insufficient. The adverse event may have occurred as a result of a pre-existing condition (a co-morbiditor) or as a result of an intervention. Moreover, a complication may have different effects in different patients depending upon the overall condition of each patient, the response of the patient to the physiological insult of the injury or procedure and the 'severity' of the complication itself. All patients should be assessed according to the American Society of Anesthesiologists (ASA) grades (Table 16.3)[13] and a record of the CEPOD category made (Table 16.4).[14] Any complication that occurs needs to be classified (if possible) so that the 'severity' can be judged. A number of health status assessments that are more extensive than the ASA grading are available, not specifically validated for orthopaedic patients but often used in the elderly and chronically ill. The *healthy-years equivalent (HYE)*,[15] and the *medical illness severity grouping system (Medisgrps)*[16] are examples of these grading systems for general health status. Severely ill and injured patients have a greater morbidity and mortality rate. Knaus *et al.*[17] demonstrated that this correlated with the disturbance of various basic physiological parameters and as a result developed the *APACHE II* scoring system for assessing these effects. Other systems are available and all show that there is a definite correlation between physiological derangement and the risk of both morbidity and mortality (see Chapter 21: Audit in intensive care). The severity of a complication itself will also be important in assessing outcome including the probability of death. Therefore, it is insufficient to record only the fact that a complication has occurred, it is necessary to record as much detail as possible about the complication including the method of diagnosis.

Minimum data set

Fundamental to audit in any specialty is the need to compare like with like. In order to do this a minimum data set common to all users is required. The Royal College of Surgeons of England publication '*Guide-lines for Surgical Audit by Computer*'[18] outlines a minimum data set in its Appendix 1. This data set was designed to be useful in all surgical specialties. The first section of the data set records basic demographic data together with consultant episode details. The next section covers the reasons for admission, including diagnosis and procedures. The third section deals with pathology reports and complications and the final section with discharge details. For a computer based audit there are relatively few fields in the data set and it should be possible to download the demographic details from the central management systems such as PAS onto the local system.

Box 16.1 outlines an 'orthopaedic' minimum data set, which is similar in structure to the Royal College data set but can be used for both paper based as well as computer based audit. Further, those fields of less importance to orthopaedic problems have not been included. A single sheet of A4 size paper can be attached to the case records of all orthopaedic patients and the details entered on the ward rounds. The data must be validated on a weekly basis by the admitting consultant. Box 16.2 outlines a similar, also simple, minimum data set, which could be used in the out-patient clinic at the initial consultation. As all orthopaedic surgeons dictate their notes either directly to a secretary or onto a dictaphone for later typing a disciplined approach would ensure that all the necessary details for both data sets can be entered without significant extra work. As computer technology becomes more widespread the computer screen should appear identical so that the secretaries can directly transfer the information.

Box 16.1 *A minimum data set for orthopaedics and trauma –*
in-patients

Demographic details	(Acquired from PAS or similar) including GP, patient details, hospital number, etc.
Consultant episode details	Date of admission
	Date of discharge
	Date on waiting list
Type of admission	CEPOD Type: Emergency
	Urgent
	Scheduled
	Elective
ASA grade	1 – 5
Diagnosis	Pre-treatment
	Final diagnosis
Co-morbiditors	
Past medical history	
Drugs/allergies	
Procedures	Date
	Surgeon and assistants (including grade)
	Details of procedure
Operative complications	Major/minor
Post-operative complications	Major/minor
Disposal	

Box 16.2 *Orthopaedic minimum data set – out-patients*

Demographic details	From PAS or similar
Date of appointment	
Provisional diagnosis	
Investigations required	
Final diagnosis	
Care plan	
Recommended procedure	Including: level of difficulty/urgency
Name added to waiting list	Date
Other disposal	

Validation

There is simply no point in gathering data if the accuracy of the data are not checked. If there is a computer based audit a clinician systems manager needs to ensure that all the fields are entered and that the detail is accurate. If a coding system is available the codes can be checked at the same time. During the initial period of installation of a computer audit system the time spent on validation may be quite extensive. However, eventually it should be possible to reduce this to only two hours or so a month once experience is gained by those entering the data (see Chapter 11).

Similarly, data entered in a paper audit must be rigorously checked on a regular basis to ensure completeness and accuracy. The easiest way this can be performed for in-patient data is to spend 30 minutes or so going through the forms at the end of the weekly consultant ward round.

Coding

Rapid access to large volumes of computer data is most effectively achieved using an alphanumeric coding system. Computer searches can also be performed by looking at key words but this is inevitably a slower process. The standard coding systems used in the UK for diagnoses (ICD-9) and procedures (OPCS-4) are grossly inadequate for use in orthopaedics and trauma. The British Orthopaedic Association established a coding committee in 1990 to develop a comprehensive coding manual and lexicon based upon the Read system. This is a long and laborious process, particularly as a lexicon of acceptable terms has to be established and the Read codes correlated with the current ICD-9 and OPCS-4 systems as Körner data still uses these. The trauma coding section was completed during 1992 and the work on the elective section commenced but will not be available for some time. Once completed this should be a comprehensive coding system which should be adopted on a national basis allowing orthopaedic surgeons to record data in a uniform fashion.

Resource management

Orthopaedic surgeons cannot ignore the resource implications of the work they do. Many orthopaedic operations involve the use of expensive implants. There is an increasing demand for orthopaedic procedures such as joint replacements. It is, therefore, necessary for orthopaedic surgeons to demonstrate the appropriateness and cost effectiveness of these procedures. This can occur only if the clinicians themselves are willing to acknowledge the resource implications and are prepared to perform cost–benefit analyses of their work. Further, increased information about the *unmet* need of the population in terms of orthopaedic operations is needed so that strategic planning for the future use of limited resources can be undertaken. The role of the Clinical Director is fundamental to these areas as the director can discuss appropriateness, cost effectiveness and future developments on an equal basis with fellow consultants and will be able to ensure that the unit presents a unified approach in its negotiations with the hospital managers.

It is self evident that at present very little information is available about the costs of individual procedures. In the USA the Medicare system developed *diagnostic related groups* (DRGs)[19] in order to control costs. A British version of DRGs is being prepared. Colter *et al.*[20] have demonstrated that DRGs are 'not capable of supporting traumatic spinal care'. Muñoz *et al.*[21] discussed various factors related to patient care in what they define as low-volume and high-volume surgeons. The DRGs were appropriate for the high-volume surgeons who had shorter lengths of stay and fewer complications but were inappropriate for low-volume surgeons whose costs were effectively much higher. Smith *et al.*[22] have highlighted a major problem that is frequently encountered in the UK, that of allocating the correct OPCS code for a procedure. This paper showed that the incorrect coding of procedures resulted in 24% of a small number of patients being allocated to the wrong DRG, which would have a major effect on resource allocation. Niinimaki *et al.*[23] have also analysed the role of DRGs in their Finnish orthopaedic practice and have found them to be unreliable. The appropriateness and accuracy of cost grouping must be properly validated before its widespread introduction. It is, therefore, necessary to gather accurate data about costs for the formulation of contracts. The purchaser–provider relationship is probably here to stay. Clinicians must be prepared to sit down with managers to devise accurate costings.

When to hold audit meetings?

Audit is a major component of the education process within all types of hospital. Therefore, regular meetings are desirable and indeed, according to the Royal College of Surgeons of England directives, weekly meetings are required for recognition of training. Further, it is desirable for juniors to learn to review their own work as an everyday, routine function and not simply when they are told to do so by their seniors. All juniors must now complete a log book of operations, which will audit the number and type of operations performed but more importantly will record the level of supervision. It is likely that reaccreditation will become a part of the continuing education process and it is, therefore, necessary for seniors to also demonstrate that their practice is effective and being kept up to date.

In hospitals where middle grade trainees are found it is useful to link the audit meetings to the postgraduate teaching programme. The meetings should be held in normal working hours. Management will have to accept a reorganisation of clinical commitments and probably a reduction in the time spent directly treating patients in order for clinicians to fulfil the requirements for both audit and teaching. All members of the orthopaedic unit must attend the meetings and each consultant's firm should be audited in rotation.

Conclusions

The development of audit in orthopaedics and trauma is still in its infancy. It is necessary for individuals and groups of consultants to develop appropriate audit methods and to discuss these methods with others in order to determine the best approach to orthopaedic problems. A minimum data set such as that shown in this chapter is required and the uniform recording of complications is needed to allow comparisons. Finally, the Clinical Directors need to lead the way in considering resource aspects of audit and ensuring that orthopaedic surgeons are armed with the necessary information in the fight for limited resources.

References

1. Keller, R. B. Personal communication.
2. Bennett, J. & Walshe, K. (1990). Occurrence screening as method of audit. *British Medical Journal*, **300**, 1248–1251.
3. The Royal College of Physicians (1989). *Fractured neck of femur: prevention and management*. London.
4. Harris, W. H. (1969). Traumatic arthritis of the hip after dislocation and acetabular fractures: Treatment by mold arthroplasty. An end-result study using a new method of result evaluation. *Journal of Bone and Joint Surgery*, **51A**, 737–755.
5. Constant, C. R. & Murley, A. H. G. (1987). A clinical method of functional assessment of the shoulder. *Clinical Orthopaedics and Related Research*, **214**, 160–164.
6. Melzack, R. (1975). The McGill Pain Questionnaire: Major properties and scoring methods. *Pain*, **1**, 277–299.

7. Liang, M. H., Katz, J. N., Phillips, C., Sledge, C., Cats-Baril, W. & the American Academy of Orthopaedic Surgeons Task Force on outcome studies (1991). The total hip arthroplasty outcome evaluation form of the American Academy of Orthopaedic Surgeons. *Journal of Bone and Joint Surgery*, **73A**, 639–646.
8. Gallus, A. S., Hirsh, J. & Hull, R. (1976). Diagnosis of venous thromboembolism. *Seminars in Thrombosis and Haemostasis*, **2**, 203–231.
9. Prandoni, P. & Lensing, A. W. (1990). New developments in noninvasive diagnosis of deep vein thrombosis of the lower limbs. *Ricerca Clinica Laboratoria*, **20**, 11–17.
10. Nelson, J. P., Glassburn, A. R., Talbott, R. D. & McElhinney, J. P. (1980). The effect of previous surgery, operating room environment, and preventive antibiotics on postoperative infection following total hip arthroplasty. *Clinical Orthopaedics and Related Research*, **147**, 167–169.
11. Peel, A. L. G. & Taylor, E. W. (1991). Proposed definitions for the audit of postoperative infection: A discussion paper. *Annals of the Royal College of Surgeons of England*, **73**, 385–388.
12. Wilson, A. P. R., Treasure, T., Sturridge, M. F. & Gruneberg, R. N. (1986). A scoring method (ASEPSIS) for postoperative wound infections for use in clinical trials of antibiotic prophylaxis. *The Lancet*, **i**, 311–313.
13. American Society of Anethesiologists (1963). New classification of physical states. *Anesthesiology*, **24**, 111.
14. Buck, N., Devlin, H. B. & Lunn, J. N. (1987). *The Report of the Confidential Enquiry into Peri-operative Deaths*. London: Nuffield Provincial Hospitals Trust and the Kings' Fund.
15. Mehrez, A. & Gafni, A. (1991). The healthy-years equivalent: How to measure them using the standard gamble approach. *Medical Decision Making*, **11**, 140–146.
16. Brewster, A. C., Jordan, H. S., Young, J. A. & Throop, D. M. (1989). Analysing in-hospital mortality and morbidity with adjustment for admission severity. *Journal of Social Health Systems*, **1**, 49–61.
17. Knaus, W. A., Draper, E. A., Wagner, D. P. & Zimmerman, J. E. (1985). APACHE II: A severity of disease classification system. *Critical Care Medicine*, **13**, 818–829.
18. Royal College of Surgeons of England (1991). *Guidelines for Surgical Audit by Computer*.
19. Bardsley, M., Coles, J. & Jenkins, L. (eds) (1989). *DRGs and Health Care. The Management of Case-Mix*, 2nd edn. London: King Edward's Hospital Fund for London.
20. Cotler, H. B., Cotler, J. M., Alden, M. E., Sparks, G. & Biggs, C. A. (1990). The medical and economic impact of closed cervical dislocations. *Spine*, **15**, 448–452.
21. Muñoz, E., Boiardo, R., Mulloy, K., Goldstein, J. Brewster, J. G., Tenebaum, N. & Wise, L. (1990). Economies of scale, physician volume for orthopedic surgical patients and the DRG prospective payment system. *Orthopedics*, **13**, 39–44.
22. Smith, S. H., Kershaw, C., Thomas, I. H. & Botha, J. L. (1991). PIS and DRGs: Coding inaccuracies and their consequences for resource management. *Journal of Public Health Medicine*, **13**, 40–41.
23. Niinimaki, T., Jalovaara, P. & Linnakko, E. (1991). Is DRG useful in orthopedics? *Acta Orthopaedica Scandinavica*, **241**, 40–41.

17

Installing audit in general practice and general dental practice

MALCOLM PENDLEBURY AND GEORGE BROWN

Introduction

The practice of medical audit, like the practice of clinical science, demands a mixture of creativity and critical analysis.[1]

In this chapter, our primary concern is to provide general medical and general dental practitioners with some methods of tackling audit in their practices, but before auditing any phenomena, it is useful to know what audit is, what auditing is for and what one is auditing. At first sight the answers to these questions may be found in *Working with Patients*[2] and the accompanying Working Paper No. 6 on medical audit.[3] Soon after publishing these papers the Government belatedly recognised that audit embraces much more than accounting; that it is a deep subtle process; that it has implications for practice management and that it is inextricably linked with professional standards and continuing professional education. The confusion that is implicit in the Government's policy is now being felt explicitly in practices that are beginning to tackle the problems of audit. Hence this chapter.

What is audit?

To audit is to estimate worth. Audit is the ugly sister of the family of assessment. Its near relatives are total quality management, appraisal, quality assurance and quality control. Marinker[4] defines medical audit as 'the attempt to improve the quality of medical care by measuring the performance of those that practice that care, by considering their performance in relation to desired standards, and by improving on this performance'. His definition raises questions about the nature of standards and whether it is always necessary to improve upon existing performance.

The process of auditing entails taking a sample of behaviour of an individual, a practice or a system, making inferences and making estimates of worth. The content of the sample may be patient records, referrals, dental treatment plans, domiciliary visits, emergency treatments, receptionists' skills, and so on. The method of sampling may be an analysis of records, direct observations, questionnaires, interviews and discussions. The audit may be conducted by oneself, a practice team, patients or peers. The process of making inferences may involve quantitative measures or qualitative descriptions. The estimates of worth may be based upon norms, ideals or achievable standards. Lurking beneath this description of the process of audit are questions of value and purpose. The process of audit itself is open to audit. The sample may be inappropriate for the purpose. The method of data collection may be inadequate, the inferences may be weak, and the estimates of worth not relevant to the purposes of the audit.

Purposes and problems of audit

There are confusions and dilemmas involved in audit in general practice medicine and dentistry. These relate to the level of the audit, the purposes of the audit and the questions of standards.

Level

Audit may be used to help a trainee, a member of the practice, the practice itself or the health system to improve or to make judgements about themselves. Herein lies a difficulty, for what is appropriate content and method for one level is not necessarily appropriate at another.

Purposes

The purposes of audit within general practice or general dental practice are judgemental and developmental. Figure 17.1 provides a simple model of the relationship before judgemental and developmental purposes.

At one end of the continuum are the judgemental purposes; these results of audit are reported to external agencies. Prescribing rates, referral rates, cervical cytology targets, number of crowns provided, are obvious examples. The judgemental data may also be used by external agencies to improve the primary health care system or to cut its costs. The two are not synonymous. The developmental purposes are used by a practice to

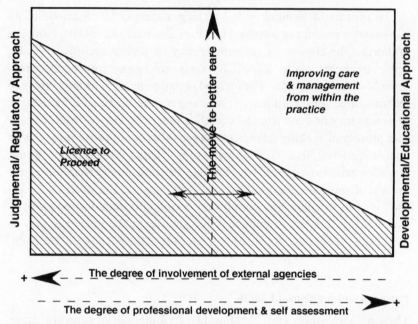

Fig. 17.1. The purposes of audit – the ratio of external (management) and internal (professional/educational) influences on improving patient care. The move to better care can be based on any mixture of regulatory and educational influences. The mixture dictates the final flavour of the audit. The developmental approach may be more palatable for the doctor/dentist. The outcome can be the same.

improve its working arrangements such as appointment systems, record keeping, requests to laboratories and so on and to identify the educational and training needs of its staff.

The continuum in Figure 17.1 is not a pure diagonal. Judgemental audit may have developmental effects. Some judgements need to be made to enable improvements to occur. However, difficulties arise if judgemental and developmental purposes are competing. A practice or practitioner may be willing to improve but unwilling to reveal its inadequacies. Neither private companies nor individuals are willing to reveal evidence that could be used against them or by their competitors. Trusts may be becoming common in the NHS but trust is not.

There remains a problem then for a health care system. If it is to improve, then monitoring is necessary. However, if that monitoring is seen as threatening to the people involved they will be reluctant to reveal information. One way of resolving the dilemma is to ensure that every practice has a quality assurance system in place. Such a system may be based upon the *Dental Practice Assessment System*,[5] the *What Sort of Doctor*[6] initiative of the Royal College of General Practitioners and the

Peer review in general dental practice[7] document recently issued by the General Dental Services Committee of the British Dental Association and the Department of Health. Extracts from the Pendlebury system are provided in subsequent sections of this chapter. If such an approach is used, the external agencies receive evidence that such a system is in place but not the detailed data generated by the system of audit. The external agencies may of course also need to receive data that are necessary for its systemic development, in particular, for its provision of hospital and community care, its pharmaceutical budget, building budgets and strategic planning such as where to site or maintain a community dental service.

Questions of standards

The question of standards presents difficulties for the healthcare system, the practice and the individual. As an example let us consider referral rates.[8] The methods of collecting referral data, the methods of calculating referral data and interpreting differences between general practitioners and general practice populations are complex issues. The standards used are the average rather than ideal or a set of explicit criteria. Data collected by the Dental Practice Board[9] gives the 'hard' measure of how many particular items of treatment are given individually, locally and nationally. These figures when combined with other data such as the target net income for dentists and the work of the Dental Rates Study Group set a fee for all items of service. The aim of this activity is to ensure that the average dentist doing the average profile of work will earn an average income. The weakness in the argument is that it becomes impossible to improve the clinical completion of any single item of treatment using a technique that involves more time without adversely affecting the dentist's income. If all dentists used rubber dam for endodontics then this would be accounted for in the fees; as it is few do and the fee for the time taken becomes inadequate. What *all* do is not necessarily correct – it is likely to be expedient.

Implicit and explicit criteria

The average norm is but a crude measure. Standards imply criteria. In the past such criteria have been implicit. The views of another professional or group of professionals were deemed sufficient even though the basis of their judgements were sometimes shrouded in mystery. The new drive towards openness requires the use of explicit criteria so that everyone may be clear what judgements are being made and on what basis. An example of explicit criteria for auditing a trainee general practitioner is given in Table 17.1 and other examples are given in subsequent sections. The advantages of explicit criteria are:

1. They give guidance on what needs to be improved to achieve the standards required.
2. They are likely to be more reliable measures.
3. They are likely to be valid measures.
4. They may be used in self or peer assessment.
5. They reveal what is valued.

However, one should be wary of assuming that explicit criteria are necessarily linked to only one standard. The same explicit criteria may fit more than one standard and explicit criteria may lead to an agreed standard rather than vice versa. In the early stages of developing audit it is often better to begin with the question: 'What counts as good practice?' (in record keeping, time management, nursing of elderly patients, consultative skills) rather than with the question 'What standards should we adopt?'

How to audit

Audit, like many research projects, requires the delineation of goals, choice of methods of data collection and analysis, estimates of time and cost involved, conclusions, reporting, and suggestions for future action. Audit differs from some research projects in its use of standards and explicit criteria. Audit may be conducted without explicit criteria just as experiments may be conducted without specific hypotheses. However, one is more likely to conduct useful audit or experiment if one knows what one is looking for. The following check-list may serve as a guide and evaluation of an audit plan (Box 17.1).

All of these steps are important but it would be naive to assume that the process is linear. Often the effort of establishing explicit criteria leads to changes of purpose. The process of developing criteria goes through a cycle of initial definition, confusion, modification and re-definition. Frequently, a group conducting an audit develop too many criteria, so it is important to run a pilot to cast out some criteria and to modify the approach and estimates where necessary. Finally, beware of being overambitious. The choice of topic is often too big, so instead choose one aspect of that topic. For example, 'What is the degree of compliance with ante-natal appointments within the practice and within areas of the practice?'. Text and

Table 17.1 *Criterion measures for the assessment of trainee general practitioners*

Criterion 1: Information gathering
This criterion is concerned with the trainee's willingness, ability and skill in gathering information necessary for diagnosis and/or decisions.

Behavioural objectives

The unacceptable trainee:
1. Follows no routine of history taking.

2. Fails to identify or does not bother to develop salient leads.
3. Will not pursue alternative hypotheses.
4. Does not seek information on clinical, psychological and social factors.

5. Records sketchily and not systematically.
6. Tends to use investigations in a 'blunderbuss' fashion.

The acceptable trainee:
1. Takes a comprehensive history, when appropriate, including clinical, psychological and social factors.
2. Records his/her information carefully.
3. Uses previous and continuing records intelligently.
4. Plans investigations and uses diagnostic services intelligently to develop diagnosis and support clinical activity.

Criterion 2: Problem-solving
This criterion is concerned with the trainee's ability and skill in using information gained.

Behavioural objectives

The unacceptable trainee:
1. Does not fully realise the implications of the data that he/she collects.
2. Is unable to interpret the unexpected result, which he/she may often ignore.

3. His/her thinking tends to be rigid and unimaginative and impedes recognition of associated problems.
4. His/her general shortcomings – rigidity of thought and lack of capacity to range round flexibly, i.e. 'diverge' when thinking over a particular problem – have an inhibiting effect on his/her problem-solving skills.

The acceptable trainee:
1. Realises the importance of unexpected findings and seeks to interpret them.
2. Understands the nature of probability and uses this to assist his/her diagnosis and decision making.
3. Takes all data into account before making a decision and routinely tests alternative hypotheses.
4. Thinks effectively – he/she has the capacity to range flexibly, or 'diverge' in the research for relevant factors in connection with the particular problem in hand, and he/she has also the capacity to focus, or 'converge', in his/her thinking on whatever factors have been decided upon as relevant.

Table 17.1 (*Continued*)

Criterion 3: Clinical judgement

This criterion is concerned with the doctor's ability to use sound judgement in planning for and carrying out treatment, and conveying his/her advice and opinion to patients.

Behavioural objectives

The unacceptable doctor:
1. Is concerned more with treatment than the overall welfare of the patient.

2. Plans treatment when not familiar with the procedures or therapy selected.
3. Shows rigid choice of treatment.

4. Tends to use set routine or 'favourite' prescriptions, whether appropriate or not.

5. Does not explain his/her proposals in terms understood by the patient.

The acceptable doctor:
1. Is familiar with the uses and limitations of the treatment he/she selected. He/she recognises his or her own limitations.
2. Considers simple therapy or expectant measures first.

3. Shows regard for the individual patient's needs, wishes and total circumstances.
4. Is flexible and will modify treatment or decisions immediately the clinical situation requires he should do so.
5. Takes patients into his/her confidence and explains his/her proposals in terms appropriate to the individual patient.

Criterion 4: Relationship to patients

This criterion is concerned with the doctor's effectiveness in working with patients.

Behavioural objectives

The unacceptable doctor:
1. Does not relate well to patients either through aloofness, discourtesy, indifference or pressures of work.
2. Has difficulty understanding his/her patient's needs.

3. Is unable to give patients confidence and may even unnecessarily alarm them.
4. Reacts poorly to a patient's hostile or emotional behaviour.

5. Does not exhibit sympathy or compassion in dealing with patients.

The acceptable doctor:
1. Gives patients confidence, affords co-operation and relieves anxiety.

2. While patients appreciate his/her interest in their well-being he/she does not become emotionally involved.
3. Is honest with the patient and his or her family.

4. Patients like the doctor and feel he/she is an easy person of whom to ask questions or with whom they may discuss problems.

Table 17.1 (*Continued*)

Criterion 5: Continuing responsibility
This criterion is concerned with the doctor's willingness to accept and fulfil the responsiblity for long-term patient care.

Behavioural objectives

The unacceptable doctor:
1. Either loses interest after initial treatment or does not spend time on follow-up care.

2. Becomes discouraged with slow progress and cannot cope with a poor prognosis.
3. Is unable to communicate hard facts to a patient or his or her relatives.

4. Uses ancillary personnel inadequately or demands greater assistance than they are competent to give him/her.
5. Fails to review a patient's case at suitable intervals.

The acceptable doctor:
1. Encourages patients to work for their own rehabilitation and shows that he/she too has the same objective.
2. Observes patient's progress and alters management and therapy as required.
3. Understands the roles of ancillary personnel and makes maximum effective use of their help.
4. Maintains a positive and consistent attitude to health and under proper circumstances to recovery.

Criterion 6: Emergency care
This criterion is concerned with the doctor's ability to act effectively in emergency situations.

Behavioural objectives

The unacceptable doctor:
1. Panics easily and loses time by ineffective action.

2. Becomes confused under pressure and has difficulty in establishing priorities.
3. Is unable to delegate appropriate aspects of care to others.
4. Is unable or unwilling to make and sustain decisions alone.

The acceptable doctor:
1. Quickly assesses a situation and establishes priorities with full regard to life saving procedures.
2. Is aware of the consequences of delay.

3. Is able to obtain and organise the assistance of others.
4. Is able and willing to make and sustain decisions alone if necessary.

Criterion 7: Relationship with colleagues
This criterion is concerned with the doctor's ability to work effectively with his/her colleagues and members of the health team.

Table 17.1 (*Continued*)

Behavioural objectives

The unacceptable doctor:
1. Has difficulty in personal relationships and lacks the ability to give and take instruction gracefully.

2. Tends to be tactless or inconsiderate.

3. Is unable to inspire the confidence or co-operation of those with whom he/she works.
4. Is unwilling to make referrals or seek consultation. Does not support colleagues in their contacts with patients.

The acceptable doctor:
1. Gets on well with perople. He/she is conscious of the need for team-work and fits in well as a member or, on occasion, as leader of a team.
2. Seeks consultation when appropriate and respects the views of others.
3. Acknowledges the contributions of others.

4. Creates an atmosphere of 'working with' and not 'working for' other people. Demonstrates self control.

Criterion 8: Professional values
This criterion is concerned with the doctor's attitudes and standards as an individual member of the medical profession.

Behavioural objectives

The unacceptable doctor:
1. Attempts to cover up his/her errors from his colleagues.

2. Is difficult to locate in emergencies and absent when required without making deputising arrangements.
3. Will not discuss medical mismanagement with patients.

The acceptable doctor:
1. Is kind, courteous, honest and humble. Reports accurately, including his/her own errors.
2. Respects the confidences of colleagues and patients.

3. Places patient care above personal considerations.
4. Recognises his/her own professional capabilities and limitations.

Based on Freeman and Byrne (1976).

publications may imply that one establishes a standard and then develops criteria to measure achievement against that standard. The process of practice is much less logical. Sometimes a standard emerges from the criteria rather than *vice versa*. Sometimes the standard is unrealistic and, just occasionally, the standard and criteria are both appropriate, they match closely and all of this is demonstrated in the pilot.

Box 17.1 *Auditing your audit*

1. Are the purposes of the audit clearly expressed and realistic?
2. Are the purposes understood by all the people involved in the audit?
3. Are the methods of data collection understood by the people conducting the audit?
4. Have explicit criteria been developed for the audit task?
5. Are these criteria linked to a standard? Will they be linked to a standard?
6. Are the criteria manageable for the task?
7. Are the methods of data analysis understood by those conducting the audit?
8. Are they appropriate for the purposes of the audit?
9. Do the conclusions arise logically from the data analysis?
10. Do the recommendations for further action take account of advantages, disadvantages and problems of the proposed change and the existing approach?
11. Are the estimates of time and cost involved realistic?
12. Do you now have a usable set of criteria and methods for repeating the audit?
13 When will you repeat the audit of this topic?

What to audit

If one were to audit every aspect of a practice then one would spend more person hours on audit than on patients. Given that only the practice expenses are to be refunded with no income to general dental practices (GDPs) for carrying out an audit and no separately identified remuneration is available for audit in general practice medicine, then one has to decide what to audit and what not to audit. Obvious items for audit are those that are now legally required and those that generate practice income.

There are two broad overlapping areas from which to select topics for audit: patient care and practice management. Each of these may be subdivided further and each has outcomes in the short, medium and long term. In health management parlance, these areas correspond roughly with Donabedian's categories of structure, process and outcome.[10] Strictly speaking, both practice management and patient care have structural and process characteristics. Practice management, which includes resources and resource constraints, has an impact upon process of patient care and upon outcomes of patient care.

Whatever topic is chosen, it is important to have developed a set of explicit criteria to apply to the task. Indeed, the process of establishing explicit criteria is probably as important as the results of the audit itself.[11] The criteria developed provide a basis for self and peer assessment for training and of course whilst developing criteria one has to think and determine what one values. In reality this is a form of practice based on postgraduate education.

However, it would be wasteful for every practice to re-invent all of its own criteria. The examples provided in this chapter are offered for consideration and modification by members of primary care teams in medicine and dentistry. Other relevant sources are, for dentists, *The Self Assessment Manual and Standards* (Faculty of General Dental Practitioners (UK) of the Royal College of Surgeons of England), the clinical audit documents issued by the Working Group on Audit in Primary Dental Care and the Dental Practice Board (DPB) Annual Reports. For doctors the most fruitful source is the Royal College of General Practitioners (RCGP) and the Registrar General's annual returns.

Auditing patient care

The first attempts at medical audit were concerned with the easily measurable rather than the highly valued. They included such items as doctor–patient ratios, number of rooms in a health centre or practice and the equipment in use.[12] The dentist practising profile issued by the DPB continues this trend comparing what is done rather than what should be done. The new general practice (GP) and general dental practice (GDP) contracts focus upon processes of patient care such as consultation rates, referral rates, prescribing rates and treatments provided. There are five basic approaches to audit of patient care: population estimates, audit trails or traces, case analyses, individual case studies and peer review. Explicit criteria may be applied to all of these.

Population estimates

Many of the contractual items such as the child capitation payments in dentistry require estimates based upon populations. Such contractual items have implications for record keeping and retrieval which in turn have implications for practice management and for monitoring practice management procedures. Computerisation of medical or dental records with appropriate software is essential for population estimates.

Audit trails and traces

For some items of care a sampling technique is all that is necessary. Traces, sometimes known as audit trails, are based upon carefully chosen samples, which will reveal a wide range of characteristics of patient care and associated practice management. An example of a suitable item for a trail is the care of the house-bound chronic sick.

Kessner *et al.*[13] suggested that two traces should be selected in an audit if one wants to obtain a broad impression of patient care in the practice. Each should be relevant to four broad age groups and both sexes. They suggest that traces should be readily diagnosable, sufficiently prevalent within the practice and part if not all of the techniques of clinical management should be well defined (the features they suggest are diagnosis, treatment, prevention and rehabilitation). Traces require explicit criteria agreed by the practitioners involved in the audit. They have features in common with performance indicators,[14] statements of competence[15] and performance evaluation guides.[16]

Clearly age–sex registers and morbidity in disease or the identification of special interests to the practice are a necessary preliminary to embarking upon an audit trail. Again computerised records with appropriate retrieval procedures are likely to be more efficient than manual methods. However, one needs to plan carefully the setting up of the computer system. Otherwise one may be record keeping by computer and auditing by hand.

Random case analysis

Random case analysis consists of selecting a set of cases, perhaps from one session, and discussing and analysing them. The procedure may reveal the range of problems tackled by a general or dental practitioner and the variety of approaches adopted. The method was initiated probably by Balint[17] and it is widely used in vocational training, in general practice medicine and general practice dentistry. Random case analysis may be augmented by the use of video and audio recordings. If these methods are used, it is important to have an agreed procedure for discussion, analysis and review of progress[18,19] and provide further details on the use of video recordings. This theme is discussed briefly under the heading of con-sultation in a later section of the chapter.

Case analyses may also be used to explore clinically significant events such as life events and emergency treatments. These may illuminate hitherto unrecognised aspects of patient care and practice management. Buckley[20] also suggests exploring 'heartsink' and 'heartlift' patients. Such investigations may reveal feelings, inner conflicts and values as well as strengths and weaknesses in patient care and practice management. Random case analysis provides a broad estimate of competence but for relatively inexperienced practitioners it may be less useful than structured case analysis in which one selects particular cases and those rare but complex demanding cases.

Individual case study

In-depth case studies may be particularly useful for examining errors, and for exploring the range of agencies involved in a case, the responses of the practice staff and the clinical care provided. Obviously one should choose a case study that has considerable clinical or practical significance.[21]

Patient perceptions

As well as the clinical aspects of patient care, there are also personal aspects that may be explored – in particular patient satisfaction with the service provided. Whilst patient satisfaction is but one aspect of patient care, it is one that can provide valuable feedback for practices and practice managers. Patient perceptions may also be sampled by family health services authorities (FHSAs), regional health authorities (RHAs) and nationally. Indeed, one of the pioneering studies in this field provided national data on patient satisfaction with their primary health care.[22]

Informal discussion with patients in the surgery in patient support groups can provide useful suggestions and points for improvement. But they run the risk of providing information one wants to hear. An alternative is to develop simple robust questionnaires that may be analysed easily.

Peer review

However, patient perceptions of quality of treatment or care are not enough.[23] The measurement of quality requires audit by fellow professionals. Such audit is best conducted by peers from within the same practice, from other practices or from a professional network. Anyone who is involved in peer review should themselves have been the subject of a peer review. The reviewers should have been provided with some training on how to audit and what to audit. They should also be aware of the particular skills required for presenting the results. If peer review is to be useful to a practice then clearly its purpose must be well defined. It must be structured and explicit. The dental practice assessment system[5] provides an

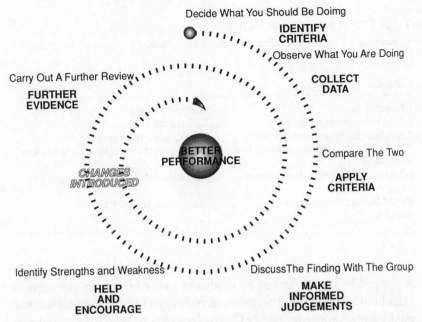

Fig. 17.2. The peer review audit path. Note: if the review system is working then the path is never a circle!

example for structured approaches to peer review, whereas Freeman and Byrne's[24] approach appears to infer more latitude. The peer review audit pathway is graphically illustrated in Figure 17.2.[7]

Performance evaluation guides

An extension of the use of explicit criteria is provided by performance evaluation guides or PEGs. The name is apt for they are devices on which one can hang one's professional judgements. The method was suggested by Hunter[25] for use in the clinical assessment of items of treatment in dentistry but it may be readily extended for use in medical tasks, the consultation and aspects of practice management. In essence the method consists of establishing explicit observable criteria and attaching a rating to each criterion. The rating may be binary – satisfactory or unsatisfactory – or much more fine grained – typical of 'a beginner', 'advanced beginner', 'adequate professional', 'competent professional', 'outstanding professional'. An example of a PEG is given in Table 17.2. Box 17.2 provides a list of common weaknesses in restorative dentistry which dentists may

Table 17.2 *A PEG for silicon based dental impressions*

Criterion	Rating					
	0	1	2	3	4	5
Choice of tray	Size and stability					
Effective material retention	No separation from tray					
Thickness of impression materials	No excessive thickness or deficiency					
All areas of importance recorded on impression	Adequate extension to show contours					
All areas of coverage demonstrates tissue contact	Absence of defects in all areas					
Reproduction of preparation margins	Margins clear and traceable					

like to use for developing their PEGs. The method may be used or developed by one person or by groups of four of five from the same or neighbouring practices. The approach provides a forum for discussing and establishing standards. The PEG produced may be used for self and peer assessment and for training purposes.

The consultation

At the heart of patient care is the consultation process. Samples of consultations drawn by topic or random case analysis or individual case study may be used. Video recordings of consultations are necessary and they are now used widely in the vocational training of doctors and dentists but are used less frequently in audits. Video recordings may also be used for training and auditing of health visitors and practice nurses and of associates in a practice.[26,18]

Video recordings are threatening so one should approach this form of audit with care. A useful starting point is to allow the person being video recorded to view his or her video recording privately but armed with a checklist (Box 17.3). Subsequently the person could be invited to choose a sample to discuss with one or two others. Then one might invite colleagues to show, analyse and discuss sections of a consultation or consultations of difficult patients, or difficult medical or dental problems. Some common errors in the consultation are shown in Box 17.4. Alternatively one may just choose a sample from a particular session of the surgery or clinic. Discussions of consultations or consultative styles often lead to discussions

---

Box 17.2   *Some characteristics of unsatisfactory restorations*

Amalgam restorations
  Major marginal overhangs
  Fractures
  Food impaction
  Active or recurrent caries
  Marginal deficiencies (enamel and amalgam)
  Absence of anatomical tooth form
  Occlusal interferences or lack of occlusion

Synthetic restorations
  Major marginal overhangs
  Food impaction
  Active or recurrent caries
  Marginal deficiencies
  Inappropriate contouring
  Poor colour match

Inlays, onlays, veneers and three-quarter crown restorations
  Under extension of margins
  Open or visible cement margin
  Perforation in occlusal surface
  Gingival overhangs
  Absence of anatomical tooth form
  Occlusal interferences or lack of occlusion

Crowns and fixed bridgework
  Under extension of margins
  Open or visible cement margin
  Perforation in occlusal surface
  Gingival overhangs
  Absence of anatomical tooth form
  Occlusal interferences or lack of occlusion
  Poor colour match
  Inflammatory tissue responses under pontics

Remember when producing a performance evaluation guide it is the presence
or quality of the criteria required for the existence of a satisfactory restoration
which should be identified and subsequently rated.

---

of practice management as well as patient management. The video
recording and discussion often encourages colleagues to learn from each
others' approach and to clarify values. Sometimes colleagues and members
of the practice team may decide to work on improving some aspect of their

Box 17.3   *The ORDERED Dental Consultation Analysis system*
           (Pendlebury 1987)

This card helps you to rate the consultation skills of a dentist. For each aspect
of the consultation listed ring the number which best represents your view.

Opening
Welcoming into the surgery including a mutual introduction
Poor   Fair   Good   Excellent
1   2   3   4   5   6   7

Rapport
Forming a social link between patient and dentist enabling fruitful
communication
1   2   3   4   5   6   7

Diagnosis
Listening, watching and leading the patient where necessary to discover the
patient's real problem or worry, including the unstated (hidden agenda)
1   2   3   4   5   6   7

Explanation
Discussing the problem with the patient using suitable vocabulary and clearly
1   2   3   4   5   6   7

Responsiveness
The recognition and follow up of clues given by the patient when explaining,
negotiating and giving treatment
1   2   3   4   5   6   7

Education
Inserting into the consultation a preventive and dental health message
1   2   3   4   5   6   7

Dismissal
A clear termination to the consultation containing a definite indication of
continuing care
1   2   3   4   5   6   7

                                                    Total score_____

What aspects were especially good?

Suggestions for improvement

Box 17.4   *Common errors in the consultation*

● Avoidance of personal issues
● Use of jargon
● Lack of precision in fact finding
● Lack of clarification
● Lack of control
● Failure to pick up verbal leads
● Failure to pick up body language cues
● Non-facilitation
● Inappropriate questions
● Single problem assumption
● Poor openings and closures

Common errors in responding

● Inappropriate statements or questions; routinised grunts
● Monotonous echoing, reflecting back every statement
● No, or rare reflection of feeling
● Inappropriate use of language (medical or non-medical)
● Over-reaching and under-reaching

consultation and to re-video a sample of consultations to explore in what ways they have improved.

Auditing practice management

Practice management is concerned with facilitating efficient, effective, equitable patient care – and how that care is perceived by patients and the community. It embraces management styles, workloads, relations with patients, relations with external agencies such as hospitals and laboratories, relations between staff, building and equipment maintenance, budgeting and accounting and patient records. Clearly not all of these can be tackled in this chapter.

Auditing enables a practice and its staff to monitor and reflect upon their performances, to adjust approaches where necessary and to identify education and training needs. Auditing practice management is a challenge that requires interpersonal skills as well as technical expertise.

The technical expertise may be subsumed under the questions:

What do we wish to audit?

What criteria will we use?

Box 17.5 *Auditing staff views*

This brief questionnaire has been designed to help the practice to explore views about work in the practice and about audit. The questionnaire will be analysed and a survey report produced. There will be a practice meeting to discuss the views expressed in the questionnaire. Please complete the questionnaire and return it by _____

1. What do you enjoy most about your work in the practice?

2. What aspects of your work is the least enjoyable?

3. What changes in your work pattern would help you to do your job better?

4. The practice may be required to audit its work. If we do an audit, which topic should be done first? (Please tick)

   Building/equipment, patient records, patient bookings, access to doctors, access to nurses, paediatric surveillance, elderly patients _____

5. If we do an audit, what suggestions do you have about how we should proceed, e.g. start with an easy, useful task.

Thank you for your help.

The interpersonal skills require answers to the questions:

How will we introduce the process of audit?
How will we conduct the audit?
How will we present the results of the audit to the members of the practice team?

It should be noted that the questions themselves imply a management style that is predominantly open, participative yet directive. Without such a management style it is unlikely that audit will lead to improvement in practice management and patient care. So as a start an audit of the staff's views of the practice might be conducted.

Auditing staff views

A brief, simple questionnaire should be designed by a small group of partners and staff. It should indicate the reasons for the survey. As a preliminary, the suggestion of conducting the survey should be discussed with all parties concerned informally and at a regular meeting of the practice staff. If the practice does not hold regular meetings then informal approaches should be made to all staff. The questionnaire should focus

---

Box 17.6 *Criteria for examining GP records:*

- Does the record contain immunisation status? (explanation needed?)
- Height and weight
- Date of last BP
- Date and results of functional assessment
- Date of cervical smear for female patients
- Are the letters in chronological order?
- Are the clinical notes legible?
- Is the medicine list up to date?
- Is there a summary of health problems?
- Current occupation

Rating on overall organisation of record 0 1 2 3 4
0 = totally inadequate, 1 = inadequate, 2 = adequate but some minor changes required, 3 = satisfactory, 4 = professionally organised.

---

upon how practice management could be improved. Some possible questions are given in Box 17.5.

Patient records

Patient records are a useful starting point for audit as record keeping is a joint responsibility for the practice team. The standard and criteria are relatively easily defined and reported. The tasks arising out of the audit are clear and the importance of accurate records for income generation, external audit and medico-legal reasons are also clear. Useful criteria are given in Boxes 17.6 and 17.7.

These checklists may be applied initially to a random sample of say 20 records, if these reveal important characteristics not covered by the check list then the original checklist should be modified. The new checklist may then be applied to a set of records based on the age–sex register, perhaps a partner's list or a random sample.

To estimate how many patient records are unsatisfactory, one can apply a simple formula to the results of a random survey.
The formula is:

$$X = \frac{N \times U}{n}$$

where X = proportion unsatisfactory, N = total number of patient records held, U = number of unsatisfactory records in the sample, and n = number of records sampled.

Box 17.7   *Practice procedures*

A. Practice management

1. Receptionist/appointment control   No ☐ Yes ☐
   a. Waiting patient monitored
   b. Dentist informed at patient's arrival
   c. Appointments confirmed
   d. Day list in each surgery

2. Appointment book   No ☐ Yes ☐
   a. Organised by dentists or surgery members
   b. Type of treatment noted
   c. Variable length appointments
   d. Lunch period identified and kept
   e. Free appointments within three weeks
   f. Reserved accommodation for emergencies
   g. Convenient hours for patients (out with 9–5)
   h. Protocol for preventative procedures
   i. System for maintaining records of training

3. Information materials   No ☐ Yes ☐
   a. Statement of practice philosophy and policies
   b. Dental health education materials
   c. Oral hygiene instructions
   d. Pre-anaesthetic and sedation instructions
   e. Post-surgical instructions
   f. Appointment cards
   g. Prescription forms other than FP14

Within limits, the bigger the random sample, the more reliable the estimate. The estimate may be used to devise a time schedule for improving patient records and for fixing a date for the next audit of patient records.

The practice or health centre building and rooms

The first impressions that a patient has of a practice is either its buildings or the receptionist's response to a phone call. The former is relatively easy and less threatening to audit. Box 17.8 provides a checklist. The rater may be a partner, member of staff, patient or colleague from outside the

Box 17.8   *Structure*

A. Facilities

1. Maximum number of dentists working in practice at any one time

2. Practice location

  a. Parking
     0   No patient parking. No public transport to practice
     1   No patient parking but public transport available
     2   Limited patient parking – one to three spaces per dentist
     3   Ample patient parking – more than three spaces per dentist

  b. Building/grounds/signs
     0   Unattractive, untidy, repairs needed
     1   Needs attention or painting
     2   Neat and clean
     3   Unusually attractive and well cared for

  c. Entrance door and hall
     0   Unattractive, messy, repairs needed
     1   Needs attention or painting
     2   Neat and clean
     3   Unusually attractive and well cared for

  d. Access for handicapped
     0   Impossible access for handicapped
     1   Difficult access for handicapped
     2   Easy access for handicapped
     3   Special provisions for handicapped

3. Reception/waiting area

  a. Size
     0   Less than two seats per dentist/hygienist
     1   Two seats per dentist/hygienist
     2   Three seats per dentist/hygienist
     3   More than three seats per dentist/hygienist

  b. Decor and furnishings
     0   Unattractive and/or repairs needed
     1   Worn or need painting
     2   Neat and clean, good repair
     3   Very attractive

  c. General atmosphere
     0   Stark, uncomfortable environment
     1   Little effort to create comfortable environment
     2   Comfortable environment
     3   A very comfortable and attractive place to be

Box 17.8 contd.

d. Dental health education material
- 0   None available
- 1   Some material but unorganised
- 2   Organised on a special table or rack
- 3   Audio visual equipment and/or educational newsletter in reception

e. Practice information leaflet (incorporating practice details and emergency arrangements)
- 0   None available
- 1   Leaflets available but unorganised
- 2   Organised on a special table or rack
- 3   Routinely given to all patients

4. Administration area/office

a. Site
- 0   Part of reception area – room for one only
- 1   Part of reception area – crowded
- 2   Part of reception area – uncrowded
- 3   Discrete area/office

b. Filing/patient records
- 0   Files spread in multiple areas
- 1   Inconvenient access
- 2   Conveniently accessible
- 3   Separate filing area

c. Computerisation of records
- 0   No computer used
- 1   Computer/wordprocessor for business administration only
- 2   Patient records excluding clinical records
- 3   Clinical records

5. Surgery

a. Size
- 0   No room available for chairside assistant
- 1   Crowded with assistant standing at chairside
- 2   Room for both dentist and assistant to operate seated
- 3   Room for more than one assistant

b. Ambience/furnishings (not equipment)
- 0   Stark, no effort to create comfortable atmosphere
- 1   Only token efforts to create comfortable atmosphere
- 2   Obvious efforts to create comfortable atmosphere
- 3   Attractive/pleasant/comfortable

c. Cleanliness
- 0   Messy and dirty
- 1   Neat, but not recently cleaned
- 2   Clean and neat
- 3   A sparkling, clean look

Box 17.8 contd.

6. Traffic flow through the practice

a. As it involves patients

0   Patient involved in congestion when in surgery
1   Patient involved in office congestion when in surgery
2   Patient not involved in congestion when in surgery
3   Patient not involved in congestion at any time

b. As it involves staff

0   Dentist and staff cannot move about office without difficulty
1   Obvious locations in practice that serve as bottlenecks to easy movement
2   Occasional crowding of some areas but no compromise to efficiency
3   Unhampered flow of personnel

practice. Often an outsider sees things that members of the practice have begun to take for granted. The outcome of the audit may require action. Indeed there is little point in auditing any aspect of practice management or patient care unless it can, potentially, lead to change.

Accessibility

Accessibility is always a compromise between the wishes of the patients and the resources of the practice. Commitment to continuing care necessarily reduces accessibility if resources are fixed. Before one can audit accessibility one needs to clarify one's values and to identify existing procedures. It may be that there is a mismatch between what one values and the procedures in use. If so, modify the procedures before carrying out an audit. If values and procedures are consistent, then carry out an audit based upon the procedures. Occasionally, one's values may be unrealistic. Difficult choices ensue. Either one accepts this mismatch or modifies one's values or one's procedures. In any modification to procedure, one should consider the advantages, disadvantages and potential problems of both the existing and the proposed changes. Changes in procedures often lead to changes in values.

These principles apply to appointments, delays, telephone access to the practice, telephone access to a doctor or nurse and to many other features of practice management and patient care.

Appointment system

Appointment systems are relatively easy to audit providing that the procedures are clear and are already agreed.

Suppose the rules of procedure are:

1. All emergencies seen the same day.
2. Appointments with own doctor must occur within five days if requested.
3. Appointment with any doctor must occur within two days.

On the basis of these rules it is relatively easy to draw up a frequency table and for the relevant date to be extracted from the appointment book and records. A similar procedure may be used to examine the incidence and frequency of night calls within the practice. Decide in a practice meeting the factors causing patients to contact the doctor or dentist out of normal surgery time. Decide which of these factors could be foreseen or predicted so avoiding a call. During the next two weeks keep a log of out of hours calls and if they fit the predicted causes change the practice procedures to avoid the need for them. You will probably find that changing surgery hours or making it easier for the patient to contact the doctor or dentist for advice will ease the need for a home visit or reopening the practice in the case of dentists.

Receptionists and patients

A common complaint of patients is the attitude of receptionists. A common complaint of receptionists is the attitude of patients and doctors or dentists. Receptionists have an important and demanding role as gate-keepers in a practice. As indicated earlier they are often the first point of contact in a practice.

Auditing a receptionist's skills is a delicate task. It is best tackled by inviting the receptionists to develop their own set of criteria, which takes account of the procedures of the practices and which enables them to conduct self and peer assessment. Some examples of criterion statements are given in Box 17.9.

Access to doctors/dentists

Every doctor or dentist has his or her own distinctive style and approach to access. Sometimes there is an agreed policy on access to the doctor or dentist; sometimes that policy is implemented and sometimes there is a random method of access to doctors or dentists. As with other aspects of

---

Box 17.9   *Auditing the receptionist's skills*

- Telephone skills – the patient is welcomed
- The patient is invited to state his/her problem
- The receptionist identifies the nature of the appointment required
- The receptionist responds in a firm but friendly manner to suggestions and requests
- The receptionist is aware of the availability of the doctor/dentist concerned
- The appointment is agreed with the patient
- The appointment is recorded in the book
- The appointment time and day are checked with the patient
- General impressions

---

audit, the first step is to agree criteria, procedures and if possible standards. On the basis of these items it is possible to audit access to the partners in the practice.

Workloads

Consultation rates and frequency of domiciliary visits vary between and within practices. It is relatively easy to extract from the appointment book the workloads of the doctors and dentists. A similar exercise is worth conducting on workloads of all members of the primary care team to establish pressure and log jams and to determine whether some changes in procedure are required. Workloads are a sensitive issue, so in carrying out such an audit one should inform the people involved of the purposes of the audit otherwise they will see the whole enterprise as a method of getting them to do more than they are able to do.

Personnel care

This category refers to all members of a primary care team. The quality of a practice is a function of the organisation and ethos of the practice and the well-being and commitment of the staff. A major neglected function of audit is to identify ways of improving the quality of the working lives of the members of the practice. Some of these ways are linked directly to changes in organisation and management style and some are associated with educational and training needs. Regular, well-organised meetings help the members of the team to keep in touch with each other and with the policy and procedures of the practice.

As well as questionnaires, one can initiate structured development interviews sometimes known as appraisal interviews or discussions. These may be between partners and staff. Most staff probably prefer development interviews with the partners or a senior partner. The purpose of the developmental interviews is to provide positive feedback, to help the interviewee to assess his or her strengths and weaknesses and to plan targets for the future, and to provide the partner with an opportunity to discuss ways of improving the organisation of the practice.

Critical incidents

So far, we have focused upon the use of guidelines, procedures and checklists to audit the on-going functions of practice management. It is also important for a practice to learn from the unexpected. Paradoxically, a procedure for learning from the unexpected may be required. Some examples of critical incidents that themselves require specific procedures are:

1. Dealing with a violent patient
2. The collapse of a patient in the surgery
3. Dealing with accidental exposure to ionising radiation following X-ray machine malfunction
4. Dealing with mercury spillage

Questions which one might ask are:

1. Did the procedure work?
2. How could it be improved?
3. What were the weaknesses?

'Near misses' and 'What if's' are also worth discussing. The discussions may yield changes in procedure and perhaps a training need. However, one should be wary of developing complex rules and procedures that are cumbersome to implement. Such procedures are unlikely to be followed.

Getting started

We end this chapter with where you should begin: with getting started on audit.

Audit is, initially, a threatening process. Many of the points outlined in earlier sections of this chapter are likely to emerge within a practice. So it is important to discuss openly with colleagues, the nature and purposes of audit in the practice. To do so you must have some plans and a willingness to accommodate other people's views. The following hints are based upon people's experience of audit and related processes.

1. *Have a practice seminar to discuss the nature and purpose of medical audit.* Provide opportunities for everyone to discuss problems and anxieties associated with the audit process. If possible, invite an outsider to lead the seminar. The person chosen may be a colleague from a practice that has successfully instituted audit or someone who is well versed in audit procedures and familiar with general practice. Insist that the leaders provide handouts, focus the discussion activities and allow some opportunities for open discussion. An example of a discussion activity is given Box 17.10.

Divide into groups of four. Each person should take on one of the following tasks – the anxieties, expectations, fears and problems of:

1. senior partner;
2. a receptionist;
3. a health visitor;
4. another partner or associate;
5. a practice nurse.

Choose a task that is different from your usual one in the practice. Make notes on what you think are likely to be hopes, fears, expectations and anxieties of a person in that role. Discuss the different perceptions of the different roles. This should be followed by a plenary discussion in which the participants pool and discuss their likely hopes, fears, expectations and anxieties.

2. *Carry out an audit on audit.* Use a simple structured questionnaire along the lines indicated above to obtain views on patient care and practice management. Invite suggestions on priorities to audit.

3. *Report back the findings of the questionnaire to all colleagues.* Indicate what actions are proposed.

4. *In the light of the questions and discussions, choose the first topic to audit.* Choose a topic that is relatively non-threatening, easy to audit, which will yield results quickly and lead to a change in practice organisation or patient care. Such a topic should, if possible, involve partners and other staff.

5. *Identify and agree criteria for conducting the audit.* The development of criteria is likely to lead to an agreed statement of standard eventually. Wherever possible keep the criteria simple, intelligible to everyone in the team and easy to use. Guidelines, checklists and rating schedules are useful

Box 17.10   *An example of focusing a discussion activity: personnel*

1. Appearance
   0 All personnel need attention to dress and grooming
   1 Some personnel need attention to dress and grooming
   2 All personnel neat and well groomed
   3 All personnel unusually neat and well groomed

2. Attitudes
   0 All staff unfriendly and unpleasant
   1 Some staff members unfriendly and unpleasant
   2 All staff friendly and pleasant
   3 Friendly and pleasant demeanour of all staff a conspicuous characteristic
     of the office

3. Continuing education – staff
   0 No member of full time staff participated in past year
   1 50% or less of staff members participated in past year
   2 Over 50% but not all staff members participated in past year
   3 All members of full time staff participated within the past year

4. Continuing education – dentist
   0 No continuing education in past year
   1 Less than 40 hours in the past year
   2 Forty to 80 hours in the past year
   3 Over 80 hours in the past year

5. Personnel management
   a. Staff meetings
      0 No staff meetings held
      1 Not scheduled but occasionally held
      2 Scheduled and usually held
      3 Weekly meetings held regularly

   b. In-service training – general
      0 No in-service training
      1 Materials available for employees' study
      2 Informal pursuit of training
      3 Formal organised training

for analysing records as well as for self assessment and direct observation.
If appropriate, repeat the audit after about three months to check what
improvements have occurred and report them to the group in a written
report.

6. *Provide a written report on the outcomes of the audit.* Have a practice
seminar on the audit in which the results are presented and discussed and

any changes in procedure that may be necessary are outlined. If things are working well within this topic then say so. Too often we neglect the positive aspects of performance of a practice team. Not all audits are appropriate for discussions at practice seminars, so use discretion in choosing what will be discussed in open forum in the practice and what is for the benefit of those involved in the audit.

7. *Invite sub-groups of the practice team to choose and work upon a topic so that they own it, and the method of auditing.* Provide some guidance on criteria, standards and checklists, but encourage them to develop the audit procedure and to organise a practice seminar if that is appropriate.

8. *Do not be over ambitious.* General practice is a myriad of activities and tasks. So after the initial phase of audit, establish priorities, time and resource allocations for the purposes of audit. An effective audit can be expensive in professional time, so when planning ensure the work can be carried out if at all possible by other members of the practice team. The local Medical Audit Advisory Group (MAAG) is available to give assistance as well as ensuring that all medical practices undertake regular and systematic audits.

9. *Remember that the process of auditing always involves personal relationships and feelings.* What may seem non-threatening to you may be threatening to the person involved in the audit. How you present the outcome of an audit is often as important as the outcome itself.

10. *Remember too that the primary purpose of audit within a practice is to help people to do their jobs and to improve the provision of health care. Good Luck!*

References
1. Marinker, M. (1990). *Medical Audit in General Practice*, p. 7. London: MSD/British Medical Journal.
2. *Working for Patients – Postgraduate and Continuing Medical and Dental Education* (1991). London: HMSO.
3. *Working for Patients, Working Paper No. 6: Medical Audit* (1989). London: HMSO.
4. Marinker, M. (ed.) (1990). *Medical Audit in General Practice*. London: MSD/British Medical Journal.
5. Pendlebury, M. E. (1990). *A Dental Practice Assessment System*. University of Nottingham.
6. Royal College of General Practitioners (1985). *What Sort of Doctor?* London.
7. Faculty of General Dental Practitioners (1992). *Clinical Audit: A Workbook.* London: The Royal College of Surgeons of England.
8. Roland, M. (1988). General practitioners referral rates: interpretation is difficult. *British Medical Journal*, **297**, 437–438.

9. Dental Practice Board, Eastbourne (1990). *Annual Report* (1988–1989).
10. Donabedian, A. (1980). *Exploration in Quality Assessment and Monitoring*, vol. 1. Ann Arbor: Health Administration Press.
11. Anderson, C. M., Chambers, S., Clamp, M., Dunn, I. A., McGhee, M. F., Sumner, K. R. & Wood, A. M. (1988). Can audit improve patient care? Effects of studying use of diagnosis in General Practice. *British Medical Journal*, **297**, 113–114.
12. Irvine, D. (1972). *Teaching Practices*, Report 15. London: Royal College of General Practitioners.
13. Kessner, D. M., Kalk, C.E &, Singer, J. (1977). Assessing health quality – the case for tracers. *New England Journal of Medicine*, **288**, 189–194.
14. Best, G. A. (1983). Performance indicators: A precautionary tale for Unit General Managers. In: *Effective Unit Management*, Wickings, H. I. (ed.), King Edward's Hospital Fund.
15. Shaw, C. D. (1990). Criterion based audit. *British Medical Journal*, **300**, 649–651.
16. Trent Dental Vocational Training Practice Assessment (1991). University of Sheffield and Trent Regional Health Authority.
17. Balint, M. (1957). *The Doctor, the Patient and the Illness*. London: Tavistock Press.
18. Pendlebury, M. E. & Brown, G. A. (1988). *The Use of Video in Dental Vocational Training*. University of Nottingham.
19. Brown, G. A. (1985). How to use and make videos in teaching. *Medical Teacher*, **7**, 83–87.
20. Buckley, G. (1990). Clinically significant events. In: *Medical Audit in General Practice*, pp. 120–143, Marinker, M. (ed). London: MSD/British Medical Journal.
21. Newble, D. I. (1983). The critical incident technique: a new approach to the assessment of clinical performance. *Medical Education*, **16**, 401–430.
22. Cartwright, A. & Anderson, R. (1981). *General Practice Revisited*. London: Tavistock Press.
23. Abrams, C. M., Ayers, C. S. & Petterson, M. V. (1986). Quality assurance of dental restorations: A comparison by dentists and patients. *Community Dental Oral Epidemiology*, **14**, 317–319.
24. Freeman, J & Byrne, P. (1976). *Assessment of Postgraduate Training in General Practice*, 2nd edn. Society for Research in Higher Education, Guildford.
25. Hunter, H. (1975). PEGS: Performance evaluation guides. In: *An Instructional Information Exchange for Dentistry in the United States*, vol. 6. *Observation and Measurement of Clinical Performance*, MacKenzie, R. S. & Harrop, R. J. (eds.). US Department of Health, Education and Welfare, Washington.
26. Pendleton, D., Schofield, J., Tate, P. & Havelock, P. (1984). *The Consultation: An Approach to Learning and Teaching*. Oxford: Oxford University Press.

18

Clinical audit in psychiatry. Models for audit in mental health

JOHN K. WING

Introduction

In general, the aims, principles and methods of audit are the same in psychiatry as in any other branch of medicine. They have been dealt with in detail in other chapters. But each specialty has its own particular profile and this chapter is mainly concerned with the problems for audit that arise when identifying and treating disorders that affect the mind as charac-

---

Box 18.1 *The range of mental disorders: International Classification of Diseases, 10th revision*

Examples from Chapter F: 'Mental and behavioural disorders, including disorders of psychological development'.

F0. Organic mental disorders, e.g. F00–F03 dementias
F1. Mental disorders due to use of psychoactive substances, e.g. F10 Alcohol, F11 Opioids
F2. Psychoses, e.g. F20 schizophrenias
F3. Affective disorders, e.g. F30 manic episodes
F4. Neurotic, stress-related and somatoform disorders, e.g. F40 phobic anxiety disorders
F5. Behavioural syndromes associated with physiological disturbances and physical factors, e.g. F50 eating disorders
F6. Disorders of adult personality and behaviour, e.g. F60 specific personality disorders
F7. Mental retardation
F8. Disorders of psychological development, e.g. F80 disorders of development of speech and language
F9. Disorders with an onset in childhood

---

teristically as, or more characteristically than, they do the body. It is also focused on the more severe and persistent disorders of adult life that are likely to be referred for specialist advice and treatment. Three factors are of particular importance.

Diagnosis

The first characteristic is that, in the absence of an abundance of precise physical indicators of disease and disability, the clinical material for diagnosis (the symptoms and signs) is derived in large part by using traditional clinical methods – taking the history, examining the 'mental state', and observing behaviour. Except when there is profound cognitive impairment (e.g. in dementia or mental handicap), much reliance has to be placed on the patient's own description of abnormal internal experiences. The underlying mental dysfunctions or impairments[1] are 'invisible' and thus can easily be ignored or denied altogether. Moreover, many of the neuropsychological mechanisms affected are closely associated with perception, arousal, mood, movement and intention, and therefore act to mediate between brain and social environment. The problem of accurate measurement of clinical phenomena becomes, in consequence, even more crucial than elsewhere in medicine.[2]

Box 18.1 lists the main categories of disorder specified in Chapter F of the tenth edition of the *International Classification of Diseases* (ICD10, 1991), shortly to be finalised by the World Health Organization (WHO). Each two-character group (F0, F1, etc.) contains disorders that may be expressed as mild to extremely severe forms, and may be transitory, recurrent or persistent. Apart from dementia, most occur during the productive years of life.

Diagnosis, though important, does not play as specific a role as in, say, neurology. As will become apparent below, some of the problems of classification faced by general practitioners are familiar to psychiatrists. Techniques such as the Read codes are fully applicable but diagnosis-related groups are not.

Disability

The second factor is clinical course. Although there is a good rate of recovery or remission in most disorders, most can also be persistent or frequently relapsing. In disorders such as schizophrenia, it is not uncommon for dysfunctions such as psychomotor slowness, thought disorder, or lack of volition, to be manifested as personality traits or changes preceding acute onset, and to persist between episodes of more

---

Box 18.2   *Conceptual levels for planning services for people with a mental illness or mental disorder*

The aim of health services is to minimise social disablement associated with mental illness and mental disability. A rational health information system should collect information at the following levels:

1. Causes of social disablement:
   Physical and psychological symptoms and impairments.
   Social disadvantages.
   Adverse self-attitudes – demoralisation.

2. Methods of preventing or minimising the causes of disablement, including treatment, rehabilitation, resettlement and care (process).

3. Service settings and service agents to identify disablement, assess causes and take action (structure).

4. Is social disablement associated with mental illness and mental disability minimised by intervention? (outcome).

---

florid symptoms such as hallucinations and delusions. In some varieties of the disorder the problem is probably developmental and the clinical course runs over the whole of a lifetime.

Some of the clinical phenomena are therefore better conceptualised as impairments or disabilities than as symptoms or signs. This problem is not, of course, peculiar to psychiatric disorders. An audit of long-term treatment for chronic schizophrenia would share some of the features of an audit of care in severe diabetes mellitus or osteoarthritis. However, the 'invisibility' of the dysfunctions, and the effect they have on psychosocial functioning and on others in the social environment, lead to features that are particularly evident in psychiatric practice. In fact, the very lack (so far) of physical indicators may have led to advances in understanding techniques of measurement, both of impairment and of relevant environmental factors, that might be adaptable for use more generally throughout medicine.

Social disablement

The first two factors, disease and disability, interact to produce disorders that have a substantial social component (see Box 18.2). Social disadvantage and social stress factors can precipitate onset or relapse, and maintain or amplify the primary dysfunctions. Self-attitudes are even more likely to be adversely affected when the disorder is within the mind than when it is somatic. Thus people who experience hallucinations are vulnerable to other mental disorders, such as depression and anxiety, as well. The social disapproval usually attached to such symptoms, and the accompanying disabilities, further increases a sense of demoralisation.

Social disablement is an amalgam of all these factors acting together. The term expresses the extent to which an individual is unable to meet personal or social expectations of performance in various fields of action and responsibility, with a consequent loss of independence. The aim of assessment, treatment, care and prevention (primary, secondary and tertiary) is to reduce social disablement to the minimum.

Quality of life is placed on the other side of the same coin as social disablement. In so far as impairments, social disadvantages and self-attitudes allow, an individual's quality of life depends, first of all, on the basic physical necessities being met, and then on the social and occupational opportunities available to exercise his or her talents and interests. If impairments to health hinder a person from making use of unimpaired talents, 'enabling' interventions are required so that these potentials can be realised. These are eminently measurable aspects of care and should therefore be matters for routine audit.

Service implications

With the exception of those who have accumulated from the past in long-stay wards, most people with mental disorders are treated in community settings most of the time. Very few treatments in themselves require an in-patient setting for their application. Admission to hospital is mainly required because of socially dangerous or embarrassing behaviour, the risk of self-harm or a need for skilled supervision that could not be given in any other setting. However, in the absence of a wide range of community alternatives where psychiatric help can be provided, the hospital ward must act as a place of shelter and protection while treatment is being given and the early stages of rehabilitation are established.

The switch from large single specialty hospitals to small psychiatric day and in-patient departments in district general hospitals, backing up what should be a broad range of community services, has emphasised the problems of mismatch, which are likely to continue to affect clinical practice for a decade to come. The problem for audit is that, as the larger hospitals run down, there is no universally accepted set of rules for setting up a structure of appropriately staffed replacement services. The problems of disease and disability do not disappear and it is in the nature of much psychiatric disorder that it can present in either mode, sequentially or simultaneously.

There is no satisfactory method of categorisation into those who need health care and those who need social care. Both types of expertise are required. But Health Authorities are charged with the responsibility of providing 'health care' to people for whom social services departments, with very different philosophies, resources and priorities, are providing 'social care', and vice versa. The House of Commons Social Services Committee's report on community care (1990) records evidence from the Royal College of Nursing that illustrates the problem. Reference was made to the absurdity of the distinction between a 'health' bath and a 'social' bath, which depends not on the reason for needing help but on what kind of professional provides it.

Part of the responsibility for care is shared with general practitioners, community psychiatric nurses, social workers and other professionals involved in day and residential centres and in domiciliary visiting. A significant portion of medical and nursing work therefore involves visiting settings that are not part of on-site hospital services at all and can be altogether outside the remit of the District Health Authority.

These are matters that public health physicians have to understand because service planning and purchasing must take account of them. General practitioners, with their very broad spectrum of care, and those involved with the care of people with long-term physical disabilities, also cannot evade the problems that arise. Psychiatrists, willy-nilly, work at the heart of this complexity at a time when many large mental hospitals are closing or moribund and responsibility for community alternatives is precariously and ambiguously divided between agencies that sometimes seem to be competing rather than co-operating.

All these complexities must be taken into account when considering the kind of health information it is desirable to collect, what service structure for a particular district is desirable, and how to assign priorities for new initiatives, for example, in purchasing arrangements.

The implications for audit are crucial. It is pleasing to note that the broadly descriptive term 'clinical audit' is gradually being adopted, in place of 'medical audit'. The new usage signifies that results have to be judged by measuring outcome in terms of the reduction of social disablement, not just by the reduction of physical disability, and not simply by the collection of administrative performance indicators. Because this entails a consideration of social disadvantage and adverse self and social attitudes to disability, this has the added attraction of ensuring that quality of life is added to quality of care as one of the central concerns of audit.

A strategy for audit in mental health

The audit strategy of the Royal College of Psychiatrists is aimed, in the longer term, at improving the quality of patient care through the scrutiny of routinely collected information about clinical work and services, and ongoing peer review (both of routine practice and of adverse events) and educational activities, which eventually become part of ordinary clinical practice and provide clinicians as well as managers with information relevant to administration and planning.

More specifically, the college aims, with the help of a dedicated clinical audit section in the research unit, to achieve five objectives, which are set out in Box 18.3.

The basic components of care that have to be audited and, if necessary on the basis of the results, improved, now tend to be called, using general systems terminology, *structure*, *process* and *outcome*. Structure includes the budget, settings and care-providers. Process is the assessment, treatment, rehabilitation, training, counsel and welfare that the carers provide. Outcome (which may include part of the course) is the change, or lack of change, in degree of impairment and social disablement brought about by process. The elements cannot easily be separated from each other but they can be illustrated by considering in more detail the second, fourth and fifth of the aims shown in Box 18.3.

Agreed clinical standards: routine or research?

Peer review and clinical guidelines; two examples

As an example of peer review of 'adverse events' we may take suicide while the patient is in hospital or shortly after discharge. A mechanism is needed to identify all such events, including scrutiny of accidental and doubtful cases, for example by liaison with the local coroner. A review should be made in each case to try to discover whether local guidelines, and others derived from a search of the literature and consultation with recognised authorities, had been applied; whether any predictive features were missed; whether any preventive action could have been taken but was not; whether the services that could have been used in preventive action were actually available. The lessons learned should be specified and introduced into clinical practice.

This case-by-case approach may or may not improve care. One way to find out is to systematise the audits, record the specifics in a standard way, review a series of such events in order to derive some general principles, promulgate guidance, and then determine whether practice has changed.

Box 18.3 *Five aims for a college audit strategy*

1. A central literature and information base, and an advisory centre, for those who wish to undertake audit locally.

2. Agreed clinical standards in some areas of particular public or clinical concern, for example because of high social or financial costs or a high public profile, or because they are very common or particularly severe or chronic.

3. Recommendations concerning standards of clinical record keeping.

4. Guidelines on the minimum structure of services required by each sub-specialty, with advice on recognising the epidemiological characteristics of higher- and lower-need districts.

5. Methods of registering data that are both user-friendly and relevant to monitoring the quality of care in a local district.

Box 18.4 *The cycle of audit and research*
(Experience at each of the following steps can inform those following until the cycle starts again)

Peer review:
'Adverse events', e.g. suicide while in hospital.
Selected topics, e.g. ECT, long-term depot medication, use of the Mental Health Act.
Random selection of cases might indicate problems of clinical management, failure to implement discharge plans, etc.

Systematisation of guidelines for selected areas of practice

Standard recording of clinical practice in chosen areas

Periodic review to discover:
Are guidelines followed?
If not, why not?

Do the guidelines actually lead to better clinical outcomes? More sophisticated experimental designs are needed in order to answer this question. The results, in turn, will inform peer review.

This kind of progressive audit may produce a local 'state of the art' standard of practice and, if repeated elsewhere, lead towards a wider consensus. It could speed up the traditional clinical process of training and clinical appraisal. But in order to address the crunch point of audit, which is not just to assess process but to discover whether outcomes are improved, rather more sophisticated designs and methods are required. In the case of suicide, of course, there is an obvious outcome, but there are problems of definition and of calculating comparative rates.

Audit of this hands-on, peer review, kind is part of 'bottom-up' research, which has substantial potential for application in specialties such as psychiatry. It speeds up the process of collecting systematic and comprehensive clinical information relevant to a particular topic. The next step is to design studies that allow comparison of outcome in groups of patients with and without selected characteristics thought to predict attempts at suicide, and in groups with the characteristics who are or are not provided with prophylactic care. In these ways audit becomes an integral part of the spectrum of clinical research as well as clinical practice (see Box 18.4).

Another topical example is ECT. Over ten years ago, the college commissioned a report on how ECT was being administered in clinics throughout the country. A detailed and critical report resulted,[3] on the basis of which a document of guidance was published.[4] A further audit was carried out in early 1991, which showed that the criticisms still applied. This time the college has acted swiftly, promulgated guidelines, set up training courses, appointed responsible clinicians in each district and inserted a question into the membership examination. A follow-up audit will assess outcomes.

Other topics for the audit-research approach

Authoritative guidelines exist in several other areas of clinical psychiatric practice. This is not to say that they must be followed. Indeed the audit-research approach may suggest that they should be scrapped or radically changed. But they provide a clinical starting point. Guidelines include those on the most effective and economic use of short-term hospital care; the assessment and prescription of health and social care for vulnerable people after discharge from hospital;[5] the best documented practice in prescribing medication as part of the long-term care of people with schizophrenia or bipolar disorders; the use of alcohol and dependence-producing drugs; and the use of the Mental Health Act.

The college research unit is interested in pursuing all these topics, the first two of which will be discussed in outline below. Other important themes are: psychiatric care for people with a mental handicap; the care of mentally disabled people who are homeless, information booklets of practical use to patients and carers; the construction of guidelines for effective interprofessional working. Specialist sections of the college are working on equivalent themes in areas such as psychogeriatrics, child psychiatry, forensic psychiatry, liaison psychiatry, mental handicap and alcohol and drug use.

The provision of a comprehensive community care structure

Epidemiology of hospital bed use

The most costly element in the provision of district psychiatric services is in-patient care. Since 1954, the number of hospital residents per 100 000 of the general population has been steadily declining. The decline has been most noticeable in the very-long-stay (over five years) group, but for many years this has been due mainly to deaths rather than to discharges. The medium-long-stay (one to five years) rate has been fairly constant at just under 40 per 100 000, and the short-stay rate similarly stable at about 60 per 100 000.

A comparative study of data from eight cumulative psychiatric case registers[6] showed that one of the most striking differences between the districts was the change in population size over time. Figure 18.1 shows that Oxford, for example, doubled its population between 1921 and 1981 and Worcester was close behind. Middle-sized industrial cities such as Cardiff, Nottingham and Southampton stayed more or less at the national average, while conurban areas such as Salford declined and the population of Camberwell in south-east London was cut by half.

This differential change in population dynamics was reflected in socioeconomic census indicators. One of these, much in use recently, is the Jarman eight-item index of deprivation,[7] also shown in Figure 18.1. The correlation between it and long-stay 'recruitment' rates in the register areas (1–2 years in hospital, age under 65) was 0.76.

It is possible to estimate from statistical trends in bed occupancy what the capacity of future accommodation for people with high-dependency needs might be. One forecast for 1991 (omitting those with a diagnosis of dementia and assuming no major change in need status) was that there would be just over 50 short-stay and 50 longer-stay residents per 100 000 national population.[8] Large old hospitals with barrack-like accommodation are not the ideal settings for care. Better housing, more conveniently situated, is needed, while retaining the virtues of open space for privacy and recreation.[9]

The estimate of the numbers likely to need high-dependency accommodation is realistic, even on the low side, but the form it should take requires imagination, based on understanding of the disabilities that create

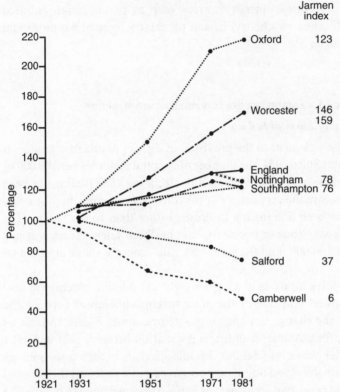

Fig. 18.1. The population of psychiatric register areas, Census 1981, as a proportion of 1921 (= 100%).

the need. In addition, the estimate is for a national average. The epidemiological characteristics of each district must be taken into account, otherwise many will be underprovided. These key questions for audit cannot be answered by examining the Körner data set. Psychiatric services are not unique in requiring a broader health information system.

Hospital closure

There are three instances where rundown to closure of a large mental hospital has been accompanied by what would now be called an audit. The first was Powick in Worcester;[10,11] the second, Darenth Park Hospital for people with a mental handicap;[12] and the third, Friern and Claybury Hospitals in the North East Thames Region, which are planned for closure. Worcester was a model because of the very gradual process of rundown coupled with the injection of substantial central funds. It was a

'Rolls Royce' experiment, difficult to replicate in districts that are more deprived and without external financial support. The final Darenth reports have not yet been published but the interim results showed no dramatic changes in the handicaps, behaviour or skills of residents, either in those who left or in those who stayed. Costs were higher in the community.[13] There was a strong impression that the major factor determining outcome was the pattern of disabilities present initially. The Friern/Claybury study is still in its early stages, during which the less handicapped are the first to leave and the balance of costs appears to be favourable.

Minimum structure for community care

Far more important, in the longer term, than the outcome for people who have accumulated as 'very-long-stay' residents in the large hospitals is the 'new' accumulation that still continues, in spite of the constraints imposed by tight admission policies. Underlying this is the problem of what pattern of community health and social services would be appropriate for the task of caring for severely mentally ill people when the large hospitals have disappeared. Most such people spend most of their time outside hospital.

At the moment, the information that would allow rational decisions to be made is not available. It is not provided by the Körner minimum data set. A list of the elements that should be considered, in every district, when reviewing general and sub-specialty needs in psychiatry, has been provided by Jenkins (unpublished).[14] This useful list is not prescriptive but it lays out a structure that can be used as part of the audit process in every district.

The next section contains a brief description of an exercise that may lead to the development of methods of data capture usable in ordinary clinical practice (thus providing clinicians with the power that information brings with it) and to results that could be used to put flesh on the structural bones in several districts with distinctive socioeconomic characteristics.

An audit of admissions to hospital

The college research unit is engaged in developing techniques for studying one of the audit problems of highest priority for psychiatry: how to combine the most effective use of scarce short-stay hospital places with adequate long-term community support for those who need it.

The reasons for the admission of two series of patients admitted during a three-month period to contrasting inner London health districts, with similar socioeconomic structure but different service patterns, have been assessed. The research instrument, which has already been piloted, contains sections on the social and clinical problems causing admission, the facilities and actions that might have been used to prevent admission if they had been available, anticipated vulnerability to readmission, and discharge plans. This last section is expanded from college guidance for good practice.[5] The results are currently being analysed.

The data will be analysed in conjunction with a structural and a sociodemographic profile for each district. Data are entered directly to a laptop computer file, and can be processed at once according to a predetermined programme, to yield individual summaries, group tables and rates. The results will be of immediate interest to clinicians, managers and directors of public health. They will show what the local problems are, what structure is available to cope with them in the period leading to admission, what care processes are required, and what vulnerabilities remain at the time of discharge. These facts can be compared with those of contrasting districts.

The research experience can also be used to simplify the technique and apply it to other areas of practice. It can then be used on a wider scale to generate health information of good quality. Another advantage is that the exercise will provide a sampling frame for the one year follow-up needs assessment study described below, including all patients thought to be vulnerable and a sample of the rest.

Techniques for measuring outcomes

The principles of need measurement

A concept central to audit, which covers all three of its elements, is that of need. It provides the link between problem assessment, care and service prescription, and the measurement of outcome. In effect, identifying a problem (say a symptom or impairment or social handicap) means specifying a potential need for one or more forms of treatment, care or welfare intervention that will remove or mitigate the problem or prevent it getting worse. 'State of the art' guidelines (ideally based on well-designed trials plus professional consensus) are used to determine the 'processes' required. This prompts a need for one or more caring agents and for settings in which the care can be given, i.e. it prompts a need for services. Matching need against provision provides a measure of unmet and met need. Re-assessment after a period of time allows the monitoring of outcome and the cycle begins again. If done systematically over a period of time, choosing target problems with high priority, information of great sensitivity, focused on important planning problems, can be collected. A simpler system derived from this cumulated experience could be incorporated into routine health information systems. Costs can be calculated for any innovations that appear indicated.

A needs assessment system designed originally for long-term attenders at day hospitals and centres[2,15,16,17] has been constructed according to these principles and is now being adapted for a wide variety of applications.

Description and classification of psychiatric symptoms

Instruments for measuring and classifying abnormal mental and behavioural phenomena have become technically sophisticated during the past 40 years. A system known as *SCAN* (*schedules for clinical assessment in neuropsychiatry*) has been developed in association with chapter F of the tenth revision of the *International Classification of Diseases* (ICD10). SCAN incorporates the tenth edition of the *Present State Examination* (PSE10) and provides descriptive profiles and scores, classification according to the rule-based criteria incorporated in ICD10 and the current American system, an account of the clinical course, and a narrative print-out. A short version will also be available.[18]

There are many simpler tools, such as the general health questionnaire, which has been widely used in general practice.[19] More recently, an instrument that can be used by lay interviewers after training has been used in large-scale population surveys in the USA.[20] This has been superseded in turn by the combined international diagnostic interview (CIDI), also for lay interviewers, which will provide a classification according to ICD10.[21]

Mental health information systems

For many years information concerning patients admitted to psychiatric hospitals was collected on the mental health enquiry (MHE) form. The material was not comprehensive, and not necessarily always accurate, but it was simple to collect and provided a useful and continuous flow of statistical data concerning the changes taking place. The Körner review of health service information[22] was told that the MHE was to be terminated for reasons of economy and asked to replace it, specifically by adding items to describe and help plan for the psychiatric services. But the Körner data set is clearly intended for acute medicine and surgery and is not adequate as a basis for financial decisions concerning the community psychiatric services. In fact there are deficiencies from any point of view. They amount to limited scope, poor quality, difficult linking and neglect of attention to outcome.

Modern mental health systems depend on domiciliary visiting by psychiatrists and nurses, close liaison with general practitioners, for example, in clinics based in health centres, reliance on clinical psychologists and social workers to carry out part of the care, the use of several kinds of day hospital and day centre (the latter often provided by voluntary organisations) and a range of non-NHS residential units, and intensive family care.[23]

Several attempts are being made in different parts of the country to set up mental health information systems that will cope with demands for planning data, including the complete spectrum of community psychiatric services, and that will be able to adapt as further innovations are introduced. So far there is no front runner, but there are several promising systems.[24]

Conclusions

The principles of audit as applied in the practice of psychiatry are basically similar to those applied across medicine as a whole. The audit of routine clinical care and of adverse events, in particular, share features that are familiar in all branches.

However, three interacting factors necessitate an approach to the audit of mental health services that has some special features. First, the lack of physical indices of the presence and severity of disease and disability means that more emphasis must be placed on the reliability and accuracy with which symptoms and impairments are described and on the psychosocial factors that influence course and outcome. Secondly, the changeover from a system based on large mental hospitals is still continuing and the build-up of alternatives has been slower than the pace of rundown. Thirdly, since most people with mental disorders are treated 'in the community', since many non-NHS personnel and settings are involved, and since the NHS and Community Care Act proposals remain to be implemented, the necessity for collecting a sufficiently broad base of information for planning is evident.

Good progress has been made in particular districts but NHS information routinely collected (for example, the Körner data set) does not reflect the scope of responsibility of the psychiatric services. New initiatives are required.

Finally, audit activities cannot be separated from research, in psychiatry as in the rest of medicine.

References

1. World Health Organization (1980). *International Classification of Impairments, Disabilities and Handicaps*. Geneva: WHO.
2. Wing, J. K. (1990). Meeting the needs of people with psychiatric disorders. *Social Psychiatry and Psychiatric Epidemiology*, **25**, 2–8.
3. Pippard, J. & Ellam, L. (1981). *Electroconvulsive Treatment in Great Britain*. London: Gaskell.
4. Freeman, C., Crammer, J. L., Deakin, J. F. W., McClelland, Mann, S. & Pippard, J. (1989). *The Practical Administration of ECT*. London: Gaskell.
5. Royal College of Psychiatrists (1989). *Guidelines for Good Medical Practice in Discharge and Aftercare Procedures*. London: RCP.
6. Wing, J. K. (ed.) (1989). *Health Service Planning and Research. Contributions from Psychiatric Case Registers*. London: Gaskell.
7. Jarman, B. (1983). Identification of under-privileged areas. *British Medical Journal*, **286**, 1705–1709.
8. Robertson, G. (1981). The provision of inpatient facilities for the mentally ill. A paper to assist NHS planners. Unpublished. DHSS.
9. Wing, J. K. (1990). The functions of asylum. *British Journal of Psychiatry*, **157**, 822–827.
10. Hall, P. & Brockington, I. (eds) (1990). *The Closure of Powick*. London: Gaskell.
11. Wing, J. K. & Bennett, C. (1988). Long-term care in the Worcester Development Project. Unpublished report to DHSS.
12. Goldberg, D. & Huxley, P. (1980). *Mental Illness in the Community. The Pathway to Psychiatric Care*. London: Tavistock.
13. Knapp, M., Beecham, J., Dayson, D., Leff, J., Margolis, O., O'Driscoll, C. & Wills, W. (1990). The TAPS Project III. Predicting the community costs of closing psychiatric hospitals. *British Journal of Psychiatry*, **157**, 661–670.
14. Jenkins, R. (1991). Towards a system of outcome indicators for mental health care. In *Indicators for Mental Health in the Population*, ed. R. Jenkins & S. Griffiths, pp. 61–86. London: HMSO.
15. Brewin, C., Wing, J. K., Mangen, S., Brugha, T. S. & MacCarthy, B. (1987). Principles and practice of measuring needs in the long-term mentally ill. *Psychological Medicine*, **17**, 971–981.
16. Brewin, C. & Wing, J. K. (1988). *The MRC Needs for Care Assessment Manual*. MRC Social Psychiatry Unit.
17. Brugha, T. S., Wing, J. K., Brewin, C. R., MacCarthy, B., Mangen, S, Lesage, A. & Mumford, J. (1988). The problems of people in long-term psychiatric day care. An introduction to the Camberwell High Contact Survey. *Psychological Medicine*, **18**, 443–456.
18. Wing, J. K., Babor, T., Brugha, T., Burke, J., Cooper, J., Giel, R., Jablensky, A., Regier, D. & Sartorius N (1990). SCAN: Schedules for clinical assessment in neuropsychiatry. *Archives of General Psychiatry*, **47**, 589–593.
19. Goldberg, D. (1978). *Manual of the General Health Questionnaire*. Windsor: NFER.

20. Robins, L. N. & Regier, D. A. (eds) (1991). *Psychiatric Disorders in America.* New York: Free Press.
21. Robins, L. N., Wing, J. K., Wittchen, H-U., Helzer, J. E., Babor, T. F., Burke, J., Farmer, A., Jablensky, A., Pickens, R., Regier, D. A., Sartorius, N. & Towle, L. H. (1988). The Composite International Diagnostic Interview. An epidemiologic instrument suitable for use in conjunction with different diagnostic systems and in different cultures. *Archives of General Psychiatry*, **45**, 1069–1077.
22. Körner, E. (Chairman) (1982). *Report on the Collection and Use of Information About Hospital Clinical Activity in the National Health Service.* London: HMSO.
23. Cooper, J. (1989). Information for planning. Case registers and Körner. In *Health Service Planning and Research. Contributions from Psychiatric Case Registers*, ed. J. K.Wing, pp.115–120. London: Gaskell.
24. Wing, J. K. (1992). *Epidemiologically-based Needs Assessment. Mental Illness.* NHS Management Executive. London: HMSO.

19

Audit in anaesthesia

D. W. RIDDINGTON AND J. F. BION

Introduction

Audit in anaesthesia involves setting standards of anaesthetic practice, monitoring the application of those standards, measuring the outcome of care, identifying strengths and deficiencies, and implementing changes that improve clinical practice. The specialty of anaesthesia is valuable for audit research because in the UK anaesthetists are the most numerous of all hospital doctors, they have more direct patient-contact time concentrated into a relatively shorter period than other speciality, the care is usually provided at a one-to-one level or higher and anaesthetic responsibilities can be clearly defined.

In the United Kingdom, audit of anaesthetic practice occurs at a national and local level. At national level the College of Anaesthetists is responsible for formal examination of anaesthetists in training and for inspecting hospitals for postgraduate training and accreditation. College tutors are appointed in individual hospitals to provide a direct link with the college and to exercise an important pastoral role for the trainees. Together with the Association of Anaesthetists of Great Britain and Ireland, the college sets standards relating to the structure of anaesthetic departments and the work which they perform. While these standards do not carry legal weight, failure to meet a basic minimum level may result in hospital accreditation for junior training being withdrawn, a powerful stimulus for corrective action. Both bodies provide a wide range of courses for continuing education and have supported national reviews of anaesthetic practice.

At a local level, audit is largely the responsibility of departments and divisions of anaesthesia. Until recently this has generally taken the form of morbidity and mortality meetings and informal review of the progress of trainees. The publication of the Government's White Paper *Working for Patients* in 1989[1] has concentrated discussions on more formal methods of assessment of the process and outcome of anaesthetic care.

History of anaesthesia audit

Hospital quality assurance can be dated from the principles established for hospital practice in the United States by the American College of Surgeons, which published five minimum standards in 1924;[2] these were based on earlier work by Dr Ernest Codman of the Massachusetts General Hospital[3] and a survey of American hospitals by the American College of Surgeons in 1919.[2] The standards covered professional organisation, qualifications and competence. In addition they required monthly meetings to review clinical work, proper documentation of clinical care, and appropriately supervised laboratory support services. By 1952 this had evolved into a formal system of hospital accreditation between other colleges and associations within North America. There is now a joint commission on accreditation of hospitals which publishes a comprehensive manual of accreditation standards for the organisation and process of medical care,[4] enforced by limiting accreditation to a three-year period that is renewable only after on-site inspection. In the United Kingdom nationwide standards have been very slow to develop because, as Secker-Walker suggests,[5] the nationalisation of the health service probably encouraged the assumption that quality of care was uniformly high. It is also likely that the tradition of charitable health care that preceded the National Health Service, and the removal thereafter of a direct link between payment and service, has tended to minimise consumer criticism and direct what there is towards the Government and away from health service professionals.

The first UK study of mortality was the report of the committee on maternal morbidity and mortality, published in 1930 by the Ministry of Health with the collaboration of the (Royal) College of Obstetricians and Gynaecologists.[6] Since 1952 the report (The Confidential Enquiry into Maternal Deaths) has been published triennially. By involving obstetric anaesthetists, these reports have influenced subsequent anaesthetic audit research, incorporating the two key elements of confidentiality and peer review. The first specifically anaesthetic survey of mortality however, was that of Beecher and Todd[7] in the USA, who surveyed prospectively nearly 600 000 incidents of anaesthetic use over a five-year period. They examined all deaths occurring in surgical patients, and separated anaesthetic causes of mortality from those attributable to surgery. Anaesthesia could be identified as a factor contributing to death in 1:1560 procedures, and causative in 1:2680. It was not until the confidential enquiry into perioperative deaths (CEPOD) was published in 1987[8] that this standard of investigation was matched.

In the UK the Association of Anaesthetists has commissioned a number of studies of mortality related to anaesthesia.[9,10,11] The first, starting in 1949, collected 1000 voluntary reports of deaths occurring over five and a half years.[9] Although it drew attention to the problem of anaesthetic mortality the study was marred by lack of structure, absence of denominator data and the purely qualitative nature of the information collected. Nonetheless, the authors were able to state that 'in the great majority of reports there were departures from ideal practice'. This was followed by Dinnick in 1964[10] who reviewed a further 600 deaths. Again no denominator information was available, but the results of this second report confirmed the finding of the first, and went on to highlight the presence of important surgical factors in high-risk patients whose deaths had been attributed to anaesthesia. Poor physical health was also identified as an independent risk factor by Dripps *et al.*[12]

In 1977 the Association of Anaesthetists, funded by the Nuffield Provincial Hospitals Trust, initiated a study of anaesthetic deaths in Britain. The objectives were to establish a system of confidential and anonymous reporting, to determine current standards for future comparative analyses, to identify factors related to anaesthetic deaths and to improve standards. Surgical collaboration was unfortunately not obtained and this made it difficult to interpret the results, published in 1982 by Lunn and Mushin.[11,13] However, the authors went on to plan a second study, this time with the participation of the Association of Surgeons. This study became the Confidential Enquiry into Perioperative Deaths, which examined factors contributing to deaths within the first 30 days following surgery in the hospitals of three Regional Health Authorities. The report,[8] published in 1987, made ten recommendations concerning quality assurance, accountability, clinical decision making and organisational issues that had direct relevance to the standards of practice of anaesthetists and surgeons. This important collaborative study was welcomed by the profession and it was agreed that the work should be expanded to cover the whole country. The National Confidential Enquiry into Perioperative Deaths (NCEPOD) continues to examine cases, and published its first report in 1990.[14] The CEPOD initiative was presented as an exemplar in the recent government document entitled *The Quality of Medical Care.*[15]

The College of Anaesthetists established an audit committee in 1988, which was subsequently expanded to become the quality of practice committee. It first reported in late 1988 when it published a brief document giving guidance on audit to anaesthetic departments.[16] This was followed by a joint study with three medical defence organisations into the incidence of brain damage following cardiac arrest associated with anaesthesia.[17]

The current activities of the committee include studies of the neurological sequelae of epidural analgesia, critical incident reporting and the involvement of anaesthetists nationally in the training of paramedical personnel.[17]

Structure, process and outcome in anaesthesia

Structure

The structure of anaesthetic services refers to the type of clinical activities provided, the number of senior and junior medical staff, their organisation and work patterns, the level of funding, anaesthetic equipment, and secretarial and clerical support.

The basic organisational unit in the practice of anaesthesia is the Department of Anaesthetics, representing the first of the requirements set out by Codman[3] and others.[2] Changes to the management structure of the NHS have altered the names, but not necessarily the nature, of this unit; departments may now be called directorates, and chairmen directors, but the system still depends on individual commitment and integrity to ensure that professional standards are maintained. The purpose of the divisional system is to provide a forum for communication between departments of anaesthesia in different hospitals in a single health district and to formulate policies agreed by all members. Standards of practice can be discussed and implemented. The extent to which this process is successful will depend, as in all political systems, on the quality of the individual members and the departmental and divisional chairmen, whose duties have been described by the Association of Anaesthetists.[18] Maintaining the divisional system is of particular importance during the period of uncertainty surrounding the introduction of new management systems and the internal market for the NHS.

In practical terms the department or division is responsible for the following activities:

- Daily administration of the department
- Education and welfare of trainees
- Equipment provision and maintenance
- Managing postoperative recovery facilities

- Quality assurance activities: guidelines and protocols
- Planning services and resource management

Administration

Undergraduate curricula rarely prepare medical students adequately to cope with management issues, and postgraduate management courses are variable in quality. This is unfortunate, because the success of any organisation depends both on the way it is run as well as the quality of the individuals within it. The chairman or director of anaesthetic services is, *de facto*, a manager and he or she should delegate to other consultants some of the activities listed above.

In each hospital there should be a consultant responsible for the daily administration of the department and theatre lists, with authority to resolve political difficulties should these arise. The trainees' on-call rota should be drawn up by a senior registrar at least two weeks in advance; the senior registrar should also allocate trainees to theatre lists, preferably under the supervision of the college tutor. Trainees' hours of work are currently under review.[19] There is a fine balance to be drawn between the needs of the service and the requirement for training. Juniors need to be exposed to sufficient numbers of emergency cases to fulfil training requirements, but excessive fatigue should be avoided. This applies equally well to consultants whose work schedules generally do not contain an allowance for recuperation. However, few fatalities in either the CEPOD report[8] or the work by Lunn and Mushin[11] could be attributed to fatigue.

Poor organisation was identified by Cooper *et al.* in 1984[20] as an important factor contributing to anaesthesia-related critical incidents and morbidity. Of 70 such incidents there were 21 in which 'a lack of structure, teamwork or general planning was evident, resulting in contributory haste, disarray, confusion etc.'. Such incidents may reflect on poor training, but they are also features of poorly administered and directed departments.

Education and welfare of trainees

Continuing postgraduate education underpins quality of care. It is the responsibility of the college tutor to ensure that the teaching given to trainees is tailored to their needs, that the number of accompanied sessions is adequate, and that study leave opportunities are taken, and are of benefit.[21] All departments should have regular weekly clinical meetings attended by all consultants and trainees, and clinical work should be organised in such a way that this is possible. This is best achieved by surgeons and anaesthetists holding their meetings at the same time; this would also allow the establishment of joint audit meetings between the two disciplines. The college tutor is an appropriate individual to co-ordinate such meetings and to monitor their educational value. An attendance record should be maintained. The proportion of consultants who attend could be regarded as a crude index of departmental quality and corporate spirit.

The progress of trainees should be reviewed systematically. Their clinical experience must be documented, preferably using the log-book recommended by the college.[16] The ratio of supervised to unsupervised operating lists is of importance, as is the type of work undertaken.[21] Trainees need to know what is expected of them and should have a designated – and available – senior colleague to call on when they need help. Theatre work should be matched to their clinical skills and not dictated by service requirements. In Cooper's study referred to above,[20] lack of appropriate knowledge, skills, or a general lack of experience could be implicated in 38 critical incidents.

Equipment

The failure of anaesthetic equipment plays a smaller part in anaesthetic-related critical incidents than does human error.[22,23] Nonetheless the work of Cooper in 1978[24] determined that human error, which is frequently the cause of both anaesthetic mortality and critical incidents, is often related to failure to use anaesthetic equipment correctly. In Cooper's study of 359 preventable incidents, 293 were attributable to human error, and of these 56 were due to errors primarily involving interactions with the anaesthetic machine. This led Cooper et al. to suggest[20] that one way of preventing these problems would be to improve the interface between operator and equipment. In part, this means developing a rational equipment procurement programme. Equipment must be uniform and safe in design, but there should be sufficient diversity for trainees to become familiar with a range of apparatus. There must be a comprehensive programme for training all staff in the use of equipment. In the next ten years improvements can be expected in information display and processing, artifact detection and alarms.

The constraints of budget, capital charging and depreciation have to be considered, with particular emphasis on the various types of service contracts available. Capital charging in the NHS involves a levy of 6% per annum payable quarterly, on all equipment owned by the directorate. The charge is based on standard valuations of the equipment, not the actual sum paid. This makes leasing arrangements very much more attractive, the costs of which will need to be incorporated in the directorate's pricing structure.

Management of recovery facilities

The CEPOD report recommends[8] that a fully equipped and staffed recovery area should form an integral part of operating theatre facilities and the service should be available at all times. The Association of Anaesthetists published guidelines in 1985[25] for those wishing to improve the recovery facilities in their hospital, providing guidance on basic recovery facilities, availability and the training of recovery nurses. The commitment of the anaesthetic department to the recovery room is important for quality control, both for the benefits that good recovery facilities bring to patient care[26] and because of the opportunities presented for training and research during the postoperative period. The absence of adequate postoperative recovery facilities is indefensible, particularly in view of the seriousness of many postoperative complications.[27]

Guidelines and protocols

Departments should ensure that there are clear guidelines for dealing with uncommon but high-risk clinical problems, such as failed intubation or malignant hyperthermia. Clear policies, preferably displayed as wall-charts, will help anaesthetists to manage complex and deteriorating situations in a structured and organised manner;[22] the Resuscitation Council's algorithm for advanced life-support is a good example.[28] It is the duty of all anaesthetists to be familiar with such protocols. Preoperative testing of anaesthetic equipment ('pre-flight checks') should also be standardised and protocol-guided.[23,29] Despite the fact that equipment failure is seldom wholly responsible for critical incidents[24] there have been serious accidents involving anaesthetic equipment that could have been avoided by appropriate preoperative testing.[9,30] This approach has been recommended for the prevention of critical incidents[20] and in the UK the Association of Anaesthetists has produced a specimen checklist for the anaesthetic machine, its vaporisers, breathing systems and the ventilator.[31] It is the responsibility of the anaesthetic department to ensure that such protocols are available and recommended standards observed.

Process

Analysis of the process of care should have well-defined aims, and should attempt to answer specific questions. As described in the chapter on intensive care audit, analysis of process requires the prior development of standards as comparators. Standards of anaesthetic practice should be developed for the following areas:

- Preoperative visiting and risk assessment
- Supervision and assistance
- Anaesthetic technique
- Monitoring
- Critical incidents
- Postoperative care

Preoperative visiting and risk assessment

Preoperative assessment and preparation of patients takes time, and for emergency cases this is sometimes compromised by a haste to operate, as the CEPOD report has identified. Cooper found that in eight of 70 critical incidents, incomplete preoperative assessment was a contributory factor.[20] Preoperative visits are important not only for the anaesthetist to assess patients and risk factors, but for the psychological reassurance derived by the patient from the consultation.[32] The effect is not the same if the assessment is made in the anaesthetic room just before induction of anaesthesia. Consultant contracts specifically allow time for preoperative assessment[33] and this is an opportunity for them to teach trainees at the bedside, a requirement for general professional training.[34]

Preoperative visits should start by ensuring that the patient has been scheduled for the right operation and that he or she understands the nature of what is involved and has consented to the procedure. The assessment of anaesthetic and surgical risk is fundamentally important. In addition to performing a general medical assessment, the anaesthetist should develop a checklist, based first on specifically anaesthetic-related matters (previous anaesthetics, family history, drug-allergies or sensitisation, airway), followed by careful assessment of organ-system function and reserve. This should concentrate particularly on the cardiac, respiratory and renal systems. Physiological reserve is often difficult to assess from the history alone and objective quantification is usually needed. Most risk factors can be reduced to the common denominator of impaired tissue oxygen delivery and the anaesthetist should look for ways of maximising delivery while minimising oxygen demand. Day-case surgery places constraints on the extent of anaesthetic assessment, and clear written guidelines must be formulated with the surgeons covering selection and exclusion of patients, the preoperative investigations required, and an 'information pack' for the patients.[35]

Methods of quantifying risk have tended to concentrate on the cardiovascular and respiratory systems. The only general method employed as a routine is the American Society of Anesthesiologists' (ASA) classification[12] (Box 19.1), though there is considerable variability in assessments made by different anaesthetists using this system.[36] The absence of a general objective measure of risk is a consequence of several factors. These are the low incidence of serious complications following anaesthesia, the difficulty of linking anaesthetic-related adverse events to the patient's pre-anaesthetic health status and the difficulty of separating anaesthetic from surgical effects on outcome. Stepwise discriminant analysis and logistic regression have been employed to quantify risk in high-risk populations.[37-40] The main factors are listed in Box 19.2. A good review of this subject can be found in Ross and Tinker.[41]

Supervision and assistance

The CEPOD report stated in its conclusions that 'There were a number of deaths in which junior (surgeons or) anaesthetists did not seek the advice of their consultants or senior registrars at any time before, during or after the operations'.[8] Anaesthetic departments must have clear guidelines defining the expected level of responsibility for each grade of trainee. All patients should be assessed both for ASA grade and urgency of procedure (emergency, urgent, scheduled, or elective as in CEPOD), and the grading should be a mandatory part of the anaesthetic form. Patients graded ASA III–V should automatically trigger consultation by the anaesthetic trainee with the duty senior registrar or consultant.

The anaesthetic operating department assistant (ODA) or nurse is one of the most important facilitators of quality of anaesthetic care in the UK. Their responsibilities are to prepare equipment for anaesthesia, to assist the anaesthetist in the conduct of the anaesthetic and to maintain supplies of drugs and disposables. The level of organisation of individual ODAs will influence theatre efficiency, particularly for busy operating lists. Experienced ODAs can contribute significantly to the safety of emergency anaesthesia given by junior trainees. They also have a useful role in cardiac arrest teams, and in intensive care units.

Box 19.1   *ASA classification of physical state*

I   Healthy patient
II   Mild systemic disease, no functional limitations
III   Severe systemic diseases with functional limitations
IV   Severe systemic disease which threatens survival
V   Moribund, not expected to survive 24 hr without surgery
      + E grade for emergency surgery

Box 19.2
Factors increasing anaesthetic risk

● Ischaemic heart disease
● Impaired myocardial function
● Pulmonary hypertension
● Obstructive airways disease
● Impaired renal function
● Co-morbidities
● ASA status IV– V
● Emergency surgery
● Male sex
● Increasing age
● Diabetes

Anaesthetic technique and monitoring

Anaesthetists, like other medical practitioners, have considerable freedom in clinical practice. The wide variety of anaesthetic drugs and techniques available makes it difficult, and perhaps undesirable, to establish rigid rules, but it is usually possible to determine broad guidelines for standard practice for most situations. The application of Crown Indemnity in the NHS since the 1st January 1990 has meant that districts and regions will now be financially responsible for the cost of medical litigation. This may result in greater standardisation of clinical practice and improvements in the availability of monitoring equipment. Whether it will also improve resources for postoperative recovery and intensive care is less certain.

Standards of minimal monitoring were proposed by Eichorn *et al.* in 1986 with the publication of the Harvard standards,[42] the application of which resulted in a decrease in malpractice claims and a consequent reduction in medical insurance premiums where the standards were observed. Concern has, however, been expressed that recommendations become *de facto* legal obligations. If a pulse oximeter or inspired oxygen alarm are described as essential items for minimal monitoring, should the operating list be cancelled if these items of equipment are missing or faulty? The adoption of some form of minimal monitoring in anaesthesia is now universally accepted at least in principle[43–45] and the additional costs per case are modest. However, other than the actuarial effects seen in North America, minimal monitoring standards have so far not been shown to influence anaesthetic morbidity, perhaps for methodological reasons. The Association of Anaesthetists published recommendations for standards of monitoring in 1988 and this publication provides an excellent framework for adoption by departments.[45] Additional monitoring will be needed when there is pre-existing medical disease, when special techniques (e.g. controlled hypotension) are used, when surgery involves the lungs, cardiovascular or central nervous systems, or when major blood loss is expected. Departments should extend the basic standard by producing recommendations for the types of high-risk patients and surgery that they undertake. However, no amount of monitoring will compensate for the ignorant, uncaring or absent practitioner. While the analogy between anaesthesia and aviation is often quoted, it should be remembered that the pilot goes down with his plane.

Postoperative care

Time is set aside for postoperative care in the workload of consultants and is a requirement for general professional training.[33,34] In some hospitals a trainee is allocated to the recovery room. This can provide both an educational opportunity and an occasion for the collection of postoperative audit data. Having set standards of practice in the recovery room, the department must be prepared to audit these standards and change them where appropriate. The precise contribution made by anaesthetists to postoperative care should be discussed with the surgeons with whom they work. While anaesthetic responsibility may strictly end with the return of the patient to the ward, the expertise of the anaesthetist in fluid management, respiratory function, oxygen therapy, analgesia and clinical monitoring may contribute substantially to the quality of postoperative care. Additionally, the appearance of the anaesthetist on the ward does much to improve communication with ward staff and improves the image of the specialty.

Postoperative visiting is crucial for audit. Seeing the patient on the ward

after the immediate recovery period provides an opportunity for anaesthetists to examine the quality of their care, as well as reminding patients
that anaesthetists are an important component of hospital care – a
necessary activity when amnesic premedication is so commonly used. In
the Survey Of Anaesthetic Practice[46] 88 % of patients were visited within 24
hours of operation, with 23 % of visits resulting in spontaneous complaint
by the patient. Of these complaints, the most prominent were operation
site pain, nausea, sore throat, headache, backache and (surprisingly)
awareness. The frequency of these complaints was magnified when the
patients were directly questioned. Individual departments should have a
standard for visiting the patients postoperatively and the anaesthetist's
work schedule should be constructed so as to facilitate this activity.

In its publication[25] on postanaesthetic recovery facilities, the Association
of Anaesthetists states that anaesthetic responsibilities continue until the
effects of the anaesthetic have worn off sufficiently for the patient to be
returned safely to the ward. The document also specifies the circumstances
and conditions under which the care of the patient can be devolved to
nursing staff. Postoperative recovery room staff should have immediate
access to an anaesthetist until the last patient has been discharged to the
ward. They should receive written care orders covering monitoring, fluids,
oxygen and drug therapy when receiving patients from theatre. Standing
orders should cover the management of the unconscious patient, airway
maintenance, respiratory and cardiovascular monitoring and support,
analgesia and criteria for fitness for discharge.

It has been tacitly recognised for many years that the management of
acute pain after surgery is inadequate in most UK hospitals. A recent
document[47] published by a working party of the Royal College of Surgeons
and the College of Anaesthetists has surveyed current information on this
subject, and makes several important recommendations, the most important of which is that hospitals should establish multi-disciplinary pain-
relief teams. Standards should be produced against which the efficacy of
pain control can be audited. Education of medical and nursing staff is an
integral part of this process, and anaesthetists should be closely involved in
a continuing educational programme.

Postoperative visiting assumes a special importance in day-case surgery.
In 1975 an editorial in The Lancet[48] condemned the early discharge of
patients following anaesthesia. The postoperative sequelae described above
assume a greater importance where the surgery has been minor and the
patients discharged early. A study in 1969[49] found the main morbidity to
be drowsiness, headache and vomiting, and in 3.9% of the patients,

sequelae lasted for more than 24 hours. It is recommended[35] that patients must be seen before discharge, the quality of recovery and pain relief assessed, potential postoperative side effects should be described, and they should be warned not to drive, operate machinery or drink alcohol for 24 hours after the anaesthetic. Departments that operate day-case facilities should introduce standards for postoperative assessment of patients and audit their findings.

Outcome

Anaesthesia is a 'facilitatory' discipline. This complicates outcome audit. The activities of physicians or surgeons can be assessed in part by examining the efficacy with which disease processes are relieved, but not so anaesthesia. Death is sufficiently common in intensive care for severity-adjusted mortality rates to be a useful outcome measure, but death due to anaesthesia alone is too rare – and therefore too coarse – an outcome measure to be useful as an index of assessing the quality of routine anaesthetic practice. Mortality only becomes a useful end-point when large populations or patients at particular risk are examined. Reference has already been made to these epidemiological studies: in the CEPOD report, anaesthesia was considered to have been wholly responsible for a fatal outcome in three out of half a million procedures. This is not to say that mortality is not useful for audit; but it may only reveal the more gross lapses of clinical practice. The approach that needs to be developed for routine anaesthetic practice should be based on morbidity and critical incident monitoring, patient satisfaction, and cost–benefit analyses; and results should be related to predicted risk, using one of the methods discussed above.

Critical incidents

Much of the work on critical incidents has been done in the USA.[20,24,50] A critical incident is a clinically significant event that, if left untreated, would have resulted in an adverse outcome. It has been shown that the vast majority of critical incidents involve human error. In his 1978 paper[24] Cooper showed that 82% of preventable incidents had human error as a contributory cause, whilst only 14% were due to overt equipment failure. Furthermore, he showed that critical incidents occurred most commonly (42%) during the middle of anaesthesia, in contrast to the 'take off and landing' philosophy; though they were also common during induction (26%). In a later paper,[20] Cooper *et al.* examined critical incidents in which the patients experienced a *substantive negative outcome* (death, cardiac arrest, cancelled surgery, or prolonged stay in recovery ward, ICU or hospital). Overall, the incidents in which a negative outcome occurred differed little in aetiology from those in which the patient suffered no harm. When the patient was graded as ASA III–V however, the risk of a critical incident causing harm was greater, presumably due to a reduced margin for error. Cooper showed that different patterns of human error could be identified, and he proposed ten strategies for their prevention, including staff training, improved supervision and better monitoring and organisation.

Identifying and avoiding critical incidents is an important part of the audit process. The quality of practice committee of the College of Anaesthetists has included in the trainees' logbook the facility to record critical incidents: consultants should do the same. Individual departments should maintain a critical incident register, analysed regularly, and containing recommendations for avoidance. The quality of practice committee is presently sponsoring a pilot study of the practical difficulties of critical incident reporting, with the intention of initiating a national critical incident reporting system.[17] As yet, the committee has not clarified the definition of a critical incident for the national critical incident register.[51]

Complications and morbidity

Complications may be considered to be adverse events that arise in part because of pre-existing disease or structural abnormalities. These frequently combine with human error or equipment failure and can result in major morbidity. Complications range from a transient bradycardia in a patient receiving beta-blocking drugs, to failed intubation with cerebral damage. Of particular importance is the first 24 hours postoperatively. A recent study of over 2000 consecutive anaesthetics has shown a 5 % serious complication rate and the authors considered that death or serious disability could have been avoided in ten patients had appropriate postoperative care been available.[27]

Secker-Walker suggests a four-point scale[5] for grading the severity of complications:

1. A transient complication not requiring treatment.
2. A potentially harmful event successfully remedied.
3. An event causing minor morbidity.
4. An event causing serious harm to the patient.

A similar classification is suggested by Lack[51] using a five-point scale that includes death. Individual departments must decide on the precise nature of the critical incidents and complications they wish to investigate, and those they wish to include in their register. Departments should review all cases in which unexpected outcomes have occurred, preferably at *joint* audit meetings with the surgeons, held at least once every four months.

It is in the area of morbidity and prevention that anaesthetists should recognise their wider potential and responsibilities. Anaesthetists are in a position to detect and modify impaired organ-system function. Indeed, the perioperative period often facilitates detailed investigation and treatment. Useful information can be gained during anaesthesia about myocardial, respiratory, and renal function. The anaesthetist who fails to identify the patient with limited renal reserve, for example, loses an opportunity to enhance renal function and may indirectly be responsible for further avoidable renal damage. The lower mortality rates associated with immediate rather than delayed operative fracture fixation may be due to earlier anaesthetic involvement and hence better resuscitation. Anaesthetists should play a more active role in the medical management of surgical patients and should examine the *indirect* results of their care more critically than hitherto.

Cost–benefit and cost-efficiency

The measurement of cost is relatively uncomplicated, if laborious: the private sector has been doing it for years. The simplest approach is for individual anaesthetists to collect detailed information for a limited period or for a limited number of cases on variable costs of drug and disposable usage for specific operative procedures. To this must be added the fixed costs: salaries of all staff involved in preoperative assessment; anaesthesia and postoperative care for that type of procedure; the anaesthetic and monitoring equipment required; the capital charge applied; and depreciation or replacement costs (10–20 % per annum depending on the item). Costs per case could then be calculated and offered to surgical directorates on a yearly contract. Additional cases would need careful calculation of the marginal costs, because to increase patient throughput might require extra medical staff. Additional weighting may be needed for emergency cases or for patients with significant intercurrent disease. Drugs account for a small proportion of total costs, most of which are salaries; but when departments hold their own budgets, the savings to be made by changing from more expensive drugs to cheaper alternatives may be used to increase study leave allocations or other educational activities. The way to prevent acrimonious disputes about clinical freedom in the use of drugs and disposables is to obtain consensus views for the department as a whole, based when possible on factual analyses. If such analyses are not available, this should encourage departments to perform their own assessments of the cost–benefit of particular drugs or procedures.

Cost-efficiency is most easily expressed as the costs per case, and as the major component of expenditure is the fixed cost, greater efficiency means a higher throughput. It is essential that measures of quality of care are combined with workload. Of greater difficulty is to relate costs to benefits or efficacy and this is why better outcome measures should be developed for anaesthesia. The absence of negative outcomes is only impressive when related to patients at risk; and quality of recovery can only be determined if patients are reviewed postoperatively.

Data collection and audit activities

Anaesthetists are perhaps as well trained as any clinical group in the acquisition and analysis of data. However, detailed information on audit or costs cannot easily be collected during a busy operating list by a single-handed anaesthetist. This is a significant problem that will not be solved by any one approach, but by gradual accommodation with a number of differing techniques. Departments should decide what information they can collect by determining the aims of the exercise, the questions that need to be answered, and the resources at their disposal. The most important initial step is to persuade every member of the department that some form of minimum data set is required. The second is to have in place the means for analysing and presenting that data. For example, it should be possible for every member of a department to record on a standard form the number of routine or emergency cases done each day, the operative procedure, the ASA grading, whether single-handed or accompanied, and adverse events. This information could be collated by the anaesthetic department secretary daily, and analysed weekly. This would give a crude index of workload, training, and short-term outcome, on which arguments for funding more developed systems could be based. The analyses should be presented monthly at departmental audit meetings. This is also an appropriate forum for setting simple standards, the monitoring of which might then gradually be incorporated in the minimum data set. Anaesthetic records of patients graded ASA III–V, all emergency cases, and all critical incidents, could be photocopied and used as the basis for review. Joint audit meetings with the surgeons should be organised regularly. The Bloomsbury audit[5] system involves standardised data forms on cards, which are completed by each anaesthetist and entered into a spreadsheet programme by the departmental secretary: the system is simple, not over-ambitious and has much to commend it.

Automated data collection

More extensive data requires a different approach. The quality of practice committee has agreed with the Computing in Anaesthesia Society a minimum data set to be collected by all junior anaesthetists.[51] This data set includes thirteen fields, covering date and time of operation, patient identity and age, ASA status, urgency of operation, procedure, and information related to anaesthetist's grade. It should be emphasised that this is a *minimum* data set and departments may want to include space for details of anaesthetic drugs and technique, monitoring used and information about outcome. Once the data set has been selected, the difficult task is getting the data from the anaesthetist into the database. The personal computer provides potential for processing large data sets and analysing inter-relationships, but it still requires commitment and time on the part of the person entering data. Automatic data entry, from monitoring equipment for example, raises the problem of data verification and the exclusion of artifact. Optical mark readers do not dispense with paper, and introduce the additional burden of having to enter data with care, often at a time when both hands are required for patient care. Hand-held computers have been employed successfully[52] by committed individuals, but the small keyboard limits applications and the devices are easily stolen or lost. Credit card techniques (smart cards) have considerable potential in conjunction with swipe readers for entering patient data, and in conjunction with a number identifying the member of staff, and an internal clock, a networked laptop computer on the anaesthetic machine is likely to be an appropriate way forward. Relational databases should be employed for writing software programs, and compatibility with hospital audit systems is essential for the future.

Closing the loop

Departments must decide on a mechanism by which the data which has been collected can used to maintain or improve good standards of training and medical care. The trainees' log book should be inspected by the college tutor at regular intervals to review their experience and supervision. The anaesthetic secretary can process data on departmental and consultant workload every month. An audit clerk is needed, however, for detailed analysis of outcomes. With the provision of sophisticated software, there are many possible aspects of anaesthetic practice that can readily be tabulated and displayed, including data on patient handling, obstetrics, resuscitation, examination results and research. This can be built into an annual departmental report showing how anaesthetic resources have been used. It must be remembered, however, that to improve standards of care, data must be used to answer specific questions.

The information obtained from these activities should be assessed by peer review at monthly audit meetings and quarterly joint meetings with the surgeons. Time must be set aside for these meetings. An attendance record should be kept. Reports and recommendations can be prepared after discussion, and presented to the hospital clinical board or management committee. Quality assurance activities will succeed if they are based on consensus and common purpose.

References

1. Department of Health (1989). *Working for Patients*. London: HMSO.
2. American College of Surgeons (1924). The minimum standard. *Bulletin of the American College of Surgeons*, **8**, 1–4.
3. Codman, E. A. (1916). Report of a Committee on hospital standardisation. *Surgery, Gynaecology and Obstetrics*, **22**, 119–120.
4. Everhart, D. (1984). Quality control in medicine in the USA. In: *Quality of Care in the Practice of Anaesthesia*, ed. J. N. Lunn. London: The Royal Society of Medicine.
5. Secker-Walker, J. (1991). Audit in anaesthesia. In: *Anaesthesia Review* 8, ed. L. Kaufman. Edinburgh: Churchill Livingstone.
6. *Report on Confidential Enquiries into Maternal Deaths in England and Wales 1952–1954* (1957). London: HMSO.
7. Beecher, H. K. & Todd, D. P. (1954). A study of the deaths associated with anaesthesia and surgery. *Annals of Surgery*, **140**, 2–34.
8. Buck, N., Devlin, H. B. & Lunn, J. N. (1987). *The Report of a Confidential Enquiry into Perioperative Deaths*. London: Nuffield Provincial Hospitals Trust and the King's Fund.
9. Edwards, G., Morton, H. J. V., Pask, E. A. & Wylie, W. D. (1956). Deaths associated with anaesthesia. *Anaesthesia*, **11**, 194–220.
10. Dinnick, O. P. (1964). Anaesthetic deaths. *Anaesthesia*, **19**, 536–556.
11. Lunn, J. N. & Mushin, W. W. (1982). *Mortality Associated with Anaesthesia*. London: Nuffield Provincial Hospital Trust.
12. Dripps, R. D., Lamont, A. & Eckenhoff, J. E. (1961). The role of anaesthesia in surgical mortality. *Journal of the American Medical Association*, **178**, 261.
13. Mushin, W. W. (1983). Mortality associated with anaesthesia: the background to the British study. In: *European Academy of Anaesthesiology Proceedings*, ed. M. D. Vickers & J. N. Lunn. Heidelberg: Springer-Verlag.

14. *National Confidential Enquiry into Perioperative Deaths Report 1989* (1990). London: NCEPOD.

15. Standing Medical Advisory Committee for the Secretaries of State for Health and Wales (1990). *The Quality of Medical Care.* London: HMSO.

16. College of Anaesthetists (1989). *First Report of the Audit Committee.* London.

17. Stoddart, J. C. (1991). College of Anaesthetists' quality of practice committee. *Anaesthesia News,* **44,** 4.

18. Association of Anaesthetists of Great Britain & Ireland (1988). *Guidelines on the duties of Chairmen of Divisions of Anaesthesia.* London.

19. Ministerial Group on Junior Doctors' Hours (1990). *Junior Doctors' Hours.* London: Department of Health.

20. Cooper, J. B., Newbower, R. S. & Kitz, R. J. (1984). An analysis of major errors and equipment failures in anaesthesia management: considerations for prevention and detection. *Anesthesiology,* **60,** 34–42.

21. Association of Anaesthetists of Great Britain & Ireland (1989). *Consultant:Trainee Relationships. A guide for Consultants.* London.

22. Gaba, D. M., Maxwell, M. & DeAnda, A. (1987). Anaesthetic mishaps: breaking the chain of accident evolution. *Anesthesiology,* **66,** 670–676.

23. Craig, J. & Wilson, M. E. (1981). A survey of anaesthetic misadventures. *Anaesthesia,* **36,** 933–936.

24. Cooper, J. B., Newbower, R. S., Long, C. D. & McPeek, B. (1978). Preventable anaesthetic mishaps: a study of human factors. *Anesthesiology,* **49,** 399–406.

25. Association of Anaesthetists of Great Britain & Ireland (1985). *Post-anaesthetic Recovery Facilities.* London.

26. Eltringham, R. J., Durkin, M. A. & Andrewes, S. (1983). *Post-anaesthetic Recovery.* Berlin: Springer-Verlag.

27. Gamil, M. & Fanning, A. (1991). The first 24 hours after surgery. *Anaesthesia,* **46,** 712–715.

28. Chamberlain, D. A. (1989). Advanced life support: revised recommendations of the Resuscitation Council (UK). *British Medical Journal,* **299,** 446–448.

29. Leading Article (1977). The Westminster Enquiry. *The Lancet,* **ii,** 175–176.

30. Brahams, D. (1989). Anaesthesia and the law: awareness and pain during anaesthesia. *Anaesthesia,* **44,** 352.

31. Association of Anaesthetists of Great Britain & Ireland (1990). *Checklist for Anaesthetic Machines.* London.

32. Derrington, M. C. & Smith, G. (1987). A review of studies of anaesthetic risk, morbidity and mortality. *British Journal of Anaesthesia,* **59,** 815–833.

33. Association of Anaesthetists of Great Britain & Ireland (1983). *Workload for Consultant Anaesthetists.* London.

34. Faculty of Anaesthetists (1987). *General Professional Training Guide.* London: Faculty of Anaesthetists at the Royal College of Surgeons of England.

35. Ogg, T. W. (1985). Aspects of day surgery and anaesthesia. *Anaesthesia Rounds,* **18,** 14.

36. Owens, W. D. (1978). ASA physical status classifications: a study of consistency of ratings. *Anesthesiology,* **49,** 239.

37. Goldman, L., Caldera, D. L., Nussbaum, S. R., Southwick, F. S., Krogstad, D., Murray, B., Burke, D. S., O'Malley, T. A., Goroll, A. H., Caplan, C. H., Nolan, J., Carabello, B. & Slater, E. E. (1977). Multifactorial index on

cardiac risk in noncardiac surgical procedures. *New England Journal of Medicine*, **297**, 845.

38. Fowkes, F. G. R., Lunn, J. N., Farrow, S. C., Robertson, I. B. & Samuel, P. (1982). Epidemiology in Anaesthesia III. Mortality risk in patients with coexisting physical disease. *British Journal of Anaesthesia*, **54**, 819–825.

39. Farrow, S. C., Fowkes, F. G. R., Lunn, J. N., Robertson, I. B. & Sweetnam, P. (1984). Epidemiology in anaesthesia: a method for predicting hospital mortality. *European Journal of Anaesthesiology*, **1**, 77–84.

40. Pedersen, T., Eliasen, K., Ravnborg, M., Viby-Mogensen, J., Qvist, J., Johansen, S. H. & Henriksen, E. (1986). Risk factors, complications and outcome in anaesthesia. A pilot study. *European Journal of Anaesthesiology*, **3**, 225–239.

41. Ross, A. F. & Tinker, J. H. (1990). Anaesthesia risk. In: *Anaesthesia* 3rd edn., ed. R. D. Miller. New York: Churchill Livingstone.

42. Eichorn, J. H., Cooper, J. B., Cullen, D. J., Maier, W. R., Philip, J. H. & Seeman, R. G. (1986). Standards for patient monitoring during anaesthesia at Harvard Medical School. *Journal of the American Medical Association*, **256**, 1017–1020.

43. American Society of Anesthesiologists (1986). Standards of basic intraoperative monitoring. *Newsletter*, **50**, 9.

44. Cass, N. M., Crosby, W. M. & Holland, R. B. (1988). Minimal monitoring standards. *Anaesthesia & Intensive Care*, **16**, 110–113.

45. Association of Anaesthetists of Great Britain & Ireland (1988). *Recommendations for Standards of Monitoring During Anaesthesia & Recovery*. London.

46. Association of Anaesthetists of Great Britain & Ireland (1988). *The Report of a Survey of Anaesthetic Practice*. London.

47. Working Party (1990). *Report on Pain after Surgery*. London: The Royal College of Surgeons of England & The College of Anaesthetists.

48. Leading Article (1975). Tottering home. *The Lancet*, **i**, 1366.

49. Fahy, A. & Marshall, M. (1969). Post anaesthetic morbidity in outpatients. *British Journal of Anaesthesia*, **34**, 44–47.

50. Flanagan, J. C. (1954). The critical incident technique. *Psychology Bulletin*, **51**, 327–358.

51. Lack, A. (1990). Anaesthetists discuss audit data collection. *Anaesthesia News*, **40**, 2.

52. Watt, J. M. & Brewin, M. (1989). Keeping the information to hand: technology versus deforestation. *Anaesthesia News*, **22**, 1.

20

Audit in intensive care
JULIAN F. BION

This review will examine audit *in* intensive care (systems of quality assurance), and audit *of* intensive care (what intensive care has achieved). An approach to intensive care audit, and the framework of the review, is given in Figure 20.1. It may be helpful to start by defining the main terms used in this chapter.

Key definitions

Intensive care is a multi-disciplinary specialty providing a comprehensive diagnostic and therapeutic service for patients with acute failure of two or more organ-systems, or with isolated acute respiratory failure. Patients with single organ-system failures may also require intensive care if their condition is unstable. A minimum 1:1 nurse:patient ratio is required, in intensive care units (ICUs) together with continuous cover by consultants and resident junior doctors.

High dependency units (HDUs) are intended to care for patients with acute failure of not more than one organ-system, excluding acute failure of the respiratory system. HDUs are not suitable places for caring for patients requiring mechanical ventilation or complex organ-system support. They have an important prophylactic role in preventing organ-system dysfunction and in treating postoperative pain following major surgery. Specialist HDUs such as coronary care, renal medicine and transplant units are often best sited within the relevant specialist clinical area, but general service HDUs (for hospital-wide work) should be placed close to the ICU in order to ensure fair access to all clinical services, and to make efficient use of existing medical management and nursing expertise. HDUs require readily available medical staff. They generally operate a 1:2 nurse:patient ratio.

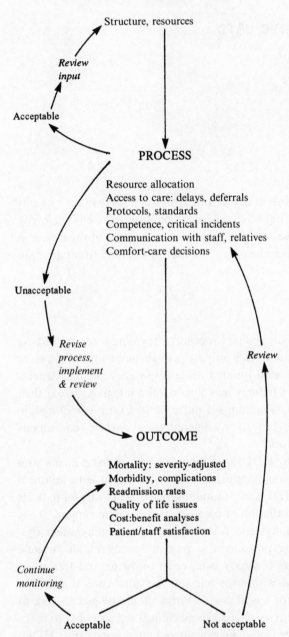

Fig. 20.1. A structure for intensive care audit.

Postoperative care units receive patients following anaesthesia and surgery and generally provide care during working hours only (08.00 – 20.00 hrs). They do not have dedicated junior medical staff because they are sited close to the operating theatre. A 1:2 nurse:patient ratio is needed during recovery from anaesthesia and to cope with a high patient throughput.

The term '*organ-system*' refers to the cardiovascular, respiratory, renal, gastrointestinal, neurological and haematological systems. The criteria for defining failure of these organ-systems are presented in Appendix I to this chapter. Failure of an organ-system implies that special measures are needed to support it, such as mechanical ventilation for respiratory failure, or dialysis for renal failure. Critical illness could be defined as a disease process causing acute failure of one or more organ-systems.

Introduction

Intensive care dates its origins from the report of the 1952 polio epidemic in Copenhagen by Professor Lassen, an epidemiologist, who reported that the mortality rate of patients with respiratory failure could be reduced, and the quality of their care improved, if they were treated in designated high-dependency areas within hospitals, received endotracheal intubation with positive pressure ventilation, and had someone present at the bedside at all times.[1] Since then intensive care has become an independent specialty in some countries, though in many it is still a subspecialty of anaesthesia, medicine or surgery. Funding of intensive care varies considerably, with the USA spending approximately 10% of its health care budget (1% of its gross national product) on intensive care,[2] whereas in Europe expenditure is much more modest;[3] France and Germany provide around 3% and the UK probably less than 1%. Despite this expenditure, there is remarkably little information on the efficacy of intensive care, particularly in the UK,[4] even though there is considerable variation between ICUs in mortality rates (in one American study[5] 8% to 40%) and in the costs of care. There are three main reasons for the lack of published reports on the efficacy of intensive care. First, using concurrent control groups is either difficult or unethical. Secondly, there are many factors that determine outcome from critical illness. Thirdly, generally acceptable standards for intensive care practice have not yet been defined. Examples of the conflicting evidence of efficacy of intensive care are provided by the report by Hook and colleagues,[6] which showed that intensive care merely delays but does not prevent death in patients with pneumococcal bacteraemia, and the report by Rogers *et al.*,[7] which showed a reduction in mortality in patients with acute respiratory failure following the introduction of an intensive care unit. These studies are difficult to interpret because they use historical mortality data. The inadequacy of this approach for a speciality such as intensive care is obvious, since the numbers of patients in specific diagnostic categories are small, many have multiple diagnoses, and disease severity varies not only within diagnostic groups but over time as well. Prior stratification for severity of illness will help to reduce bias[8-10] and requires the development of suitable measures. These difficulties are to some extent now being addressed. The results of research are likely to have a significant impact on intensive care practice, in particular on the structure and process of care, both of which affect outcome.

Structure and funding of intensive care

Medical training

In Australia and many European countries, intensive care is a specialty in its own right, with a system of accreditation and examination, and a career structure. In the USA, all the major specialties have their own systems of accreditation in intensive care and it has not been possible to produce a unified discipline. In the UK, intensive care has hitherto developed as a service rather than a specialty, with the major input from anaesthetists who frequently give their time without sessional recognition. This is now changing, with the establishment in several centres of directorships of intensive care.

Intensive care training has always been part of the Faculty (now College) of Anaesthetists' requirements for higher professional training (HPT); and in 1984 the Royal College of Physicians also decided to include intensive care experience as a recommendation for HPT. Both colleges recognise the importance of developing multi-disciplinary intensive care. It does not yet form a required part of surgical training, but most surgeons would regard it as a useful attribute. Members of all three colleges contribute to the joint advisory committee on intensive therapy, which advises the Department of Health on the placement of senior registrar posts in intensive care. The Intensive Care Society is engaged in establishing standards of care[11] and systems of audit for the UK as a whole, and a recently completed study comparing ICUs in the UK with those in the USA[12] has shown that British units perform on average as well as those in the USA, but receive only the most severely ill patients. Less seriously ill patients requiring intensive monitoring and high dependency care are not being admitted, presumably because they cannot get access because resources are limited. This suggests that opportunities for prevention of critical illness are being lost.

An aspect of intensive care practice that is generally overlooked by health care planners is its educational role in teaching junior medical and nursing staff to identify patients on ordinary wards who are at risk of organ-system failures and to apply appropriate resuscitative measures. This highly cost-effective form of medical education will not realise its potential unless intensive care develops as a specialty, and this requires the same resources as any other clinical discipline in terms of medical manpower, management, and audit.

Number of beds

Publications on the subject of ICU provision commonly fail to distinguish between the geographical size of a unit and the number of beds that are actually open. When the distinction is made, it is rare for the nurse:patient ratio to be described in detail. An ICU bed does not merely refer to a geographical space containing a bed, it means an ICU-trained nurse, medical staff, equipment and support services. Moreover, referral patterns or bed occupancy are not accurate reflections of need, as this can only be determined by measuring the number of patients in a hospital who would have benefitted from intensive care had that service been made available to them. Research in this area would need to address the problem of influencing a system merely by studying it. However, no official report on this subject has even attempted to record the number of refused or deferred admissions to intensive care.

In the UK current Department of Health policy for intensive care is described in Building Note 27 (1970, revised 1974). This recommends that hospitals should provide 1–2% of the total acute beds as ICU beds, with the average district general hospital having a six to eight bedded ICU. This recommendation appears to have been based on opinion rather than fact. A postal survey by the Medical Architecture Research Unit in 1988[13] showed that the average acute bed allocation for intensive care was 1%, but the study did not examine whether this provision was adequate. The mean bed occupancy was 61%, but this measure is often an approximation, is dependent on referral patterns and does not necessarily reflect clinical need. A recent survey by the Association of Anaesthetists of Great Britain and Ireland[14] states that an ICU of less than four beds, fewer than 200 admissions per year, a bed-occupancy rate of less than 60%, and that stands empty for more than 50 days a year, is 'almost inevitably inexpert and uneconomic'.

Calculations to determine the appropriate number of ICU beds for a hospital must take into account the type of work that hospital performs, the presence or absence of high-dependency and postoperative recovery facilities, current bed usage, modifications of work practices as a result of changes in funding, teaching obligations, and future expansion of medical techniques that have potential intensive care needs. It is rare for these considerations to be taken into account in the development of services that do not directly demand postoperative intensive care, and a good example is a recent review of resource allocation for chronic renal failure units,[15] which omits any comment on the requirement for intensive care support services for patients with chronic renal failure. Such patients occupy 8–10% of the ICU bed-days in the author's hospital.

A substantial proportion of intensive care work involves emergencies and cannot therefore be planned in advance. This results in peaks and troughs in admissions and a consequent need for a small surplus of beds to cope with busy periods. This is particularly true of hospitals with a busy accident and emergency (A&E) department on site. If the number of ICU beds is inadequate to cope with peak demand, patients will either receive sub-standard care, or will have to be transferred to other hospitals. This practice is safe when a specialist transport team is available,[16] but unsafe when it is not,[17] as is usually the case in the UK.

Based on US data[18] the number (n) of ICU beds required for a hospital serving a known population is given by the formula below, with 75% as the ICU allocation and 25% for high-dependency care:

$$n = 75\% \text{ of } \frac{45/1000 \times \text{total population}}{365 \times \text{desired occupancy}}$$

Miranda et al.[19] have suggested that this formula is flawed because the figure of 45/1000 will need revision according to clinical practice. Moreover, the desired bed occupancy will be influenced by flexibility of working practices both within a given ICU and between different units. A bed occupancy of 90% will mean that on average there will be no free beds available on 37 days per year. This would result in an unacceptable number of deferred or refused admissions. It is the author's experience that the maximum average bed-occupancy rate should be around 70% to allow for periods of peak demand; this conforms to the recommendations of the Intensive Care Society[11] and exceeds the even more conservative figure of 60% recommended by a BMA working party in 1967.[20] Bed occupancy should be calculated not by a census at a particular time during the 24-hour period, but by recording duration of stay for each patient. Duration of stay of 12–24 hours should be counted as one day, because considerable work is generated during the admission and discharge of a patient.

A simple approach for a hospital providing a wide range of surgical and medical specialties would be to allocate 2 % of acute general hospital beds to intensive care. A further 0.5–1 % might be required to accommodate the activities of a busy A&E department, and if complex surgical or medical patients were attracted to the hospital by consultants with particular expertise in certain areas. Additional resources would be needed for specialty regional or supra-regional programmes such as transplantation, cardiac surgery, burns and trauma.

In addition, 0.5–1 % of acute *general* beds should be designated as general HDU beds, to be sited close to, and managed by, the intensive care unit. There are no Department of Health recommendations about size or structure, and the precise resource allocation will depend upon the type of work (particularly surgical) that is undertaken, the number of emergency admissions, and the particular requirements of certain specialities for high-dependency care rather than intensive care. HDU beds must be considered in relation to the number of ICU beds available. If the number of ICU beds is inadequate to cope with peak demand, then greater pressure will be placed on HDU beds. HDUs also serve a vital role as step-down units, giving ICU patients who are recovering from acute illness time to adjust to independent self-care.

Demographic changes throughout Europe and the planned expansion of degree nurses, will result in a reduction in the numbers of nurses working on ordinary wards. It is likely that there will be a proportionate increase in the requirement for high-dependency care, so that scarce resources are used efficiently. In this context, it is crucial that health care planners and managers recognise the cost-efficacy of high-dependency care: prevention is cheaper than cure. The absence of postoperative care facilities in many hospitals in the UK, in conjunction with the lack of sufficient HDU or ICU beds, has resulted in avoidable deaths in the last few years, and has meant that patients who needed relatively simple prophylactic care end up receiving expensive intensive care with a higher mortality rate.

A well-equipped postoperative recovery ward must form part of the theatre suite or suites. This should also function as a holding area where patients who have received their premedication on the ward can be cared for while awaiting transfer to the anaesthetic rooms. This will minimise wasted time between cases. It should be possible to provide short-term respiratory support (four hours maximum) and analgesia for patients for up to 12 hours. Such areas should not, however, try to function as HDUs.

The aim should be to provide a high throughput of patients during normal working hours and to minimise nursing requirements at night.

Staffing

The intensity and costs of care are related in large part to the high ratio of nurses and medical staff to patients: salaries are the largest component of hospital budgets.[21] In the United Kingdom the Intensive Care Society recommends[22] that there should be a minimum of one nurse to each patient. This translates into a *minimum* of 6.5 whole-time-equivalent (WTE) nurses per bed. In practice, the precise ratio will depend on bed occupancy rates, turnover, the size of the unit, casemix complexity, the volume of data collection and administrative work required of each nurse, their level of experience, and the number of trainee nurses needing supervision. Methods of calculating the number of nurses required are given by the Intensive Care Society (UK).[11] Automated data collection and intelligent monitoring systems will help to increase nursing efficiency, but at present there should be one nurse for each patient, and a supernumary senior nurse for every four beds. High-dependency care can function effectively at half this level.

The medical staff must be able to provide 24-hour consultant cover offering a comprehensive specialist clinical service, 24-hour cover by supervised resident junior medical staff capable of providing high-level organ-system support, and a medical response time of less than one minute for emergencies occurring in the unit.

Support staff should include a full-time technician, a ward clerk, a physiotherapist, a secretary, and a half-time audit clerk. ICUs exceeding twelve beds will need additional staff. Units holding their own budget will of course need a business manager, perhaps shared with another discipline such as anaesthesia. Technicians and ward clerks relieve the nursing staff of a considerable administrative burden, and substantially improve the efficiency of the unit, particularly in the areas of equipment maintenance and stock taking. Close links should be maintained with the laboratories and nutrition team or dietician. Cleaning staff are part of the ICU team and the work should not be delegated to inexperienced individuals.

Geography

Whatever the size of resource eventually provided, flexibility of use of that resource will be of considerable importance in determining the efficiency with which it is used. Geographically isolated units will not be able to share resources, and there will therefore be a higher proportion of unoccupied bed-days than for an integrated and centralised system. Intensive care, general high-dependency care, operating theatres and postoperative recovery should as far as possible co-exist in the same area of the hospital. This allows for the most flexible and efficient distribution of medical and nursing staff, the co-ordination of care and training, and the provision of equipment and laboratory services. Large acute-care areas could be subdivided into units of specialty interest, in order to maintain natural clinical groupings and corporate identities.

Specialty HDUs are often best sited within their clinical areas to ensure continuity of medical care, and for nurse training. However, if multiple organ failure supervenes specialist intensive care is needed. This cannot be provided in the HDU on a part-time basis with inadequate numbers of inadequately trained staff. The patient should be transferred to the ICU. Specialist HDUs should create formal links with the ICU to ensure that their medical and nursing staff learn to exercise a preventative role.

Management

If an organisation is to be successful, it requires structure, efficient systems of communication, individuals with clearly defined responsibilities, a specific set of aims and values (a 'culture'), a system of internal review, and direction. Intensive care units are no exception. ICUs should be managed by a responsible and experienced clinician working closely with the senior nurse, exercising budgetary control with the help of a business manager, and with secretarial support. In large hospitals, centralised intensive and acute care facilities could be divided into areas of specialist interest, under the overall managerial control of a director of intensive and acute care services. Postoperative recovery units could be placed either under theatre or intensive care management, with day-to-day supervision by anaesthetists, who should establish with nursing staff protocols for the care of patients using this facility.

Budgeting

There is a strong argument for making intensive care a 'core-funded' specialty, at least for the emergency admissions. Emergency admissions are in effect all those patients whose admission to the unit was not, or could not have been, booked 24 hours in advance. This would help to protect the budget of primary clinicians who might be faced with major unplanned expenditure if one of their patients needed intensive care, to the detriment of their elective medical work. Similarly, it would avoid the risk of clinicians deciding not to refer their patients for intensive care because of anticipated high marginal costs.

There are various methods of determining charges for intensive care services: detailed collection of costs on each patient, the use of surrogate measures such as diagnosis-related groups and workload scores, or a combination of the two. The private sector (which has the luxury of only treating elective, non-emergency cases) combines standardised charging for diagnosis or procedure and a daily room charge, with detailed information on all drugs and disposables. This could be applied to the public sector, provided that the demands of emergency work are understood, and the additional work engendered for nursing staff is taken into account. Bar-code readers will be useful for recording drug and disposable usage, but currently available portable instruments are insufficiently reliable. Smart-cards and swipe readers are an alternative, but the fact remains that data will not be collected in an emergency by nursing staff working under pressure.

Charges per bed must include an element for the opportunity cost of keeping a bed open even if it is unoccupied; if the ICU workload is predictable and stable, then the cost of the previous year's unoccupied bed-days can be spread over the charges set prospectively. An empty bed still requires medical and nursing staff, and a crude estimate would therefore set the opportunity cost of an empty bed at 70 % of the cost of an occupied bed. Gilbertson and his colleagues have shown that the cost of salaries, radiology services, equipment, and administration was 60 % of the total ICU budget.[23] The simplest way of dealing with this problem is to agree with other hospital directorates what their likely ICU bed usage will be for the year and to charge them the 'opportunity cost' of keeping that bed open. When the bed is occupied by a patient from a given directorate, additional costs for drugs and disposables are then calculated each day. Actual bed usage should be determined monthly and charges reviewed at the end of the financial year. Underusage could not be refunded, because payments are made for the opportunity to use the bed; but directorates using more than their allocated resource could re-imburse those using less.

Audit of process and outcome: standards and comparators

It is generally accepted that the process of medical care – the way in which care is provided – affects outcome. This is, however, an hypothesis that can be difficult to prove, because so many factors are involved and because so few medical procedures have been subject to rigorous validation. In consequence clinicians have tended to avoid process audit and concentrate on outcome instead. In practice, both methods should be used, as they will reveal different aspects of medical care.[24] Although the relationship between the two is not clear, it seems likely that given a choice between a high-quality process of care with a poor outcome, or poor process with a good outcome, most people would choose the latter.

Neither process nor outcome audit can be conducted without standards for comparison. Standards are comparators: that is, they are systems of measurement, which range from compliance with simple clinical protocols (e.g. hand-washing, documentation, pressure area care), to relatively sophisticated physiological scoring systems. It is in this latter area that intensive care has made significant contributions, with the development of scoring systems for measuring severity of illness.

Scoring systems

Severity of illness is an important concept because it is the first of three determinants of outcome from critical illness. The second is the extent of physiological reserve (previous health and age), and the third the specificity and timing of treatment. Severity of illness can be defined as 'the extent to which a disease process has affected physiological, psychological, or functional homeostatic mechanisms'. If a validated measure of illness severity is not incorporated in analyses that relate quality of care to outcome, the analyses will be flawed.[25] Scoring systems are constructed by calibrating them against a defined outcome event. This must be of sufficient frequency to be useful, relevant to the concept of 'severity' and free of observer bias. In intensive care mortality is a sufficiently frequent event to be a useful outcome measure, but this is not appropriate for general anaesthetic practice or medical disciplines where death is much less common; here scoring systems have used morbidity, functional disability, and quality of life as outcomes, except for high-risk groups. Costs may also be used as outcomes for measures of therapeutic intensity.

There are many severity scoring systems available for intensive care (Table 20.1). In general, scores are obtained by summing (or otherwise processing) a number of weighted variables selected for their predictive power. It is however important not to confuse the process of measurement (deriving the score) with that of prediction (applying it for a specific purpose). Scoring systems are useful because clinicians vary in their ability to assess both severity of illness and the degree to which their patients have responded to treatment.[57-59] Scoring systems provide an objective unitary

Table 20.1 *Selected scoring and classification systems*

Title and clinical area	Acronym	Theoretical basis	Reference
Intensive care			
Acute physiology and chronic health evaluation	APACHE	Physiological	Knaus 1981 (26)
APACHE second version	APACHE II	Physiological	Knaus 1985 (27)
Therapeutic intervention scoring system	TISS	Therapeutic activity	Cullen 1974 (28)
Omega	—	Therapeutic activity	Loriat 1988 (19)
Project of research in nursing	PRN	Nursing activity	Tilquin 1987 (29)
Simplified acute physiology score	SAPS	Modified APACHE II	Le Gall 1984 (30)
Organ system failures	OSF	Physiology + therapy	Knaus 1985 (31)
Sickness score	—	% change in APACHE II	Bion 1988 (32)
Riyadh intensive care programme	RIP	APACHE + OSF	Chang 1988 (33)
Mortality prediction modelling	MPM	Binary variables	Lemeshow 1988 (34)
Physiologic stability index	PSI	Physiological	Yeh 1984 (35)
Paediatric risk of mortality	PRISM	Derived from PSI	Pollack 1988 (36)
Hypoxic-ischaemic coma outcome	—	Clinical neurology	Levy 1985 (37)
Trauma			
Glasgow coma scale	GCS	Clinical neurology	Teasdale 1974 (38)
Paediatric GCS	—	Clinical neurology	Reilly 1988 (39)
Abbreviated injury scale	AIS	Anatomical	AAAM 1985 (40)
Injury severity score	ISS	Anatomical	Baker 1974 (41)
Triage index	TI	Physiological	Champion 1980 (42)
Trauma score	TS	Physiological	Champion 1981 (43)
Trauma score (revised)	rTS	Coded TS	Boyd 1987 (44)
Injury severity score + revised trauma score	TRISS	Combined	Boyd 1988 (44)
Paediatric trauma score	PTS	Physiological	Tepas 1988 (45)
DEFinitive methodology	DEF	MTOS TRISS statistics	Champion 1983 (46)
Burns			
The burn index	—	Burn area + age	Fuller 1980 (47)
Cardiology			
Coronary prognostic index	CPI	Clinical + lab tests	Norris 1969 (48)
Anaesthesia			
Goldman cardiac risk index	CRI	Clinical	Goldman 1977 (49)
American Society of Anesthesiologists status	ASA	Clinical grading	Dripps 1961 (50)
Critical incident analysis	—	Error reporting	Cooper 1984 (51)
Functional quality			
Sickness impact profile	SIP	Functional ability	Bergner 1981 (52)
Uniscale	—	Subjective reporting	Spitzer 1981 (53)
Karnofsky index	—	Physical activity	Hutchinson 1979 (54)
Others			
Sepsis score	SS	Clinical/physiological	Elebute 1983 (55)
Severity of illness index	—	Casemix	Horn 1986 (56)

measure of many different variables and prevent clinicians from attributing undue weight to any one in particular. They are of considerable importance for stratification for research, for the assessment of quality of care and for reducing prognostic uncertainty. Detsky *et al.*[60] have shown how prognostic uncertainty affects costs in intensive care, with the highest charges being incurred by the patients with the most uncertain outcomes. The costs of intensive care will need to be justified in the new internal market proposed by the UK government for the health service. Diagnosis-related groups will not be adequate for this purpose.[61] Similarly, crude mortality rates are an inappropriate measure of quality of care and variability in cost–benefit ratios between clinicians or units can only be explained if severity of illness is incorporated in the analysis.

In this review reference will be made to applications of the following scoring systems: the acute physiology and chronic health evaluation II system (APACHE II)[5,27,62] and related methods;[16,32,34,35] the injury severity score (ISS), trauma score (TS), and TRISS systems;[41,43,44] organ-system failures (OSFs);[31,63] mortality prediction modelling (MPM);[34,64] the Glasgow coma scale (GCS)[9,38,39,65-67] and the therapeutic intervention scoring system (TISS).[28,68] More detailed reviews of scoring systems are provided by Bion[69] and Miranda *et al.*[70]

It is the APACHE II and related SAPS methods that have obtained widest acceptance. In many ICUs data collection is delegated to the junior medical staff, and while this is acceptable, it does require constant supervision by a committed and experienced senior clinician. Problems are commonly experienced with the diagnostic categories for APACHE II, with determining the Glasgow coma score in sedated or potentially encephalopathic patients, and with the timing of data collection in relation to the influence of therapy ('lead-time bias'[71]). This last factor must be taken into account if outcome results are to be compared between units: the duration and place of therapy preceding admission to ICU must be clearly recorded, because prior intensive therapy will correct abnormal physiology, lower the score, and give a falsely optimistic predicted survival rate. Cross-stratification using a less therapy-sensitive method would help in this respect; OSFs or the MPM may be appropriate measures.

Protocols

It is easy to produce written standards and protocols, but difficult to implement and maintain them. Success is more likely if the standards are produced by consensus amongst all staff involved in intensive care, if specific individuals are charged with the development and monitoring of those standards, if staff retention is high, if standards become part of the culture of the unit and if there is responsible medical and nursing leadership of the unit. It is best to allow written policies to grow, rather than to produce a comprehensive, unreadable, and unread, document *ab initio*. Policies should include the areas defined in the list below (Box 20.1). New medical staff in particular should have these policies explained to them. Standards should not be limited in scope by inadequate resources, but should be used to identify deficiencies in structure and funding. They should not be seen necessarily as coercive or proscriptive: junior medical and nursing staff find written standards helpful in understanding their role in patient management. There must be some system for monitoring compliance with protocols. This is best done by the ICU consultants and senior nurses as a routine part of clinical work. The quality of care can only be maintained if those responsible for setting standards are seen to apply them to their own practice. Formal review should be conducted at weekly clinical meetings.

Written protocols are particularly important for the diagnosis of brain-stem death, for the medical management of potential organ donors and for the psychological support of their families. Intensive care units are the main source of solid organs for transplantation. ICU staff have a duty to ensure that organs are requested whenever possible. The survey by Gore *et al.*[72] showed that in 6% of brain-stem dead patients consent was not requested from relatives, a relatively small proportion. However, Salih and colleagues[10] have identified a much larger pool of potential donors amongst patients dying of acute cerebrovascular disease who were never referred to the ICU in their hospitals. They propose that these patients should be admitted to intensive care for elective mechanical ventilation so that organ donation can then be requested. The implementation of such a practice has been shown to double the organ donation rate.[73] While this approach makes practical sense in that it increases the chances of salvaging something good from personal tragedy, the ethics have not been publicly debated; neither has the effect on ICU staff morale or resources. Many ICUs are already hard-pressed to find space for the living.

Ensuring quality of care

The elements of good quality that are relevant to the process of care can be summarised as the 'four Cs': *competence, compassion, communication* and *costs* (as resource allocation). Clinicians and nurses have a direct influence on these factors, and this is where the training and supervision of junior staff are so important. Scoring systems, protocols, and standards are

---

Box 20.1   *Written ICU policies*

- Clinical responsibility for patient care
- Admission and discharge decisions
- Inter- and intra-hospital transfers
- Communication
- Support of relatives and staff
- Infection prevention and control
- Specific drug use (e.g. sedation regimens, antibiotics)
- Specific procedures (e.g. flotation catheters, X-rays)
- Prescription responsibilities
- Treatment limitation orders
- Brain death and organ-donation requests
- Record keeping
- Audit

---

crucial for assessing and monitoring quality of care, but what actually matters to individual patients and relatives is that they receive appropriate treatment delivered by competent and compassionate staff, at the minimum financial and psychological cost compatible with the best outcome. 'Appropriate' treatment might of course mean not admitting someone with an incurable disease, and the 'best' outcome could be a painless death. To ensure that the criteria of the 'four Cs' are met, standards of care have to be incorporated in an analytical framework that will help staff to provide the right treatment at the right time. Readers might like to consider the outline approach given in Appendix II, and revise it for their junior staff as they consider appropriate.

Markers of clinical competence

The items listed in Box 20.2 include certain measures that also fall into the category of outcome audit. Readmission rates and post-discharge mortality are not only potential markers of ward care, but may also indicate premature discharge from the ICU, or a lack of HDU facilities. Acute renal failure occurring after admission to the ICU means one of two things: either the underlying disease process has not been reversed, or the quality of organ-system support is inadequate. Critical incident monitoring was devised in the 1940s for aviation,[74] has been applied usefully in anaesthetic audit,[75] and has recently been described for intensive care audit[76] to show that most critical incidents are a consequence of human error (80%), and rarely result in serious consequences for the patient.

Box 20.2   *Markers of clinical competence*

● Severity-adjusted mortality rates
● Readmission rates
● Post-discharge mortality
● Critical incidents
● Complications/morbidity rates, such as:
    ● Acute renal failure occurring *after* ICU
      admission
    ● Cross infection rates
    ● Pressure sores

Confidentiality and a non-punitive approach are important if voluntary reporting is to be useful.

Monitoring resource allocation

This refers not to the costs of providing care (an outcome measure), but to the way in which intensive care resources are used. Obviously the two are related, but the emphasis is different. The data required will form part of a larger ICU information system, but can be considered at this point in relation to quality of care. Information systems are still very expensive, and until more resources are provided for intensive care audit the volume of data that can be collected will be limited. Minimum data are listed in Box 20.3.

Relating process to outcome in intensive care: costs and benefits

There are several outcome events that are relevant to intensive care (Box 20.4). Mortality has the advantage of being sufficiently frequent to be useful, easy to recognise, and cheap to document. All ICUs should be able to give absolute figures for both unit and hospital mortality rates. The ratio may give a crude estimate of prematurity of discharge from the unit as discussed above and of quality of care on the wards. Little further information can be derived without stratification for severity of illness and relating observed mortality rates to the expected rate for each severity band. Long-term survival and quality of survival should also be recorded and assessed, but this requires funding and the work cannot be undertaken without proper support. The same remarks apply to the routine detailed measurement of expenditure, though crude estimates of cost can be derived using surrogate measures such as the TISS or Omega systems.

Box 20.3 *Minimum data set for monitoring resource allocation*

● Source and diagnostic category of patient
● Age spectrum and percentage with chronically impaired health
● Emergency or elective admission
● Duration of mechanical ventilation
● Ratio of days of mechanical support to length of ICU stay
● Percentage of shifts where nurse:patient ratio was 1:1
● Percentage of readmissions
● Use of laboratory services

Box 20.4 *Outcome events*

● ICU mortality
● Hospital mortality
● Treatment limitation orders
● Six-month and one year survival rates
● Quality of survival indices
● Morbidity
● Costs (expenditure)
● Satisfaction

Once audit structures of the type outlined above are in place, it becomes easier to determine the efficiency and efficacy of intensive care, and to interpret the results of analyses.

Does intensive therapy improve survival?

This is not as naive a question as it may appear. There are still clinicians who regard the intensive care unit as an ante-chamber to the post-mortem room, occasionally with justification, and many of the procedures that constitute intensive care have not been independently validated.[77] Patients die despite intensive care because of one or more of three limiting factors: First of all, the severity of the acute illness may have irreversibly damaged the capacity for tissue repair. Secondly, the capacity for recovery is limited by chronically reduced physiological reserve. Finally, our understanding of the disease process, and hence the specificity of treatment, may be limited by our current state of knowledge. Knaus *et al.*[27] have shown how severity scoring can reveal the effect of the third factor, by plotting the relationship between physiological disturbance (APACHE II score) and mortality rates for three disease processes: sepsis, congestive heart failure and diabetic coma. Their study shows that understanding pathophysiology improves therapeutic potency, and the more specific the treatment the greater the potential for reversing life-threatening illness. Other studies have shown that the greater the extent of physiological correction, the better the chances of survival[32,33,78], providing further circumstantial evidence that organ-system support saves lives if it is combined with appropriate definitive treatment.

An alternative approach is to examine the outcome of patients who were denied access to intensive care because facilities were not available[79,80] or whose admission was delayed.[81] These three studies (the first two of which relate to neonatal intensive care) suggest that survival rates are increased if critically ill patients receive prompt intensive care. A study by Franklin *et al.*[82] has shown that the introduction of an intermediate care unit (HDU) reduced the death rate on ordinary wards by 25% and the incidence of cardiac arrests by 38.8%; although this study did not stratify the base population for severity of illness, the conclusion that high dependency care exerts a useful prophylactic effect is reasonable.

Does the process of care affect outcome from critical illness?

Outcome can be used as a way of identifying deficiencies in process. For example, pressure sores are well-recognised as a guide to the adequacy of nursing care. APACHE II scoring can reveal differences in survival rates between intensive care units with different management structures. In a study of thirteen hospitals,[5] the ICU with the highest observed:expected mortality ratio had no defined policies for patient care, poor communication and working relationships between staff, and no clinical or nursing direction, in marked contrast to the units in hospitals with a better performance. PSI scoring has been used to demonstrate that employing an intensivist can improve the efficiency and efficacy of paediatric intensive care,[83] and a retrospective study using APACHE II scoring has shown similar results for adult intensive care.[84] TRISS (the combination of the RTS and ISS) has been presented graphically to enable unexpected outcomes (non-survivors predicted to live, and *vice versa*) to be identified for further examination.[44,85] The coronary prognostic index has recently been used to show that outcome following myocardial infarction has improved between 1969 and 1983 despite the absence of any reduction in severity of illness;[86] possible explanations include improvement in treatment modalities, or failure of the index to account for a better chronic health status of the patients.

APACHE II scoring has been used to examine the process of care given to critically ill patients undergoing secondary transport to a centralised intensive care unit; such patients can be transported without physiological deterioration between hospitals provided that they are attended by experienced medical staff.[16] A separate study showed that complications during non-specialist transport are related to the inexperience of the attendants and not the severity of illness of the patients.[17]

Does intensive care merely enhance short-term survival?

APACHE II and TRISS scoring systems have been used in conjunction with measures of function to determine whether the process of intensive care has an impact on quality of life following discharge. In a study of 337 patients, Sage and his colleagues analysed 140 of 254 survivors who responded to a questionnaire about their quality of life.[87] They used the *sickness impact profile* (SIP) and *uniscale* as measures of function and life quality respectively, and found that the worst outcomes were associated with the highest TISS scores and total costs of hospital stay and to some extent with APACHE II score. They also found that while increasing age predicted post-discharge mortality, older survivors considered that they had a better quality of life than the younger ones. Chronic health status before admission also predicted life quality and survival following discharge, as others have shown.[88-90] Mahul *et al.*[90] have shown that for 295 survivors aged more than 70 years, the mortality at discharge from intensive care was 26.7%, rising at one year to 49%. Compared with an age-matched healthy population, mortality rates were increased five times for the first five months following discharge and three times for the second six months. Of the 103 survivors at one year, 70% had regained their previous health, 10% had improved, and 20% were worse; the *simplified acute physiology score* (SAPS) predicted long-term survival, but not quality of life. Zaren[91] followed up 980 Swedish patients for two years after discharge, and found that after six months life-expectancy was similar to that of age-matched controls. These studies suggest that the severity of acute physiological disturbance is the prime determinant of short-term (six month) survival, while impaired physiological reserve places constraints on the quality of that survival.

What determines resource allocation in intensive care?

Nursing salaries account for a large part of the fixed costs of intensive care, and the efficient use of nurses is therefore an important part of minimising those costs. Nursing dependency scores are still not well developed and can be cumbersome to use. They have been employed to demonstrate differences in perceived severity of illness and the distribution of nursing staff.[92,93] Miranda has proposed a model relating SAPS to TISS that identifies three levels of intensive care and the associated nursing ratios required,[70] but this model does not take into account the non-linearity of the relationship between severity of illness and the level of therapeutic support required. More work is required in this area.

Scoring systems may help clinicians to predict which patient groups will consume the most resources.[8] Cullen[28] has used TISS to show that survivors need less therapy as time passes, while the non-survivors continue to require high levels of support. Similar results have been obtained for critically ill children.[35] For neonatal intensive care, birthweight is a useful predictor of cost.[94] Length of ICU and hospital stay will influence costs[8,95] and severity indices can explain much of the variability that appears between diagnostic groups[61] in general hospital practice.

It is the emergency admissions who subsequently die who cost the most in intensive care. It is these patients who have the highest APACHE II and TISS scores. This relationship is not apparent for elective admissions,[87] who have generally received extensive therapeutic support before admission (lead-time bias). The relationship between severity of illness and costs is non-linear[95] and to some extent may reflect cultural attitudes to monitoring and the level of care. Diagnostic related groups (DRGs) have been shown to underestimate the true costs of caring for critically ill patients by a considerable margin.[96,97] Prognostic uncertainty is associated with high costs, as the study by Detsky *et al.*[60] showed, and clinicians should be aware of the marginal costs of caring for patients with known poor outcomes. A disease process with a mortality rate of 90 % means that nine non-survivors will have to be treated in order to obtain one survivor, and the costs of that survivor's care will include the costs of all ten patients. Gilbertson *et al.*[23] have shown that the costs per survivor of acute combined respiratory and renal failure were £67 000, but for all their survivors of intensive care the costs were £12 000, a relatively modest figure when compared with the current cost of other high-technology procedures such as cardiac surgery (around £4500) or liver transplantation (in excess of £30 000).

The adequacy of intensive care resources can be determined to some extent by looking for evidence of rationing: refused or deferred admissions, transfers, and premature discharges are useful data, though referral patterns do not of course detect the absolute need for intensive care. An additional method has been proposed by Stambouly *et al.*,[98] which looks for evidence of an inverse relationship between severity of illness and bed occupancy. They also proposed as a measure of efficiency the ratio between the number of patient-days provided to patients requiring unique ICU therapies, divided by the total number of patient-days. This approach requires very clear definitions of what is meant by low-risk 'monitor-only' patients and fails to include the nurse:patient ratio.

Can we identify groups of patients for whom intensive care is inappropriate?

There are broadly two groups of patients for whom intensive care brings no benefits: those who will die no matter how skilled the treatment; and those who would have survived equally well had they received standard ward care. The use of scoring systems to determine access to intensive care or duration of treatment has caused more anxiety than is justified, particularly when one considers the variability of clinical assessment.[57-59] Such systems assist, but do not substitute for, clinical judgement; and like any other form of medical technology they should be interpreted with caution. However, their use has been proposed as a method of reducing expenditure by identifying patients who cannot benefit from intensive care.[99,100] In this respect, Knaus has employed two useful phrases. The first is that, for the family of the patient kept alive by technology but for whom there is no hope of meaningful independent existence, this may indeed be 'a fate worse than death', and scoring systems may provide support for decisions to withdraw treatment. The second is that a prediction of death of 50% means that the clinician (or scoring system) is 'maximally uncertain' about the outcome, a strong indication that treatment should be pursued vigorously.

There are several studies comparing the predictive power of individual clinicians and nurses with that of the APACHE II score or its modifications, with varying results.[32,101-105] While such comparisons are of interest, it should be remembered that clinicians usually have the added advantage of observing the response to resuscitation before predicting outcome, whereas the APACHE II score, like many other scoring systems, is a static measure of the worst values in the first 24-hour period. This diminishes its predictive power, particularly when applied to single organ-system impairment such as left ventricular failure[106] or when used for making individual rather than group judgements about therapy.[107] APACHE III will probably address some of these problems by measuring response to treatment, the approach adopted by Bion[32] and by Chang.[33] As referred to earlier, the timing of data collection is important with physiologically based systems: data collected after treatment has started will increase the number of patients incorrectly predicted to survive by lowering the scores.[71] Chang and colleagues have compared dynamic risk modelling with clinical predictions, and have shown an advantage for the former.[102] The observation that incorporating diagnostic weights actually reduced prognostic power of the APACHE II system in a UK study[103] strengthens the arguments for using dynamic models that measure change in score with time.[32] It should also be remembered that measurement (deriving the score) is not the same thing as prediction (a specific application): the APACHE system is a valid measure of severity of illness, but in diabetic coma is a useless predictor of mortality because insulin now interferes (fortunately) with the relationship between the two.

Certain diagnostic groups have such a poor outcome from intensive care that a case could be made for excluding them altogether. Haematological malignancy in adults, in conjunction with respiratory failure and a high APACHE II score is an example;[108] similar results using the PSI have been reported for children.[109] The risks and benefits of intensive care should be discussed with these patients and their families prospectively, when they are receiving treatment for the underlying disease and not deferred until critical illness supervenes.

Is advanced chronological age an arbiter? Several studies have shown that premorbid health status is closely related to outcome[88,89,106,110] and it is likely that this is a more important determinant than age *per se*. Biological age and physiological reserve are interlinked. The health of the population from which the study group was drawn may explain differences in the studies that have examined the relationship between chronological age and outcome.[90,91,111-113] Chronological age is a reasonably good marker of biological age for large groups[27] but as predictors of outcome, previous health and functional independence are more important.[114]

Severity scoring can help to identify groups of low-risk patients who probably did not need intensive care,[83,84] but it may be less reliable when used prospectively to define criteria for admission to intensive care.[115] Organ-system failures are probably a more reliable guide to therapeutic dependence, and are less sensitive to the effects of therapeutic interventions. Patients at risk of developing an organ-system failure should receive high dependency care, particularly if they already have reduced physiological reserve. Adverse prognostic factors include physiological instability on admission to hospital, particularly in the presence of co-morbid diseases, the development of complications with progression of the disease after admission, and acute dyspnoea in patients with chronic pulmonary disease.[116] More precise criteria must wait until we have better methods of measuring severity of illness and physiological reserve.

Is auditing intensive care a useful exercise?

The etomidate story provides an example of the value of measures of severity of illness. Etomidate is a short-acting hypnotic that was licensed for intravenous anaesthesia during surgery, but which came to be used for long-term sedation of critically ill patients in intensive care. In 1983, the medical staff of an intensive care unit in Glasgow noted a near-doubling of mortality rates in their multiple trauma patients. By using the injury severity score they showed that the excess mortality was *not* a consequence of an increase in severity of injury.[117] This negative finding directed attention towards alternative explanations,[118] leading to the identification of the potent adrenocortical suppressant effect of etomidate.[119]

Scoring systems have also been used to audit the number of laboratory tests ordered in a paediatric intensive care unit, showing a relation with severity of illness.[120] The same paediatric scoring system has been used to show that differences in clinical practice between the USA and France result in similar outcomes,[121] and to demonstrate the beneficial effect on resource allocation and survival rates of employing a trained paediatric intensivist.[82] The study by Knaus *et al.*[5] referred to above is further evidence that severity-adjusted audit can identify deficiencies in process that adversely affect outcome. Other examples include the variability of decisions to withdraw therapy,[122] the wasteful use of parenteral nutrition,[123] the useless treatment of severely ill patients with haematological malignancy,[104] the expensive treatment of trauma patients who subsequently die,[100] and the unnecessary admission to intensive care of low-risk patients.[99,124] Differences have also been identified between hospitals in the use made of intensive care, suggesting inconsistencies in the selection of patients by clinicians.[125] Only one study[126] has examined the effect of providing clinicians with risk estimates based on the APACHE II score, and this showed a small but significant increase in the number of treatment-withdrawals.

Audit in intensive care embraces a wide range of activities that in general should form part of routine good clinical practice, and that require only modest resources, without the need for expensive computing systems. Providing evidence of the efficacy, and in particular the cost-efficacy, of intensive care, is less easy, however. For this purpose automated data collection systems are now being developed. These will make more efficient use of nursing time, and will also process some of the information needed for risk stratification, measurement of expenditure, and long-term follow up. Such systems cannot be funded on existing inadequate resources. Quality control costs money.

Appendix I   *Organ–system failures: definitions* Knaus *et al.*[32]

Cardiovascular failure: One or more of the following:

Heart rate	<55/min
Mean arterial blood pressure	<50 mmHg
Ventricular tachycardia or fibrillation	
Serum pH	<7.25 despite a P_aCO_2 <50 mmHg

Respiratory failure: One or more:

Respiratory rate	<5/min or >49/min
PaCo2	>49 mmHg
AaDO2	>349 mmHg [$A_aDO_2 = 713(F_iO_2 - P_aCo_2 - P_aO_2$]

Dependent on mechanical ventilation or CPAP after 3rd ICU day

Renal failure: One or more:

Urine output	<480 ml/24hrs (<7 ml/kg/24 hrs)
Serum urea	>35.7 μMol/l (>100 mg%)
Serum creatinine	>308 μMol/l (>3.49 mg%)

Haematologic failure: One or more:

WBC	<1000 cmm
Platelets	<20 000 cmm
Haematocrit	<20% (Hb <6gm)

Neurological failure:

Glasgow coma scale	<7 in the absence of sedative drugs

Notes: This system has not been validated or calibrated for paediatric intensive care. It is assumed that physiological derangements are a reflection of a disease process and not consequent upon a transient – and physiologically insignificant – misapplication of a drug, such as nitroprusside producing profound vasodilatation for a brief period.

Appendix II   *A structured approach to the critically ill patient*

1. Initial analysis:

Name the disease	*What is the primary diagnosis? History, examination.*
Define the pathological process	*Effect of disease on organ-system function. Trend analysis: rate of change.*
Place both in context of previous health status & medical history	*Effect of physiological reserve, co-morbidities, and age on expression of disease process. Has the patient made a known preference for treatment limitation?*
Review current therapy and response	*Is treatment appropriate? What effect has it had? What should be the next step?*

2. Initial action:

Provide appropriate organ support (OSS)	*Is oxygen delivery (DO_2) adequate, and is tissue oxygen consumption (VO_2) appropriate, for each organ-system?*
Perform investigations	*Confirm or refute the primary diagnosis, and determine the adequacy of organ-system support.*

3. Pause for thought:

Obtain and review results	*Do not wait for results: go and get them.*
Communicate with referring team	*Communication underlies good practice. Discuss results of tests, and appropriate action. Is diagnosis correct?*

4. Definitive action:

Establish new care plan	*In conjunction with referring team, ICU nurses.*
Apply definitive treatment	*Directed against the underlying disease. Refine OSS.*
Inform and involve relatives	*Must be spoken with each day by ICU consultant or SR, in preference to nurse.*
Documentation	*Keep a daily record of all the steps listed above.*

5. Repeat steps 2–4

In a continuous cycle.

References

1. Lassen, H. C. A. (1953). A preliminary report on the 1952 epidemic of poliomyelitis in Copenhagen with special reference to the treatment of acute respiratory insufficiency. *The Lancet*, i, 37–41.
2. Berenson, R. A. (1984). *Health Technology Case Study*: 28 *ICUs*. Congress of the United States Office of Technology Assessment.
3. Bams, J. L. & Miranda, D. R. (1985). Outcome and costs of intensive care. *Intensive Care Medicine*, 11, 234–241.
4. King's Fund Panel (1989). *Intensive Care in the United Kingdom*. London: King's Fund.
5. Knaus, W. A., Draper, E. A., Wagner, D. P. & Zimmerman, J. E. (1986): An evaluation of outcome from intensive care in major medical centers. *Annals of Internal Medicine*, 104, 410–418.
6. Hook, E. W., Horton, C. A. & Schaberg, D. R. (1983). Failure of intensive care unit support to influence mortality from pneumococcal bacteremia. *Journal of the American Medical Association*, 249, 1055–1057.
7. Rogers, R. M., Weiler, C. & Ruppenthal, B. (1972). Impact of the respiratory intensive care unit on survival of patients with acute respiratory failure. *Chest*, 62, 94–97.
8. Chassin, M. R. (1982). Costs and outcomes of medical intensive care. *Medical Care*, 20, 165–179.
9. Teasdale, G., Knill-Jones, R. & van der Sande, J. (1974). Observer variability in assessing impaired consciousness and coma. *Journal of Neurology, Neurosurgery, and Psychiatry*, 41, 603–610.
10. Salih, M. A. M., Harvey, I., Frankel, S., Coupe, D. J., Webb, M. & Cripps, H. A. (1991). Potential availability of cadaver organs for transplantation. *British Medical Journal*, 302, 1053–1055.
11. Standards sub-committee recommendations. *Standards for Intensive Care Units*. London: The Intensive Care Society (UK), Biomedica Ltd.
12. Knaus, W. A. (1991). Presentation to the intensive care society (UK) meeting, Swansea.
13. Dixon, R., Myers, F. & Rawlinson, C. (1988). *Intensive Therapy and Coronary Care Units: Postal Survey Report*. London: Medical Architecture Research Unit; Polytechnic of North London.
14. Association of Anaesthetists of Great Britain and Ireland Working Party (1988). *Provision for Intensive Care*. London: Association of Anaesthetists.
15. King's Fund Project Paper Nr 83 (1990). *Management and Resource Allocation in End-stage Renal Failure Units*. London: King's Fund Project.
16. Bion, J. F., Edlin, S. A., Ramsay, G., McCabe, S. & Ledingham, I.McA. (1985). Validation of a prognostic score in critically ill patients undergoing transport. *British Medical Journal*, 291, 432–434.
17. Bion, J. F., Wilson, I. H. & Taylor, P. A. (1988) Transporting critically ill patients by ambulance: audit by sickness scoring. *British Medical Journal*, 296, 170.
18. US Department of Health and Human Services (1979). *Planning for General Medical and Surgical Intensive Care Units: A Technical Assistance Document for Planning Agencies*. HRP-0101101, Washington.
19. Miranda, D. R., Williams, A. & Loirat, Ph. (eds) (1990). *Management of Intensive Care: Guidelines for Better Use of Resources*. Dordrecht: Kluwer Academic Publishers.

20. British Medical Association (1967). *Intensive Care. Planning Unit Report No* 1. London: BMA.
21. Wilson, L., Prescott, P. A. & Aleksandrowicz, L. (1988). Nursing: a major hospital cost component. *Health Services Research*, **22**, 773.
22. Working party recommendations (1990). *The Intensive Care Service in the UK*. Intensive Care Society (UK).
23. Gilbertson, A. A., Smith, J. M. & Mostafa, S.M (1991). The cost of an intensive care unit: a prospective study. *Intensive Care Medicine*, **17**, 204–208.
24. Brook, R. H. & Appel, F. A. (1973). Quality of care assessment: choosing a method for peer review. *New England Journal of Medicine*, **288**, 1323–1329.
25. Green, J., Wintfeld, N., Sharkey, P. & Passman, L. J. (1990). The importance of severity of illness in assessing hospital mortality. *Journal of the American Medical Association*, **263**, 241–246.
26. Knaus, W. A., Zimmerman, J. E., Wagner, D. P., Draper, E. A. & Lawrence, D. E. (1981). APACHE – acute physiology and chronic health evaluation: a physiologically based classification system. *Critical Care Medicine*, **9**, 591–603.
27. Knaus, W. A., Draper, E. A., Wagner, D. P. & Zimmerman, J. E. (1985). APACHE II: A severity of disease classification system. *Critical Care Medicine*, **10**, 818–829.
28. Cullen, D. J., Civetta, J. M., Briggs, B. A. & Ferrara, L. C. (1974). Therapeutic intervention scoring system: a method for quantitative comparison of patient care. *Critical Care Medicine*, **2**, 57–60.
29. Tilquin, C. (1987). *Equipe de Recherche Operationnelle en Sante*. Succursale, Montreal: Departement d'Administration de la Sante. Universite de Montreal.
30. Le Gall, J. R., Loirat, P., Alperovitch, A., Glaser, P., Granthill, C., Mathieu, D., Mercier, P., Thomas, R. & Villers, D. (1984). A simplified acute physiology score for ICU patients. *Critical Care Medicine*, **12**, 975–977.
31. Knaus, W. A., Draper, E. A., Wagner, D. P. & Zimmerman, J. E. (1985). Prognosis in acute organ-system failure. *Annals of Surgery*, **202**, 685–693.
32. Bion, J. F., Aitchison, T. C., Edlin, S. A. & Ledingham, IMcA. (1988). Sickness scoring and response to treatment as predictors of outcome from critical illness. *Intensive Care Medicine*, **14**, 167–172.
33. Chang, R. W. S., Jacobs, S. & Lee, B. (1988). Predicting outcome among intensive care unit patients using computerised trend analysis of daily APACHE II scores corrected for organ system failure. *Intensive Care Medicine*, **14**, 558–566.
34. Lemeshow, S., Teres, D., Avrunin, J. S. & Pastides, H. (1987). A comparison of methods to predict mortality of intensive care unit patients. *Critical Care Medicine*, **15**, 715–722.
35. Yeh, T. S., Pollack, M. M., Ruttimann, U. E., Holbrook, P. R. & Fields, A. I. (1984). Validation of a physiologic stability index for use in critically ill infants and children. *Pediatric Research*, **18**, 445.
36. Pollack, M. M., Ruttimann, U. E. & Getson, P. R. (1988). Pediatric risk of mortality (PRISM) score. *Critical Care Medicine*, **16**, 1110–1116.
37. Levy, D. E., Caronna, J., Singer, B. H., Lapinski, R. H., Frydman, H. & Plum, F. (1985). Predicting outcome from hypoxic-ischemic coma. *Journal of the American Medical Association*, **253**, 1420–1426.

38. Teasdale, G. & Jennett, B. (1974). Assessment of coma and impaired consciousness. A practical scale. *The Lancet*, **ii**, 81–84.
39. Reilly, P. L., Simpson, D. A. & Thomas, L. (1988). Assessing the conscious level in infants and young children: a paediatric version of the Glasgow coma scale. *Child's Nervous System*, **4**, 30–33.
40. American Association for Automotive Medicine (1985). *The Abbreviated Injury Scale (AIS)* – 1985 *Revision*. Des Plaines, Illinois: AAAM.
41. Baker, S. P., O'Neil, B., Haddon, W. & Long, W. (1974). The injury severity score: a method for describing patients with multiple injuries and evaluating emergency care. *Journal of Trauma*, **14**, 187–196.
42. Champion, H. R., Sacco, W. J. & Hannan, D. S. (1980). Assessment of injury severity: the triage index. *Critical Care Medicine*, **8**, 201–208.
43. Champion, H. R., Sacco, W. J., Carnazzo, A. J., Copes, W. & Fouty, W. J. (1981). Trauma score. *Critical Care Medicine*, **9**, 672–676.
44. Boyd, C. R., Tolson, M. A. & Copes, W. S. (1987). Evaluating trauma care: The TRISS method. *Journal of Trauma*, **27**, 370–378.
45. Tepas, J. J., Ramenofsky, M. L., Mollitt, D. L., Gans, B. M. & DiScala, C. (1988). The pediatric trauma score as a predictor of injury severity: an objective assessment. *Journal of Trauma*, **28**, 425–429.
46. Champion, H. R., Sacco, W. J. & Hunt, T. K. (1983). Trauma severity scoring to predict mortality. *World Journal of Surgery*, **7**, 4–11.
47. Feller, I., Tholen, D. & Cornell, R. G. (1980). Improvements in burn care, 1965 to 1979. *Journal of the American Medical Association*, **244**, 2074–2077.
48. Norris, R. M., Brandt, P. W. T. & Lee, A. J. (1969). Mortality in a coronary-care unit analysed by a new coronary prognostic index. *The Lancet*, **i**, 278–281.
49. Goldman, L., Caldera, D. L., Nussbaum, S. R. *et al.* (1977). Multifactorial index on cardiac risk in noncardiac surgical procedures. *New England Journal of Medicine*, **297**, 845.
50. Dripps, R. D., Lamont, A. & Eckenhoff, J. E. (1961). The role of anesthesia in surgical mortality. *Journal of the American Medical Association*, **178**, 261.
51. Cooper, J. B., Newbower, R. S. & Kitz, R. J. (1984). An analysis of major errors and equipment failures in anesthesia management: considerations for prevention and detection. *Anesthesiology*, **60**, 34–42.
52. Bergner, M., Bobbitt, R. A., Carter, W. B. & Gibson, B. S. (1981). The sickness impact profile: development and final revision of a health status measure. *Medical Care*, **19**, 787–805.
53. Spitzer, W. O., Dobson, A. J., Hall, J., Chesterman, E., Levi, J., Shepherd, R., Battista, R. N. & Catchlove, B. R. (1981). Measuring the quality of life of cancer patients: a concise QL – index for use by physicians. *Journal of Chronic Diseases*, **34**, 585.
54. Hutchinson, T. A., Boyd, N. F., Feinstein, A. R., Gonda, A., Hollomby, D. & Rowat, B. (1979). Scientific problems in clinical scales, as demonstrated by the Karnofsky index of performance status. *Journal of Chronic Diseases*, **32**, 661–666.
55. Elebute, E. A. & Stonor, H. B. (1983). The grading of sepsis. *British Journal of Surgery*, **70**, 29–31.
56. Horn, S. D. & Horn, R. A. (1986). Reliability and validity of the severity of illness index. *Medical Care*, **24**, 159–178.
57. de Saintonge, D. M. C., Kirwan, J. R., Evans, S. J. W. & Crane, G. J. (1988). How can we design trials to detect clinically important changes in disease severity? *British Journal of Clinical Pharmacology*, **26**, 355–362.

58. Jachuk, S. J., Brierley, H., Jachuck, S. & Willcox, P. M. (1982). The effect of hypotensive drugs on quality of life. *Journal of the Royal College of General Practitioners*, **32**, 103–105.

59. Poses, R. M., Bekes, C., Copare, F. J. & Scott, W. E. (1989). The answer to 'What are my chances, Doctor?' depends on whom is asked: Prognostic disagreement and inaccuracy for critically ill patients. *Critical Care Medicine*, **17**, 827–833.

60. Detsky, A. S., Stricker, S. C., Mulley, A. G. & Thibault, G. E. (1981). Prognosis, survival, and the expenditure of hospital resources for patients in an intensive-care unit. *New England Journal of Medicine*, **305**, 667–672.

61. Horn, S. D., Bulkley, G., Sharkey, P. D., Chambers, A. F., Horn, R. A. & Schramm, C. J. (1985). Interhospital differences in severity of illness: problems for prospective payment based on diagnosis-related groups (DRGS). *New England Journal of Medicine*, **313**, 20–24.

62. Wagner, D. P., Knaus, W. A. & Draper, E. A. (1986). Physiologic abnormalities and outcome from acute disease. Evidence for a predictable relationship. *Archives of Internal Medicine*, **146**, 1389–1396.

63. Pine, R. W., Wertz, Lennard, E. S., Dellinger, E. P., Carrico, C. J. & Minshew, B. H. (1983). Determinants of organ malfunction or death in patients with intra-abdominal sepsis. *Archives of Surgery*, **118**, 242–249.

64. Lemeshow, S., Teres, D., Avrunin, J. S. & Pastides, H. (1987). A comparison of methods to predict mortality of intensive care unit patients. *Critical Care Medicine*, **15**, 715–722.

65. Jennett, B., Teasdale, G., Braakman, R., Minderhoud, J. & Knill-Jones, R. (1976). Predicting outcome in individual patients after severe head injury. *The Lancet*, **i**, 1031–1034.

66. Morray, J. P., Tyler, D. C., Jones, T. K., Stuntz, J. T. & Lemire, R. J. (1984). Coma scale for use in brain-injured children. *Critical Care Medicine*, **12**, 1018–1020.

67. Murray, G. D. (1985). Use of an international data bank to compare outcome following severe head injury in different centres. *Statistics in Medicine*, **5**, 103–112.

68. Cullen, D. J. (1977). Results and costs of intensive care. *Anesthesiology*, **47**, 203–216.

69. Bion, J. F. (1991). Scoring systems in intensive care. In *Recent Advances in Anaesthesia and Analgesia* 17, ed. A. Adams & R. Atkinson. London: Churchill Livingstone.

70. Miranda, D. R. & Langrehr, D. (1990). National and regional organisation. In *Management of Intensive Care. Guidelines for Better Use of Resources*, ed. D. R. Miranda & D. Langrehr. Dordrecht: Kluwer Academic Publishers.

71. Dragsted, L., Jorgensen, J., Jensen, N-H., Bonsing, E., Jacobsen, E., Knaus, W. A. & Qvist, J. (1989). Interhospital comparisons of patient outcome from intensive care: Importance of lead-time bias. *Critical Care Medicine*, **17**, 418–422.

72. Gore, S. M., Hinds, C. J. & Rutherford, A. J. (1989). Organ donation from intensive care units in England. *British Medical Journal*, **299**, 1193–1197.

73. Feest, T. G., Riad, H. N., Collins, C. H., Golby, M. G. S., Nicholls, A. J., Hamad, S. N. (1990). Protocol for increasing organ donation after cerebrovascular deaths in a district general hospital. *The Lancet*, **335**, 1133–1135.

74. Flanagan, J. C. (1954). The critical incident technique. *Psychology Bulletin*, **51**, 327–358.

75. Cooper, J. B., Newbower, R. S., Long, C. D. & McPeek, B. (1978). Preventable anesthesia mishaps: a study of human factors. *Anesthesiology*, **49**, 399–406.
76. Wright, D., Mackenzie, S. J., Buchan, I., Cairns, C. S. & Price, L. E. (1991). Critical incidents in the intensive therapy unit. *The Lancet*, **338**, 676–678.
77. NIH Consensus Development Conference (1983). Statement on critical care medicine. *Journal of the American Medical Association*, **250**, 798–804.
78. Pilz, G. & Werdan, K. (1990). Cardiovascular parameters and scoring systems in the evaluation of response to therapy in sepsis and septic shock. *Infection*, **18**, 253–262.
79. Sidhu, H., Heasley, R. N., Patterson, C. C., Halliday, H. L. & Thompson, W. (1989). Short term outcome in babies refused perinatal intensive care. *British Medical Journal*, **299**, 647–649.
80. Powell, T. G. & Pharoah, P. O. D. (1987). Regional neonatal intensive care: bias and benefit. *British Medical Journal*, **295**, 690–692.
81. Purdie, J. A. M., Ridley, S. A. & Wallace, P. G. M. (1990). Effective use of regional intensive care units. *British Medical Journal*, **300**, 79–81.
82. Franklin, C. M., Rackow, E. C., Mamdani, B., Nightingale, S., Burke, G. & Weil, M. H. (1988). Decreases in mortality on a large urban medical service by facilitating access to critical care. An alternative to rationing. *Archives of Internal Medicine*, **148**, 1403–1405.
83. Pollack, M. M., Katz, R. W., Ruttimann, U. E. & Getson, P. R. (1988). Improving the outcome and efficiency of intensive care: the impact of an intensivist. *Critical Care Medicine*, **16**, 11–17.
84. Brown, J. J. & Sullivan, G. (1989). Effect on ICU mortality of a full-time critical care specialist. *Chest*, **96**, 127–129.
85. Spence, M. T., Redmond, A. D. & Edwards, J. D. (1988). Trauma audit – the use of TRISS. *Health Trends*, **20**, 94–97.
86. Hopper, J. L., Pathik, B., Hunt, D. & Chan, W. W. (1989). Improved prognosis since 1969 of myocardial infarction treated in a coronary care unit: lack of relationship with changes in severity. *British Medical Journal*, **299**, 892–896.
87. Sage, W. M., Rosenthal, M. H. & Silverman, J. F. (1986). Is intensive care worth it? – an assessment of input and outcome for the critically ill. *Critical Care Medicine*, **14**, 777–782.
88. Yinnon, A., Zimran, A. & Hershko, C. (1989). Quality of life and survival following intensive medical care. *Quarterly Journal of Medicine (New Series 71)*, **264**, 347–357.
89. Goldstein, R. L., Campion, E. W., Thibault, G. E., Mulley, A. G. & Skinner, E. (1986). Functional outcomes following medical intensive care. *Critical Care Medicine*, **14**, 783.
90. Mahul, Ph., Perrot, D., Tempelhoff, G., Gaussorgues, Ph., Jospe, R., Ducreux, J. C., Dumont, A., Motin, J., Auboyer, C. & Robert, D. (1991). Short and long-term prognosis, functional outcome following ICU for elderly. *Intensive Care Medicine*, **17**, 7–10.
91. Zaren, B. & Bergstrom, R. (1989). Survival compared to the general population and changes in health status among intensive care patients. *Acta Anaesthesiologica Scandinavica*, **33**, 6–12.
92. Lee, T. H., Cook, F., Fendrick, A. M., Shammash, J. B., Wolfe, E. P., Weisberg, M. C. & Goldman, L. (1990). Impact of initial triage decisions on nursing intensity for patients with acute chest pain. *Medical Care*, **28**, 737–745.

93. Thompson, J. D. (1984). The measurement of nursing intensity. *Health Care Financing Review*, **6S**, 47.
94. Tudehope, D. I., Lee, W., Harris, F. & Addison, C. (1989). Cost-analysis of neonatal intensive and special care. *Australian Paediatric Journal*, **25**, 61–65.
95. Rapoport, J., Teres, D., Lemeshow, S., Avrunin, J. S. & Haber, R. (1990). Explaining variability of cost using a severity-of-illness measure for ICU patients. *Medical Care*, **28**, 338–348.
96. Bekes, C., Fleming, S. & Scott, W. E. (1988). Reimbursement for intensive care services under diagnosis-related groups. *Critical Care Medicine*, **16**, 478–481.
97. Kreis, D. J., Augenstein, D., Civetta, J. M., Gomez, G. A., Vopal, J. J. & Byers, P. M. (1987). Diagnosis related groups and the critically injured. *Surgery, Gynaecology and Obstetrics*, **165**, 317–322.
98. Stambouly, J. J., Pollack, M. M. & Ruttimann, U. E. (1991). An objective method to evaluate rationing of pediatric intensive care beds. *Intensive Care Medicine*, **17**, 154–158.
99. Henning, R. J., McClish, D., Daly, B., Nearman, H., Franklin, C. & Jackson, D. (1987). Clinical characteristics and resource utilisation of ICU patients: implications for organization of intensive care. *Critical Care Medicine*, **15**, 264.
100. Fischer, R. P., Flynn, T. C., Miller, P. W. & Rowlands, B. J. (1985). The economics of fatal injury: dollars and sense. *Journal of Trauma*, **25**, 746–750.
101. Kruse, J. A., Thill-Baharozian, M. C. & Carlson, R. W. (1988). Comparison of clinical assessment with APACHE II for predicting mortality risk in patients admitted to a medical intensive care unit. *Journal of the American Medical Association*, **260**, 1739–1742.
102. Chang, R. W. S., Lee, B., Jacobs, S. & Lee, B. (1989). Accuracy of decisions to withdraw therapy in critically ill patients: clinical judgement versus a computer model. *Critical Care Medicine*, **17**, 1091–1097.
103. Marks, R. J., Simons, R. S., Blizzard, R. A. & Browne, D. R. G. (1991). Predicting outcome in intensive therapy units – a comparison of Apache II with subjective assessment. *Intensive Care Medicine*, **17**, 159–163.
104. Brannen, A. L., Godfrey, L. J. & Goetter, W. E. (1989). Prediction of outcome from critical illness. A comparison of clinical judgement with prediction rule. *Archives of Internal Medicine*, **149**, 1083–1086.
105. McClish, D. K. & Powell, S. H. (1989). How well can physicians estimate mortality in a medical intensive care unit? *Medical Decision Making*, **9**, 125–132.
106. Fedullo, A. J., Swinburne, A. J., Wahl, G. W. & Bixby, K. R. (1988). APACHE II score and mortality in respiratory failure due to cardiogenic pulmonary failure. *Critical Care Medicine*, **16**, 1218–1221.
107. Hopefl, A. W., Taafe, C. & Stephenson, G. C. (1989). Failure of APACHE II alone as a predictor of mortality in patients receiving total parenteral nutrition. *Critical Care Medicine*, **17**, 414–417.
108. Lloyd-Thomas, A. R., Wright, I., Lister, T. A. & Hinds, C. J. (1988). Prognosis of patients receiving intensive care for life-£threatening medical complications of haematological malignancy. *British Medical Journal*, **296**, 1025–1029.
109. Sivan, Y., Schwartz, P. H., Schonfeld, T., Cohen, I. J. & Newth, C. J. L.

(1991). Outcome of oncology patients in the pediatric intensive care unit. *Intensive Care Medicine*, **17**, 11–15.

110. Slater, M. A., James, O. F., Moore, P. G. & Leeder, S. R. (1986). Costs, severity of illness and outcome in intensive care. *Anaesthesia and Intensive Care*, **14**, 381–389.

111. McClish, D. K., Powell, S. H., Montenegro, H. & Nochomovitz, M. (1987). The impact of age on utilization of intensive care resources. *Journal of the American Geriatric Society*, **35**, 983–988.

112. Wu, A. W., Rubin, H. R. & Rosen, M. J. (1990). Are elderly people less responsive to intensive care? *Journal of the American Geriatric Society*, **38**, 621–627.

113. Ridley, S., Jackson, R., Findlay, J. & Wallace, P. (1990). Long term survival after intensive care. *British Medical Journal*, **301**, 1127–1130.

114. Anonymous (1991). Intensive care for the elderly. *The Lancet*, **338**, 209–210.

115. Franklin, C. M., Rackow, E. C., Mamdani, B., Burke, G. & Weil, M. H. (1990). Triage considerations in medical intensive care. *Archives of Internal Medicine*, **150**, 1455–1459.

116. Sax, F. L. & Charlson, M. E. (1987). Medical patients at high risk for catastrophic deterioration. *Critical Care Medicine*, **15**, 510–515.

117. Watt, I. & Ledingham I.McA. (1984). Mortality amongst multiple trauma patients admitted to an intensive therapy unit. *Anaesthesia*, **39**, 973–981.

118. Ledingham, I.McA. & Watt, I. (1983). Influence of sedation on mortality in critically ill multiple trauma patients. *The Lancet*, **i**, 1270.

119. Lambert, A., Mitchell, R., Frost, J., Ratcliffe, J. G. & Robertson, W. R. (1983). Direct in vitro inhibition of adrenal steroidogenesis by etomidate. *The Lancet*, **ii**, 1085–1086.

120. Klern, S. A., Pollack, M. M. & Getson, P. R. (1990). Cost, resource utilization, and severity of illness in intensive care. *Journal of Pediatrics*, **116**, 231–237.

121. Davis, A. L., Pollack, M. M., Cloup, M., Cloup, I. & Wilkinson, J. D. (1989). Comparisons of French and USA pediatric intensive care units. *Resuscitation*, **17**, 143–152.

122. Zimmerman, J. E., Knaus, W. A., Sharpe, S. M., Anderson, A. S., Draper, E. A. & Wagner, D. P. (1986). The use and implications of *Do Not Resuscitate* orders in intensive care units. *Journal of the American Medical Association*, **255**, 351–356.

123. Chang, R. W. S., Jacobs, S. & Lee, B. (1986). Use of APACHE II severity of disease classification to identify intensive-care-unit patients who would not benefit from total parenteral nutrition. *The Lancet*, **i**, 1483–1487.

124. Wagner, D. P., Knaus, W. A. & Draper, E. A. (1987). Identification of low-risk monitor admissions to medical-surgical ICUs. *Chest*, **92**, 423.

125. Zimmerman, J. E., Knaus, W. A., Judson, J. A., Havill, J. H., Trubuhovich, R. V. & Draper, E. A. (1988). Patient selection for intensive care: a comparison of New Zealand and United States Hospitals. *Critical Care Medicine* , **16**, 318–326.

126. Knaus, W. A., Rauss, A., Alperovitch, A., Le-Gall, J. R., Loirat, P., Patois, E. & Marcus, S. E. (1990). Do objective-estimates of chances for survival influence decisions to withhold or withdraw treatment? *Medical Decision Making*, **10**, 163–171.

21

Medical audit: lessons from the USA

ROBERT B. KELLER

Introduction

This chapter will describe the development of quality assurance (audit) measures and outcomes research in the United States. Over the past two decades a number of problems have developed in the US health care system, many of which have provided a strong stimulus to push participants toward a vigorous assessment of the quality, appropriateness and effectiveness of medical care in this country.

Health care in the United States is recognised as generally being innovative and of high quality. The financing mechanisms in our system have encouraged vast amounts of research and technological innovation. It is well known that the US system is the most expensive in the world, spending $2051 per capita as opposed to $758 in England and $1483 in Canada (calculated in US dollars for 1987).[1] It is also recognised that while we provide abundant medical care for most of our citizens, some 37 million Americans are at great risk because they have no health insurance coverage.

We have also learned that much of the care we provide may not be necessary, appropriate, or effective. As a result, we appear to be expending too many resources on care for many people while a large number go without even minimal levels of care. The United States expenditure of 11.6% of gross national product on medical care is the highest in the world, and costs continue to inflate at a rate faster than the rest of our economy. Although not all policy makers agree, there is a strong feeling that the current level of spending is too high and the US economy cannot continue to allocate increasing resources on health care and still remain competitive in the international marketplace. Many solutions have been proposed, including a complete overhaul of the health care financing

339

system, perhaps adopting national health insurance similar to that of Canada.

In the meantime a number of alternative solutions have been proposed and implemented, all of which focus on the cost of care. The development of *health maintenance organizations* (HMOs), prospective payment to hospitals under the Medicare system (*diagnostic related groups* – DRGs) and complex systems of cost control such as pre-admission authorisation, second surgical opinions and concurrent review have all been instituted. The *health care financing administration* attempts to monitor physician and hospital performance in the Medicare program through state based *professional review organizations* (PROs), spending over $250 million annually on that activity alone.

Cost shifting, a phenomenon by which health care costs which are unfunded or under funded are transferred from one group to another, has become a major problem in the US. In addition to those who cannot pay, large public programmes such as Medicare and Medicaid do not pay their total share of costs to providers. These costs are shifted to the private sector resulting in major increases in health care costs beyond those actually incurred by this group. This problem has driven business and insurers to attempt to find ways of decreasing their burden – usually by decreasing and limiting insurance coverage, subscribing to managed health care programs, self insurance, and shifting costs to the individual.

Physicians in the US feel trapped in an economic system that they did not create and one in which their ability to practice medicine as they think best is becoming progressively limited. The Federal Government's new Medicare reimbursement system (resource-based relative value scale),[2] while generally endorsed by the medical profession, has caused great concern and the medical profession remains concerned about continued federal efforts to limit physician fees.[3]

In short, no one is very happy about the current state of the American health care system. There are no simple answers. While some cost-cutting efforts may have been marginally effective, overall costs have continued to rise.[4] Given that new technology, an aging population, and the AIDS epidemic will require increased funding, we are unable to even calculate what we ought to be spending on health care in the US. In the face of this escalating problem are there any solutions in sight? For at least one segment of this problem there does seem to be an opportunity to respond to some of the many challenges confronting medical care in the United States.

There is powerful evidence that much of what we do in medicine may be inappropriate and excessive. Marked geographic variations in utilisation of medical and surgical care have demonstrated that physicians lack certainty about much of what they do and what the outcomes of their treatments are.[5] The cost tag applied to this problem alone is very high. Wennberg *et al.*[6] have calculated that (in 1982) the variations in medical care utilisation between the cities of Boston, Massachusetts and New Haven, Connecticut resulted in $2647 in Medicare reimbursements for Boston residents as compared to $1561 for New Havenites (41 % higher in Boston).

We feel that the dilemmas in health care demonstrated by the Boston–New Haven example need resolution and unlike some issues, there are potential solutions. This chapter focuses on our approach and its relevance to other health care systems.

Medical audit in the USA

'Audit' can take many forms. Typically, it has been carried out in hospitals through such activities as morbidity and mortality conferences, tissue conferences, quality assurance committees, etc. In the United States peer review organisations carry out audit of Medicare beneficiaries utilizing a variety of mechanisms such as pre-admission certification and quality measurement 'screens' to check specific cases for admission criteria, length of stay, complications, readmission and mortality. Many other audit or utilisation techniques, both public and proprietary, have been developed to measure hospital and physician quality. The major driving force underlying many of these systems is the attempt to save money.

This type of review is done at the 'micro' level. That is, assessment is carried out on individual cases and physicians. While such forms of audit may be useful in assessing quality and appropriateness of care provided to individual patients, unit case review is limited in scope. It does not assess general patterns of utilisation. It may not indicate if the care provided was necessary or the best choice of several alternatives. It does not measure the patients' preferences of choice of treatment, and it does not measure the long-term outcome of treatment intervention.

Small area analysis (SAA) is a very different form of audit. This methodology is based on epidemiology and considers rates of health care provided to people based on their area of residence. It permits an accurate measurement of the overall utilisation of care in specific geographic areas. The type and level of care can then be compared to other areas within states, countries, and between nations. We will focus on this form of audit, discussing its development in the US and abroad and how the fact of marked variation in practice patterns has lead to the development of a major programme in outcomes research in the United States.

Small area analysis

The concept of *small area analysis* (SAA) was pioneered by Wennberg and Gittelsohn.[7] The method is based on epidemiologic measurements of health care. 'Small areas', or hospital market areas, are defined as groups of towns (or other geographic zip code units) within which are located one or more hospitals that provide the plurality of in-patient hospital discharges of local residents. Standard discharge data sets, containing essential demographic and medical information such as diagnoses, operations, length of stay, type of discharge and costs, are computerised. It is then possible to calculate per capita rates of various diagnoses and procedures and to compare those rates to average rates for the state, region and nation.

By measuring the medical care provided to populations in this manner it is possible to assess accurately how much and what kind of care people are receiving. Studying individual physician or hospital rates of care does not provide this information because the denominator – the size of the population served – is unknown.

When Wennberg and his associates began to analyse data in this way, the findings were surprising. They learned that there are marked variations in the utilisation of health care for most medical and surgical causes of hospitalisation. For a few conditions, such as heart attack, hip fracture, gastrointestinal bleeding, and hernia repair, rates of admission are quite consistent across areas. However, almost all elective surgical procedures show wide variations; and medical diagnoses (such as pulmonary disease, gastroenteritis, medical back problems, etc.) demonstrate variations which are even greater than surgical admissions.[6]

These variations persist after careful analysis and adjustment for age, sex and other factors. In other words, they are real and they indicate a remarkable degree of inconsistency in the delivery of health care. Similar research has been carried out in Canada, Great Britain, and Scandinavia. These countries demonstrate similar patterns, indicating that variations are not driven by the structure or financing of the health care system.[5]

Variations are calculated by establishing an average rate of admission for a given region and comparing each area to that average. However, one should not conclude that the average rate is the correct rate. In fact the 'right rate' is most difficult to determine. It does seem apparent in the US, at least, that very often high rates of utilisation are indicative of excessive utilisation. Experience in Maine supporting this finding will be further described. The Boston–New Haven analysis mentioned previously indicates that overall residents of Boston utilize 53 % more medical care than people residing in New Haven[6] – a remarkable difference in resource utilisation with no obvious differences in patient outcome.

Why are there variations?

A number of possible explanations for practice pattern variations have been proposed. First, there may be errors in the data themselves. Small area analysis is carried out using large computerised databases, and there are opportunities for various coding and input errors. There are techniques to check the accuracy of data and more mature data systems appear to be quite accurate.

Secondly, there may be differences in the populations and disease incidence that are not corrected for in analysis of the database. For example, an area with endemic tuberculosis would be expected to produce much higher admission rates relative to that condition than an area where the incidence was very low. If this was not recognised, incorrect conclusions could be drawn.

Thirdly, there may be significant differences in health care resources from one area to another. The availability of hospital beds, physicians and other health care workers appears to positively influence utilisation. Work in Maine, not yet completed, and the previously noted Boston–New Haven analysis, both suggest that available resources may be a powerful factor in producing their own demand.

Fourthly, and perhaps the most important, is physician 'uncertainty' about the best way to treat and manage most conditions in medicine. Variations in practice patterns make clear the fact that the decision to admit or operate on a patient is made in very different ways and with different frequency among physicians. While there are financial incentives for American surgeons to do surgical procedures, variations are noted to exist in financing systems such as the US Veterans Administration, the military services and HMOs where physicians are salaried and personal income is independent of the volume of surgery performed. Thus, variations cannot be entirely explained on the basis of physicians' desire for financial reward. Further, variations in admissions for non-surgical conditions are even more marked than those for surgery.[6] The financial incentive theory is even more suspect here, in as much as physician reimbursement for these conditions does not differ markedly with the site of treatment. It appears that, in spite of fairly standardised medical education and specialty training, board certification and continuing medical education, there remains a remarkable lack of consensus and consistency among practitioners as to the best way to treat and manage the majority of medical and surgical problems that we confront on a daily basis.

A problem and an opportunity

Variations in practice patterns provide physicians with both a problem and an opportunity. The problem lies in the fact of variations. When confronted with marked differences in medical admissions and surgical rates that can be explained only on the basis of physician uncertainty and differing use of hospital and medical care facilities, the profession has two choices. It can ignore the problem and accept the consequences of corrective actions others will take – generally actions that doctors do not like because they involve increasing regulation and may not contribute in any way to the quality of medical care. The alternative is for physicians to accept and acknowledge that variations present a major challenge to the medical profession. We must concede that we practice medicine in very different patterns and work toward resolving the issues that have been raised.

By assuming a pro-active role, physicians have a great opportunity to resolve issues of uncertainty, improve quality of care, control costs and maintain a pre-eminent role as advocates of patient care and medical quality. Many of the problems that surround health care in the US and elsewhere are beyond the control of physicians. But dealing with practice variations is very much within the profession's capability.

Outcomes research

As medical groups and researchers in the US have attempted to study and deal with variations and uncertainty, a new field of 'outcomes research' has developed. This new form of health services research focuses on patient oriented, quality of life measurements of various treatments. Roper has described the essential elements of this process as the *'effectiveness agenda'*.[8]

Evaluation of the current medical literature indicates that it tends to be 'process' oriented and often lacks essential statistical controls and standards.[9] The result is a scientific literature that may not provide practitioners with the information they need and this may add to the uncertainty and variations that are observed. Outcomes research focuses directly on patients' perceptions of their care and outcomes and less on the process of care.

The Federal Government has undertaken a major initiative in this area. A new agency in the US Public Health Service, *The Agency for Health Care Policy and Research* (AHCPR), has been created to carry out wide-ranging research into the effectiveness of many aspects of medical care. Among its several missions is the funding of outcomes research projects.[10] These projects will carry out in-depth research into the benefits and outcomes of many aspects of medical care. For example, the currently funded major multi-centre *Prospective Outcomes Research Teams* (PORTS) will study cataract, heart attack, heart surgery, prostatism, low back pain and knee arthritis, hip arthritis and hip fracture, gall bladder disease, diabetes and pneumonia. In addition to carrying out small area analysis, database research, literature reviews, and prospective patient outcome studies, the PORT teams are expected to develop decision analytic models and disseminate new information.

Another initiative of the AHCPR is the development of practice guidelines with a goal towards providing the profession with current advice to assist in patient care. Guidelines are under development by AHCPR, the American Medical Association, and many medical specialty societies. It is recognised that for much of medical care, truly effective guidelines must await outcomes research.

The Maine Medical Assessment Foundation (MMAF)

The work of the Maine Medical Assessment Foundation provides an example of using medical audit to deal with the issues and concepts discussed previously. In the mid 1970s Wennberg, Hanley and Soule began to study small area variations in the state of Maine.[11] This work confirmed earlier research by Wennberg,[12] but in this instance Dr Hanley went beyond the data analysis and began to search for ways to encourage physicians to respond to the issues raised by variations. The result was the development of the *Maine Medical Assessment Program* (later incorporated as the MMAF).

One of the early lessons learned by Hanley and his co-workers was that understanding and dealing with variations was best done through specialty physician study groups. The complexity of modern medicine makes it difficult for broad-based physician groups such as hospital medical staff, county medical societies, etc. to deal with complex medical issues. Specialty groups on the other hand easily understand the clinical conditions and problems under focus and can come to the grips with the issues raised by variations. The specialty study group model has worked well, and the foundation continues to work with existing groups and add new ones.

Presenting information about practice variations is challenging and often threatening to doctors. Practitioners are unaware of their rates of medical activity in comparison with peers. Although the data are not presented in a form specific to single individuals, participants in these sessions quickly recognise how their practices rank against others. There is a learning curve for each study group, and significant initial doubt, anxiety, and resentment is common.

The Maine programme has emphasised that study group activities are confidential and educational. Over time a significant degree of trust has developed between practising physicians and the foundation. Once that trust is gained doctors become willing participants in the process. The importance of gaining the trust and confidence of physicians in this process cannot be over-emphasised. While it is admitted that the state-wide average rate does not represent the 'right rate' it does become obvious to physicians that unexplained wide variations in rates simply do not make sense, regardless of their cause. Once doctors understand and accept this evidence they are almost always eager participants in the process.

Each study group carefully analyses the data presented. Explanations are sought. Frequently, study groups request refinements of ICD9-CM codes and other details that can be abstracted from the database. The clinical conditions under study are discussed and debated. There may be disagreement about the clinical management of certain conditions. Questions may be raised about differing needs of communities, differences in the infrastructure of the local health care system that may influence practice patterns and other factors. More often than not, no clear explanation of the variations can be developed.

This portion of study group activity is known as 'feedback' and is an essential ingredient in the process. Bringing groups of specialists together, educating them about variations, convincing them that the variations are real, and encouraging peer discussion and debate in a non-threatening, non-regulatory, confidential atmosphere has had a remarkable and almost consistent effect. Physicians who are high outliers consistently and rapidly alter their practice patterns and utilisation rates begin to drop. It appears

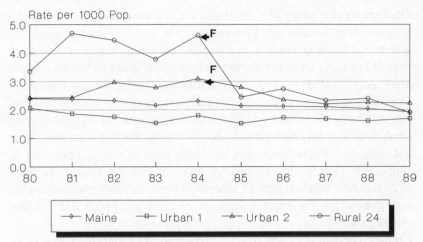

Fig. 21.1. Hysterectomy 1980–1981 – three Maine areas. F = feedback.

that outliers are not comfortable in that role, and almost regardless of their feelings about whether their practices are appropriate or not, they alter their practice patterns.

Other attempts at feedback of information to physicians have not been as successful. Development of consensus panel practice guidelines and providing that information to physicians has not consistently changed practice patterns. A group of Canadian physicians agreed that guidelines for caesarian section were acceptable and appropriate. Had these guidelines been followed, C-section rates should have dropped, but follow-up data analysis showed that rates of this procedure in fact increased.[6]

What then is different about the process developed by the Maine Medical Assessment Foundation? We believe that the essential elements relate to the fact that physicians are included in the process rather than being subjected to the process. Many forms of medical audit focus on the doctor from a distance and they frequently are regulatory and punitive in their approach. We give physicians the data, and we provide all the supporting information that we have available. They understand that we do not have all the answers but they understand that the variations are not logical and that they demand their attention. Practitioners thus become a part of the process and they respond well to it.

Examples

The following section summarises the work of several study groups and illustrates graphically the results of their efforts.

Obstetrics/gynaecology The obstetrics/gynaecology study group has had a long-standing interest in hysterectomy – a highly variable condition wherever it has been studied. In the early 1980s hysterectomy rates varied fourfold or more from the highest to lowest rate areas in Maine. Careful analysis by the study group of all potential causes led to the conclusion that variations were driven primarily by physician uncertainty about the best way for both physicians and patients to deal with the various uterine conditions that may be treated by hysterectomy. Participating physicians did come to the conclusion that very high rates of surgery could not be supported. During this process of analysis and discussion, feedback occurred. As noted in Figure 21.1 rates of surgery have dropped toward the state average and these rate changes can be consistently related to episodes of feedback.

Urology The urology study group noted significant variations in the rate of transurethral prostatectomy (TURP) in Maine. In addition it was discovered that mortality rates for men undergoing apparently uneventful, uncomplicated TURP were significantly higher at one year postoperatively than in a similar population not undergoing surgery. The explanation for this difference in mortality is not yet clear. As a result of this finding an outcomes study of Maine residents undergoing prostatectomy was undertaken. This was the first of this new form of patient oriented, quality of life outcomes research. The results of this project have been published elsewhere.[13] A majority of Maine urologists participated in this study. As a result of the sentinel effect of the study and the coincident out-migration of several urologists the overall rate of TURP fell significantly (Figure 21.2).

Orthopaedics/neurosurgery The orthopaedic/neurosurgery study group has studied lumbar disc herniation among other conditions. Like most other elective surgical procedures, significant variations are noted – almost fourfold over a number of years. Using the methods previously described, information regarding variations and other factors was fed back to physicians in a series of meetings. As illustrated in Figure 21.3, rates in a large urban area were noted to rise rapidly from a long-term rate that had been slightly under the state average. Careful evaluation of all possible causes revealed the only explanation for this abrupt change to be the arrival of three new surgeons in the community.

In this instance members of the study group, aware of the lower incidence of disc surgery in their communities and feeling that their rates were appropriate, could not support the high surgical rates in the community under focus. However, surgeons from this community dis-

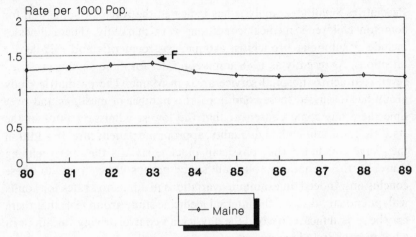

Fig. 21.2. Prostatectomy 1980–1989 – Maine statewide trend. F = feedback.

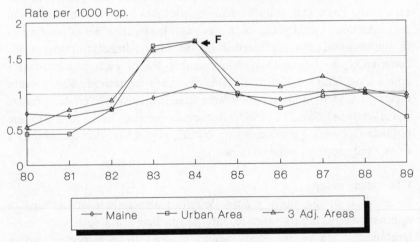

Fig. 21.3. Lumbar disc excision 1980–1989 – urban area plus three adjacent areas. F = feedback.

agreed and felt their practices were appropriate and that results of their care were excellent. In spite of this defensive attitude, Figure 21.3 demonstrates the prompt alteration in practice patterns that took place and which has persisted ever since. This episode illustrates well the effect of peer pressure and the apparent discomfort physicians feel as 'outliers'. Feedback never went beyond the confidential and educational discussion of the data and clinical management of disc herniation carried out among a group of peers. No other management or regulatory process has been necessary, yet the change in practice patterns has persisted for five years.

Paediatrics Small area analysis has indicated that rates of admission for common children's medical conditions vary markedly. These illnesses include pneumonia, bronchitis, asthma, gastroenteritis and middle ear infections. As recently as 1988 admission rates for these diagnoses varied seven fold across hospital service areas in Maine. The paediatric study group has discussed these conditions at a number of meetings and over time there has come consensus that the lowest admission rates in the state are consistent with high quality, appropriate patient care. In addition they have concluded that physician practice style is the overwhelming cause of the variations. Not all study groups have come to these conclusions. Indeed, in examining variations in admission rates for adults with pulmonary disease, the internal medicine study group feels that there may be several factors beyond the physician's control driving variations in adult pulmonary admission rates.

Figure 21.4 shows the results of the paediatric feedback process in one area of the state. This example demonstrates that behaviour modification may take time. Initially, feedback was provided by the chief of paediatrics in the hospital. Having learned of the high admission rates in his community, he began to post a monthly list of each paediatrician's admissions. This was partially effective until he retired. Rates again increased, and the study group became directly involved. Even that process has taken time and only in 1989, after several meetings and a review of one physician's hospital practice by an outside expert, did this community's rates finally approach the state rate.

Other study groups

In addition to the study groups described above there are groups in ophthalmology, family practice, internal medicine and substance abuse treatment. Each of the study groups is lead by a respected, active practitioner in that specialty. Members of the study group are chosen on the basis of their professional competence and esteem and on the basis of geographic distribution. Practitioners representing high, median and low rates of admissions are recruited.

Each study group pursues its agenda somewhat differently, but underlying all study group activities is the assurance to practitioners that the information they deal with is confidential and educational and will not be used in any public, punitive or regulatory way. It has taken time to convince Maine doctors that the Maine Medical Assessment Foundation really does function this way. In the US there are many regulatory systems that operate on the premise that the doctor must prove that he or she is

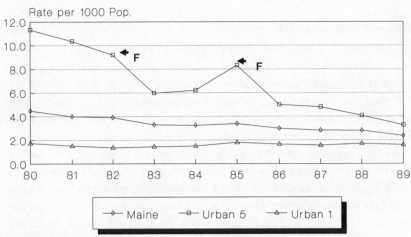

Fig. 21.4. Paediatric medical admissions 1980–1989 – two urban areas.

right. Not unexpectedly, physicians do not like that approach and tend to be suspicious of any group or individual who appears to be scrutinising what they do.

At this point, the foundation has high credibility in the state and has achieved strong support from the medical community and medical societies. However, we know that each time a study group is developed, participating physicians must be guided through a process of education, and suspicion and hostility must be overcome. Once that is accomplished practitioners become strong supporters of the process of small area analysis and feedback. Additionally, as a result of their participation in this process, they understand the issues of physician uncertainty and the inconsistencies in medical practice. They become eager participants in the outcomes research agenda that has developed in the United States.

In addition to the completed prostatectomy outcomes study,[13] the Obs/Gyn study group is currently involved in the 'Maine Women's Health Study' – a project analysing the outcomes of operative and non-operative treatment of various benign uterine conditions. The orthopaedic/ neurosurgical group is participating in a prospective study of patients with herniated lumbar disc and spinal stenosis who will be treated with and without surgery, and the family practice study group has developed a data-based analysis technique to study the birth outcomes of Medicaid and low-income mothers. We feel that the high level of voluntary participation in these outcome studies relates strongly to the sense of trust, interest and active participation that Maine physicians have developed in the study group process.

National medical specialty societies

Specialty medical organisations across the US have been quick to recognise the importance of practice pattern variations, physician uncertainty, and the cost and quality issues that are raised as a result of them. They have followed the development of the federal initiative in outcomes and effectiveness research and are eager to be involved in working with the PORT teams and other researchers.

As an example, the American Academy of Orthopedic Surgeons (AAOS) has established a council on health care policy and committees in quality assurance, outcomes research and practice parameters. The AAOS feels that it should support the national research agenda, facilitate and co-ordinate outcomes research, and work with PORT teams studying orthopaedic topics. Academy members and staff sit on the advisory panels of the PORTS and are interested in evaluating and disseminating new information and practice parameters and guidelines as they are developed by investigators. The academy views participation in the 'effectiveness agenda'[4] as an important part of its mission in orthopaedic leadership and education.

At the same time the Federal Government and its agencies look to national specialty societies for consultation, support and assistance in this effort. It is recognised that in order to be truly effective, the new information generated by outcomes research must be disseminated to practising physicians in ways that will result in real change in practice patterns. The support of major national medical organisations will be essential in establishing the credibility and importance of this new information and in devising methodologies to assist in effectively implementing change. It would appear that all parties in health care – government, regulators, payers, patients, and providers have, for the moment, at least, agreed that they must co-operate in the effort to deal with runaway costs and lack of access to medical care for many US citizens, while simultaneously maintaining and improving appropriateness and quality of care.

Conclusion

Medical audit or quality assurance takes many forms. The evolution of small area analysis has revealed large differences in the practice of medical care in all health care systems that have been studied. Patterns of over and under utilisation of health care raise serious questions about the effectiveness and appropriateness of the practice of medicine. This evidence also points to deficiencies in current techniques of medical audit. If audit procedures were accomplishing their goals effectively, one would not expect to see such inconsistencies in practice.

In the United States this problem is heightened by rapidly increasing costs of care and lack of access and underservice for many citizens. Evaluation of practice pattern variations and outcomes research offer the opportunity to deal with some of the issues of cost and quality. The Maine Medical Assessment Foundation has developed a model through which physicians have become active participants in dealing with issues of practice pattern variations and conducting outcomes research projects. The US Government has responded to these issues with the development of the Agency for Health Care Policy and Research, and US medical specialty organisations are taking an active role in support of this effort.

Physicians have the opportunity to play a major role in this effort. If the '*effectiveness agenda*' is to work, doctors must recognise the problems that confront the profession, participate in outcomes research and be willing to modify their practice patterns as new information develops. Problems of quality and appropriateness of care exist in all organised health care systems. The crisis in cost of care in the United States has stimulated the development of important new methods and strategies to begin to deal with these issues. These techniques may be of value to physicians in other countries.

Acknowledgement: This work is supported in part by grant no. HS 06813-01 from the Agency for Health Care Policy and Research.

References

1. Blendon, R. J., Leitman, R., Morrison, I. & Donelan, K. (1990). Satisfaction with health: systems in ten nations. *Health Affairs*, **9**, 185–193.
2. Hsiao, W. C., Braun, P., Yntema, D. & Becker, E. R. (1988). Estimating physicians' work for a resource based relative value scale. *New England Journal of Medicine*, **319**, 835–841.
3. Iglehart, J. (1986). Canada's health care system. *New England Journal of Medicine*, **315**, 202–206.
4. Shroeder, S. (1990). Preface. In *Medicare: A Strategy for Quality Assurance* 1990, vol. 1, pp. ix–xi, ed. K. N. Lohr. Washington DC: National Academy Press.
5. McPherson, K., Wennberg, J. E., Hovind, O. B. & Clifford, P. (1982). Small area variations in the use of common surgical procedures: an international comparison of New England, England and Norway. *New England Journal of Medicine*, **307**, 1310–1314.

6. Wennberg, J. E., Freeman, J. L. & Culp, W. J. (1987). Are hospital services rationed in New Haven or over-utilized in Boston? *The Lancet*, **i**, 1185–1189.
7. Wennberg, J. E. & Gittelsohn, A. M. (1973). Small area variations in health care delivery. *Science*, **182**, 1102–1109.
8. Roper, W., Yordy, K., Hackbarth, G. & Krakauer, H. (1988). Effectiveness in health care: an initiative to evaluate and improve medical practice. *New England Journal of Medicine*, **322**, 1197–1202.
9. Gartland, J. J. (1988). Orthopaedic clinical research. Deficiencies in experimental design and determinations of outcome. *Journal of Bone and Joint Surgery*, **70A**, 1357–1364.
10. Agency for Health Care Policy and Research (1990). *AHCPR Program Note OM90–0059*. Rockville, MD.
11. Wennberg, J. E., Gittelsohn, A. M. & Soule, D. N. (1975). Health care delivery in Maine I: patterns of use of common surgical procedures. *Journal of the Maine Medical Association*, **66**, 123–130.
12. Wennberg, J. E. & Gittelsohn, A. M. (1982). Variations in care among small areas. *Science*, **246**, 120–134.
13. Wennberg, J. E., Mulley, A. G., Hanley, D. F., Timothy, R. P., Fowler, F. J., Roos, N. P., Barry, M. J., McPherson, K., Greenberg, E. R., Soule, D. N., Bubolz, T., Fisher, E. & Malenka, D. (1988). An assessment of prostatectomy for benign urinary tract obstruction. Geographic variations and the evaluation of medical care outcomes. *Journal of the American Medical Association*, **259**, 3027–3030.

22

Quality control in health care: the Dutch experience

MICHAEL B. LAGAAY

Introduction

Quality control has become a familiar word in health care in the Netherlands in the last ten years, as it has elsewhere in the Western world. The self-evident way in which medical practitioners meet their obligations towards their patients on the strength of the Hippocratic oath is apparently no longer a sufficient guarantee of the best possible treatment. There would appear to be pressure to keep a critical eye on the work of medical practitioners, both within the profession itself and also on the part of representatives of patients or those who regard themselves as such. Such a state of affairs has probably arisen not so much as the result of any failing on the part of medical practitioners, but because of a changed cultural pattern in the Western world. Regulated quality control in medicine is a phenomenon typical of those parts of the world where medical care is in abundant supply. Where medical care is scarce, doctors few, and work done on a more individual basis, there is neither the opportunity nor the funds and consequently perhaps not even the inclination to make arrangements to monitor doctors. Similarly, quality control is an issue that arises more commonly in (intramural) hospital care where groups of consultants work, rather than in general practice where medical practitioners operate on an individual basis.

A quantifiable record of treatment in medicine is not always easy. The results of surgery lend themselves most readily to this, for it is here that the body of the patient is directly affected and the conditions prior to and subsequent to the operation can be compared as a tangible outcome of medical intervention. In this field feedback is possible between the desired and achieved result.

The attitude of the doctor in carrying out treatment is more difficult to define. It certainly represents a quality aspect of health care and in the perception of the patient is often more important than the immediate state of health subsequent to contact with the doctor. Social developments, certainly in countries such as the UK and the Netherlands, are prompting government and professional associations to concern themselves increasingly with the number of hours being worked, including the hours being worked by doctors. Continuation of this trend will inevitably hasten the disappearance of the personal patient–doctor relationship. Instead, patients will find themselves being treated by a group of doctors. The result will be external quality control aimed at groups of doctors. At the same time doctors themselves will become more aware, through the common patients they are treating, of the way in which their colleagues are practising their profession. In the Netherlands, consultants as a group have themselves been preoccupied with the subject of quality for years. Forms of audit play a role in this context. Recently, the government and insurers have sought to become involved in these aspects of health care. The way in which an endeavour is made to promote and monitor quality by Dutch consultants is described below after a very brief sketch of the organisation of health care in the Netherlands. Specific attention will be given to the experiences of surgeons who have embarked on a special aspect of quality monitoring, namely a kind of peer review system called 'visitatie' in Dutch. The plans of the other parties referred to will be dealt with at the end of this section.

Health care in the Netherlands

A brief sketch of the organisation of the Dutch health care system is required to understand the activities and organisation of quality control in the Netherlands. Practically all Dutch residents are medically insured. Depending on income level, they are either compulsorily insured under the '*Ziekenfonds*', the premium for which is partly paid by the employer or by social insurance funds or, in the case of those with a higher income, through private health insurance.

The type of insurance is more or less irrelevant to the quality of treatment. The absence of a national health service in the Netherlands has meant that there are practically no private clinics. All hospitals in the Netherlands admit both compulsorily insured (about 70%) and privately insured (about 30%) patients. Practically all doctors in the Netherlands are members of the KNMG (*Royal Dutch Medical Association*), which looks after the professional, medical but also the social interests of medical practitioners and sees to contacts with the Government and insurers and can therefore be regarded as a kind of union. Consultants are members of the LSV (*National Specialist Society*), a subsection of the KNMG comprising societies of the 29 accredited specialties in the Netherlands. Each medical specialty has its own association, which concerns itself with medical science and research, training aspects of the discipline and, increasingly now, with relationships between consultants and the Government and insurers. The fact that practically every consultant is a member of the appropriate association makes it in principle easier in the Netherlands to take initiatives and reach agreements on the quality of health care. Another major contributory factor is that all consultants in hospitals belong to the medical policy staff, which initiates a common medical policy for the entire hospital.

Lastly, many consultants work in an associate practice and for those with a teaching qualification this associateship is a prerequisite. Such forms of co-operation again, in principle, make it easier to take initiatives and to arrive at agreements on quality in health care.

Definitions

Quality can be defined as the degree of correspondence between the goals set and goals achieved in the provision of care, while avoiding unnecessary use of resources. It is a question of applying the existing knowledge in health care in the correct fashion. For this both quality promotion and quality monitoring are needed. Activities that promote quality are those that encourage the provision of good quality such as postgraduate teaching and the formulation of guidelines and protocols. Quality monitoring implies a feedback between the goal set and the goal achieved. How are agreements which have been made or objectives set actually complied with or achieved in practice? Quality monitoring also implies corrective action should this prove necessary. Items under this heading include examinations, keeping records of complications and mortality figures, consultation, auditing and supervision. The terms quality promotion and monitoring are often used interchangeably and are not always easy to separate. In this chapter stress will be on what happens in the Netherlands in monitoring the quality of specialist health care.

Quality monitoring in Dutch hospital health care

There are three ways in which those in the Netherlands seek to monitor quality: *auditing*, '*visitatie*' and *re-registration*. In 1979 the *National Organization for Quality Assurance in Hospitals* (CBO) was set up as an initiative of the LSV and the joint hospital governing boards. The aim was to encourage and give guidance in monitoring and promoting quality in activities relating to medical treatment in hospitals in the Netherlands. This active organisation has done much in the last decade to formalise quality promotion in hospitals by medical specialists.

Many internal hospital audits have been supervised by the organisation and it is partly thanks to these activities that the majority of hospitals in the Netherlands have guidelines (agreements, protocols), for example for blood transfusion policy, analysis of jaundiced patients and first aid for accident patients. Hospitals executives can appeal to the organisation in setting up and working out an internal hospital audit.

Furthermore, since 1982, the organisation has organised national consensus meetings whose findings have now been recorded in more than 30 reports (see Box 22.1). These guidelines are available to every medical practitioner in the Netherlands and are thus an aid to quality control. All these guidelines are described as generally accepted policy and therefore as a yardstick of good care. The guidelines drawn up subsequent to such consensus meetings are explicitly not regarded as compulsory regulations for Dutch doctors. It is not the idea that the Government and/or the insurers should use these guidelines to check the medical treatment provided. The voluntary nature of the consensus meetings serves to promote rather than monitor quality. They can be used as a guide for hospital audits. For example, six years after a first consensus on skin melanoma a second consensus meeting was arranged. A review of reporting by pathologists and a survey of the manner of treatment have revealed a clear improvement. This is regarded as quality promotion brought about as a result of a jointly formulated guideline.

Another of the many activities of the CBO is the two-monthly newsletter. This is sent to all doctors in the Netherlands and contains brief reports of audit activities as well as summaries and comments on relevant articles from the world literature.

'Visitatie'

Consultants in the Netherlands are trained on the basis of rules drawn up by the profession itself. Visitaties are carried out to check whether these rules are implemented. A group of three consultants and a resident visit a hospital to ascertain whether the group of consultants meets the criteria that are conducive to a good training climate. Whether or not the teaching qualification is extended or granted to a consultants' joint practice depends

Box 22.1   *Topics reported upon by national consensus meetings*

1. Blood transfusion
2. Thoraco-lumbar vertebral injury
3. Mammography
4. Severe brain injury
5. Melanoma of the skin
6. Thrombocyte-transfusion
7. Solitary thyroid node
8. Prevention of decubitus ulcers
9. Osteoporosis
10. Diabetic foot
11. Diagnosis of deep venous thrombosis
12. Non descended testis
13. Treatment of decubitus ulcers
14. Prevention of herpes neonatorum
15. Treatment of haemophilia
16. Follow up of colon polyps
17. Cholesterol
18. Diagnosis of a pathological node in the neck
19. Diagnosis of atopic syndrome
20. Total hip prosthesis
21. Follow up of colon cancer
22. Diagnosis of dementia
23. Sport and heart disease
24. Prevention of deep venous thrombosis
25. Prevention of hospital infections
26. Diagnosis of pulmonary cancer
27. Diagnosis and treatment of hypertension
28. Food and allergy
29. Otitis media
30. Melanoma of the skin

on the report of the visitatie committee. Visitaties take place every five years, or earlier if a new trainer is appointed or if shortcomings were due for rechecking after an agreed period. Thus the quality control of the training takes place by colleagues from the same discipline.

Visitatie of non-teaching surgical consultants

The Association of Surgeons of the Netherlands started peer reviews of non-teaching clinics in 1989 on the grounds of the internal and external pressure for quality control referred to earlier and supported by the experiences with visitaties of teaching practices. A surgical practice in a hospital may voluntarily apply for a visitatie. This is carried out by a teaching surgeon and by a non-teaching surgeon both appointed by the Association of Surgeons of the Netherlands. In the course of their review they take due note of aspects such as co-operation within the practice, which results from meetings, reports and guidance of junior doctors; the size of the practice in relation to the number of surgeons and junior doctors; and the organisation of patients' treatment, which results from the transfer of data, continuity of treatment and regulation of duty periods. After almost two years' experience with this external quality assessment of non-teaching clinics by visitatie the reports of 30 clinics have been evaluated. The interaction between a group of surgeons determined by the level of co-operation, mutual assistance, locum arrangements and transfer was often given a positive score but left something to be desired in a quarter of the cases. Meetings by surgeons to discuss indications for operations and findings were seldom common and thus too few. Internal quality control through discussion of complications, necrology and interdisciplinary transfer was equally insufficient in the majority of the clinics reviewed. Record-keeping on clinical and out-patient data invariably scored positively. Finally, a worrying aspect was that the guidance and instruction of junior doctors/housemen were regarded as inadequate in more than half of the surgeons' practices.

A survey carried out among the 30 surgeons' practices reviewed produced 18 replies. Sixteen regarded the energy invested as useful, and seven had changed the form of their practice in response to the review. Half had discussed the report with the hospital governors. All of them said they would appreciate a repeat in due time. The standards for a well- functioning surgeons' practice, the data to be assessed, the procedures to be followed and the method of reporting have been adjusted accordingly.

Hospital visitatie

The LSV regards it as its responsibility to co-ordinate and encourage the developments with regard to visitaties. Following the example of the Association of Surgeons of the Netherlands a visitatie of hospitals is planned. This review will include the following components:

It will be carried out voluntarily.
No sanctions will ensue.
The review serves to monitor and promote quality.

The emphasis is not on a measurement of quality on which basis sanctions might follow. The accent is on providing advice as to how quality can be monitored and promoted. An endeavour will be made to carry out an integral assessment of the functioning of the joint specialties that will be complementary to the internal quality monitoring in the hospital. The quality assessment of each specialist category will remain for the time being in the hands of the individual medical associations.

As regards the criteria, a numerical check on the basis of data from various national health care records is not being considered. The review will concentrate primarily on the total process of mechanisms for monitoring and promoting quality and on the process of medical treatment, but not on the results of the treatment.

These criteria have been subdivided into:

1. the functioning of the medical consultants
2. the functioning of the medical staff
3. consultative structures
4. reporting
5. committees.

Roughly the following criteria are assessed:

1. The functioning of all consultants in a particular discipline, in a practice or in another co-operative association or individually.
2. Reporting (keeping a medical file).
3. The compiling of an annual report for each specialty.
4. Institutionalised inter- and intra-disciplinary discussions.
5. The functioning of the medical staff.
6. The relationship of the medical staff to the hospital governors, the nursing staff and GPs in the region.
7. The functioning of a number of committees, such as the audit committee, the accident committee, the medicines/drugs committee, the patient complaints committee, the infection committee, the complications committee, the necrology committee, and the intensive care committee, with particular reference to the assignment, composition, frequency of meeting, annual reports, reports, guidelines, etc. of the committee.

It is expected that these reviews will primarily serve as a stimulus to consultants in the Netherlands. Meanwhile a number of pilot hospital reviews have taken place.

Re-registration

Registration as a medical consultant in the Netherlands immediately allows the specialist to put himself forward as a candidate for a full post as a consultant in a hospital. The English registrar–consultant system does not exist in the Netherlands. Registration takes place after a training of four to six years has been completed and in accordance with the rules that have been drawn up by the 'Centraal College'. This college, a subsection of the KNMG, comprises medical professors, teaching consultants and a number of representatives from hospital governing boards and from the government. Training and registration is supervised by the SRC (*Specialisten Registratie Commissie*); this includes the aforementioned visitaties of teaching clinics.

Up to now this has meant that specialists were accredited for life. The realisation is gradually dawning that regular checks on the functioning of medical practitioners is all part of quality monitoring. After almost ten years of preparations and debate a system of recertification was introduced on 1 January 1991. As of that date a specialist who has not practised the specialty for which he is registered for five years can be deleted from the register of accredited specialists.

In the eyes of many Dutch medical consultants the change has been a revolutionary one. For the time being, therefore, moves in this matter have been marked by cautious manoeuvring. After detailed preparations and in consultation with the medical associations, minimum criteria have been formulated that have to be met to remain registered. The basic factor in continuing to be an accredited specialist is the time during which one practices one's specialty. The number of patient-related hours per week need to be known, the time allocation between in-patient and out-patient work and any interruption in the work in the preceding five years. What is referred to as a re-registration with a proviso is possible for specialists no longer working in the curative field. To be re-registered a specialist must complete a questionnaire stating the number of hours he/she has devoted to patient care in the preceding five years and is doing currently. No one has worked out how these data can be checked, though arrangements have been made for arbitration in the case of differences of opinion on the information provided. This will be done in accordance with the rules drawn up for training.The hospital visitaties described above will undoubtedly exert an influence. Consequently, the re-registration system is provisionally being based on minimum quantitative criteria drawn up by the profession itself. Qualitative criteria such as attendance at conferences, postgraduate teaching and active participation in internal assessment are equally likely to play a role. The American accreditation system is regarded as a model.

It will be evident that the acceptance of the principle of re-registration as an accredited specialist is a very radical step towards quality control of the individual specialist. Loss of accreditation means loss of one's post in the hospital, inability to invoice insurance companies, and termination of contracts entered into on the basis of a consultant's title.

Quality control by third parties

Other bodies besides medical consultants are thinking about developing systems to check the quality of health care.

Proposals have been put forward by the *National Council for Public Health* to arrive at the certification of institutions, the latter being based on the check of internal hospital quality systems (for example audit). The *Medical Inspectorate of Public Health* systematically supervises all health care institutions and all members of the medical profession (not only medical practitioners) to obtain a more general impression of the quality of care.

A pilot project is being run in eight hospitals based on the *Guide to Accreditation of Canadian Health Care Facilities* to assess how internal quality care can be promoted in hospitals through external inspection by an 'independent' accreditation authority. All these plans for checks are still in the development phase and no demands have yet been set. We will now have to be alert to ensure that with the advent of growing interest in quality control from all quarters excessive interference and overlapping do not make for a situation in which everyone is busy checking everybody else and attention to the individual patient is jeopardised. This is why it is a good thing that medical consultants in the Netherlands have taken active steps to develop internal quality control.

Conclusion

Primary responsibility for the quality of the health care provided rests with the medical practitioners and the institutions. A consensus exists on this in the Netherlands. It is the job of insurance companies to make sure that qualitatively good care is feasible and is promoted. Through the growing influence of the users of care (patients' associations) their co-responsibility for the quality of the care provided is increasing. The government should create the conditions to enable the parties to live up to their responsibilities with regard to the quality of care. The government is responsible for establishing the basic level of health care, as laid down in the constitution.

Thus, there are four groups preoccupied with promoting the quality of health care. All of these parties want to draw up criteria. If basic criteria for the quality to be achieved have to be drawn up, by far the most preferable course is to have these drawn up and checked by those providing the care, the medical practitioners. Once this has been achieved, others, notably the Government, can decide on the criteria as formulated by the medical profession.

To summarise, the work of consultants is assessed in the Netherlands at three levels:

1. At the individual level during training when the quality of the trainer and the teaching institution is checked by visitaties.
2. By the system of re-registration that has been introduced where a check is made to see whether the consultant is keeping his or her experience, and in the second instance his or her know-how, up to scratch. There is also internal quality monitoring in hospitals through the medical policy staff, audit and protocols.
3. There is also external quality control of hospitals through visitaties. In this instance an opinion is formed on the functioning of departments or functional units within the hospital as well as the functioning of individual medical consultants. Audit of the medical aspects by visitatie in the Netherlands is the responsibility of the relevant medical association. Visitatie regarding more general aspects of the functioning of consultants in the medical policy staff of the hospital is the responsibility of the LSV.

Thanks to the level and efficiency of the organisation of Dutch consultants it has been possible for them to be in at the beginning of all of the developments connected with quality assessment.

23

Medical audit: experience from Sweden
KARL-GÖRAN THORNGREN

Introduction

When efforts are made to audit results in medical health care there is often a lack of measures describing the outcome of a certain treatment for the continued function and rehabilitation of the individual in relation to health care consumption. Measures of results and control of productivity comparing larger regions within a country or comparing countries are also lacking. Through uniform follow up of major diseases the efficiency of different hospitals and regions can be evaluated and awareness of treatment results and improvement will be facilitated.

The most resource-consuming groups in orthopaedics are hip fractures and arthroplasties of the hip and the knee. The evaluation of the effectiveness of the treatment is hampered by the lack of control of the treatment provided. To meet these demands orthopaedic audit has been started with prospective multi-centre studies of hip fractures, hip arthroplasties and knee arthroplasties covering all Sweden. The three registers differ in outlines and performance and will therefore be described separately. The hip fracture audit has its focus on the operation, and rehabilitation and resource consumption within the first months after the fracture, whereas the arthroplasty audits concentrate on long-term revisions. These studies have been initiated with the support of the Swedish Orthopaedic Society.

Hip fractures

The 'Swedish multicentre hip fracture study' was commenced in January 1988 with the intention to cover the entire country. The project covers hospitals with different geographic location and size. Within each region at

365

MULTICENTER
HIP FRACTURE
STUDY

co-ordinator prof. K-G Thorngren
Lund University Hospital
S-221 85 Lund, SWEDEN

Patientcard

1. ⌊_1_⌋ **FORM**

   HOSPITAL CODE
2. ⌊__⌊__⌊__⌊__⌊__⌋ (or NAME of hospital..)

3. ⌊__⌋ **OPERATING DEPARTMENT,** 1. orthopedic, 2. general surgery, 3. other

4. ⌊__⌊__⌊__⌊__⌊__⌊__⌊_–_⌊__⌊__⌊__⌊__⌋ **DATE OF BIRTH-SOCIAL SECURITY NUMBER;** the first six
                                                                 digits show year, month and day.
5. _____ **NAME OF PATIENT**

6. ⌊__⌋ **SIDE OF FRACTURE**   1 = left, 2 = right.

7. ⌊__⌋ **SEX**   1 = male, 2 = female.

8. ⌊__⌊__⌊__⌊__⌊__⌊__⌋ **DATE OF ADMISSION** (year, month, day)

9. ⌊__⌊__⌊__⌊__⌊__⌊__⌋ **DATE OF OPERATION** (year, month, day)

10. ⌊__⌊__⌊__⌊__⌊__⌊__⌋ **DATE OF DISCHARGE** (year, month, day)

11. ⌊__⌋ **ADMITTED FROM:** 1. own home   6. acute hospital
                            2. convalescent home   7. other
12. ⌊__⌋ **DISCHARGED TO:** 3. fullservice unit with meals,   8. not admitted, taken care
                               home for the elderly   of in another department
                            4. geriatric department, rehabilitation clinic   (which ....)
                            5. long-term care institution, nursing home   9. unknown

13. ⌊__⌋ **MARITAL STATUS AT PRESENT:** 1. not married, 2. married, 3. divorced, 4. widow/er

14. ⌊__⌋ **LIVED ALONE AT THE TIME OF FRACTURE:** 1 = yes, 2 = no.

15. ⌊__⌊__⌋ **HOME HELP AT THE TIME OF FRACTURE:** Number of hours/week (none = 0)

16. ⌊__⌋ **TYPE OF**   1. undisplaced cervical (Garden I–II)   4. trochanteric twofragment fracture
         FRACTURE   2. displaced cervical (Garden III–IV)   5. trochanteric multifragment fracture
                           3. basocervical   6. subtrochanteric

17. ⌊__⌊__⌋ **PRIMARY OPERATION** (method of operation, for alt. see the back of the form)

18. ⌊__⌋ **REOPERATIONS DURING THE PRIMARY ADMISSION PERIOD:** 1 = yes, 2 = no (Note that if "yes"
         the reoperation form 3 should be completed)

19. ⌊__⌋ **GENERAL LOCOMOTOR ABILITY BEFORE THE FRACTURE:**
         1. could walk alone out of doors   5. could not walk but was sitting in a chair
         2. could walk out of doors only accompanied 6. always bedridden
         3. could walk alone indoors but not out of doors 9. unknown
         4. could walk indoors only accompanied

    Which **WALKING AIDS** did the patient use indoors?

20. ⌊__⌋ **BEFORE THE FRACTURE**   1. can walk without aids   5. two tripods
                                            2. one stick (crutch or tripod, hemiwalker) 6. rollator/walking-frame
21. ⌊__⌋ **2 WEEKS AFTER THE OPERATION**   3. two sticks   7. wheelchair
         (or at discharge if earlier than 2 weeks) 4. one stick + one tripod   8. does not walk

22. ⌊__⌋ Could the patient **DRESS-UNDRESS (ADL)** before the fracture. 1 = yes, 2 = no

23. ⌊__⌋ Could the patient manage **ADL** two weeks **after** the operation (or at discharge if earlier than two
         weeks) 1 = yes 2 = no

24. ⌊__⌋ **DEAD** in hospital. 1 = yes (date should be given in item 10 above), 2 = no

25. ⌊__⌊__⌋ I ....   26. ⌊__⌊__⌋ II ....   27. ⌊__⌊__⌋ III ....

28. ⌊__⌊__⌋ IV ....   29. ⌊__⌊__⌋ V ....   30. ⌊__⌊__⌋ VI ....
         (Items 25–30 permit the department to enter parameters of their own choice)

The form completed by .... position .... telephone: ....

Lidbergs, Skurup 22004

Fig. 23.1. Registration form 1 for the Swedish multicentre hip fracture project.

least one county hospital, one central hospital and the regional hospital were included, but in most regions the project started with considerably more hospitals. To date about two thirds of the Swedish hospitals participate and the goal is to include all within the next few years.

Forms

The follow up forms were compiled with criteria that had proven most decisive in previous Swedish hip fracture studies. This was performed by a discussion group of five researchers from different parts of Sweden, who were well experienced in hip fractures. The hip fracture audit covers both technical data and data on the patient's function, well being and resource demands, such as place of residence, need for institutional care, walking ability, activities of daily living (ADL) performance, pain and consumption of home help.

The audit consists of three separate printed forms. Form 1 (Figure 23.1), covers data from the treatment period at the operating department. Preferably it is filled in by the nurses at the orthopaedic ward because they have direct access to all necessary data, collected at admission from the patients, their relatives or from health care personnel in other institutions. Such information is anyhow routinely collected to facilitate nursing and rehabilitation of the patients, but the information is, apart from this audit, not uniformly registered. The hip fracture form can thus, apart from the audit registration, be used as a page of standardised patient file. Consequently, form 1 is printed on double self-carbonating paper. One page goes into the file, and one goes for computer registration. It contains, apart from preoperative functional parameters, data concerning fracture type, operation and time in hospital, as well as function at two weeks after the operation (or at discharge if earlier than two weeks).

Form 2 is a patient inquiry. It concerns the place of residence during the first four months after the fracture, as well as walking ability, pain and ADL capacity at precisely four months after the fracture. The different places of residence after discharge from the operating department are of particular importance for tracing the 'treatment chain' of the patient. With this information it is possible to create a detailed graph (Figure 23.2) showing the residence changes day by day up to four months after the fracture. Previous studies on hip fracture rehabilitation[1,2] have shown that with an active rehabilitation attitude most improvements are gained within this period. Thereafter little change in place of residence and functional parameters is to be expected.

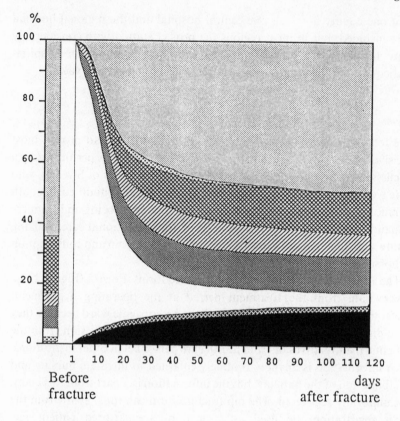

Fig. 23.2. Type of residence at different periods before fracture as well as up to four months after fracture. Based on 3715 patients in Sweden.

At the orthopaedic ward the patients have already received their form and instructions from the nurses on how to fill in and return it. If the form is not received a reminder is sent out and then usually the district nurse or the district physiotherapist aids in collecting the information. For patients treated in institutions the staff there report by filling in and returning form 2.

Form 3 is a reoperation report. This form is only used if some complication that needs operation occurs. As a reminder, all patient files are marked on the envelope once they belong to the hip fracture register. The reoperation form covers reasons for and type of reoperation, as well as place of residence and walking ability of the patient.

Routines for data reports

Sweden has a distance from south to north of 2000 km and contains 8.5 million inhabitants. Approximately 17 000 hip fractures occur per year. To handle a problem of this size a decentralised system was organised for reporting data. Every participating department received a special data program for personal computers. The computer program was written specifically for the project, but it is now possible to modify a commercially available PC-program. The program shows the forms on the screen, making it easy to enter data. It is self-instructing and some data analysis is possible, e.g calculation of mean value for age and time spent in hospital. Cross tabulation of data is also important. The program makes it possible for the participating departments to make their own calculations and to check for completeness of data sets at regular intervals. By cross-checking with operation files 'missing data' items on individual patients and 'missing patients' can be found. Regularly (every 3–6 months) disc copies are sent to a regional centre (there are seven dispersed throughout Sweden), which send data to the main centre in Lund. Every half year a report is sent out from Lund to all participating departments with calculations from their own data, as well as the average calculations from all Sweden for comparison.

Of all types of disease treated by some kind of surgery, hip fractures constitute the group that consumes most bed resources throughout the whole treatment chain. A more uniform pattern of hip fracture treatment throughout the country would lead to better treatment and better cost efficiency. The hip fracture audit aims at both better results and a uniformity of measures for comparison of quality of care, and for the creation of a high and consistent level of care, provided by different hospital units throughout Sweden.

Knee arthroplasties

In 1975 the Swedish Orthopaedic Society started a nationwide computer survey known as the Swedish knee arthroplasty project. Knee arthroplasties are reported for computer filing. This project is mainly concerned with medical information. At entry, data on the diagnosis, the type of replacement, type of cement, antibiotic prophylaxis, any complications and length of hospital stay are registered. Participating units use their own indications for arthroplasty, choice of prostheses and revision and their own criteria for complications. Each patient is now followed up by questionnaire at three, six and ten years after operation. Questions concerning any revisions or complications make this necessary. All patients who reported that they were not satisfied with the operation were seen by the surgeon at a follow up.

In Sweden about 3000 knee arthroplasties are performed per year. This project has been highly centralised since its start. All participants report on special forms to Lund where the computerisation is performed. Until recently the project used a large-scale central computer (UNIVAC 1100/80 – Lund University Computing Centre). It has now been reconstructed for personal computer (PC) use for the following reasons:

1. The access to data was much more complicated with a central computer.
2. A special computer operator was given a request for calculations and a pile of paper was sent to the investigator for further mental digestion.
3. The modern PCs (IBM or MacIntosh) now have the capacity to handle this large amount of numerical material allowing the investigator to do direct calculations, statistics and presentations in numerical or graphical form.
4. The direct access to data saves time and avoids mistakes.

Thus, the knee arthroplasty project has turned to the same type of data computing as the hip fracture project.

The type of data collected has changed during the period. The initial detailed reports with functional outcome and analysis of radiographs as well as a one year follow up, have, due to the workload and the problem of missing data, been transformed to a registration of reoperations (survival of the knee). Furthermore, there was previously no consensus as to the method of reporting failure rates for the arthroplasties, especially the knee arthroplasties. As failure rates are time dependent, the life table technique or survivorship method has been advocated.[3]

Comparison of results is only valid if uniform definitions are used. No generally accepted radiographic or clinical criteria for failure have yet been defined. One way of defining failure is to use the only definite endpoint for an arthroplasty – its revision because of some complication. This definition has been used in survivorship studies of prostheses of both the hip and the knee. For multi-centre studies of arthroplasties it is necessary to use an endpoint that is easy to define, and only revision with removal, addition or exchange of prosthetic components meets this criterion. On the other hand evaluation of a prosthetic survival study has the limitation that some complications, such as those after a hinge arthroplasty, are more often treated conservatively than those after a surface replacement. Furthermore, a large surgical unit may perform more revision operations because of more experience, special interest and better equipment and choice of prostheses. A lower complication rate would then be counteracted by the wider indications for revision. This may possibly explain why no correlation was found between the number of procedures at each centre and the failure rate in the evaluation of 8000 cases from the nationwide multi-centre investigation of knee arthroplasties in Sweden.[4]

Hip re-arthroplasties

In 1979 the Swedish Orthopaedic Society started a prospective national recording of reoperations after total hip replacement in Sweden. Registration and continued follow up of primary hip arthroplasties was considered too extensive a project to undertake (at present, 10 000 arthroplasties are performed per year in Sweden). Instead, all reoperations for hip arthroplasties were registered. The entry point used was thus the same as that used for follow up of the knee arthroplasties. The total hip replacement project has been highly centralised since its start. Complete hospital records of all reoperated hip replacements were routinely sent to a co-ordination centre in Gothenburg. From these, the required data were transferred to a standardised computer form for subsequent entry into the database. The form contained 132 variables. To be able to fill in the computer form, it was necessary to have access to complete case records, including the discharge summary, operative report and out-patient records. In addition, information was obtained from temperature charts, anaesthetic charts, radiologists reports, laboratory reports, results of any bacteriological cultures and pathology, and bone scintigraphy reports.

The data were entered into the computer at Gothenburg University Computing Centre using a double-entry technique in order to eliminate registration errors at an early stage. One of the same system operators was responsible for both programming and data processing. In collaboration with a biostatistician, a statistical program was developed that is used for comparative analyses. The data forms were returned to the participating departments and if needed corrections were made. In this elaborate procedure only a few persons participated in the registration and completion of the computer form. Therefore, there was reason to believe[5] that between 1979 and 1986 the case records were assessed uniformly in this study.

The registration of reoperated hip arthroplasties has given a large amount of highly interesting information on different types of prostheses as well as patient-related parameters, influence of surgeon and type of hospital.[5] However, the registration of only reoperations has disadvantages. Direct comparisons between the primary and the reoperation material was impossible because there was no prospective study of primary arthroplasties. Therefore, the statistical analyses had to be based on data from each patient's reoperation in relation to average information about primary material during a given year.

Recently, it has been planned to expand the hip re-arthroplasty project with a simplified registration of all primary hip arthroplasties, as well as to keep a numerical registration of all other types of arthroplasty performed in Sweden. In addition, some years ago a separate registration of all shoulder arthroplasties was started in Stockholm.

Motivation

It is necessary to build up audits that can be prospectively used over many years and that will facilitate the daily work. Some general aspects and lessons can be drawn from the Swedish experience of medical audit. Motivating the different departments to participate is of vital importance. Motives differ in different places and times. The first major motive is the facilitation of everyday routine medical work. The audit form can be used as a standardised part of the patient's file, thereby simplifying routines. Less unstructured type-written text and thereby less secretarial work is needed. It is also easier to find this information in the file at a later date, e.g. at out-patient follow up visits.

The second main motive is its usefulness for administrative purposes, e.g. yearly activity reports, to support resource claims in discussions with administrative authorities and to receive funding. It is preferable that the profession itself outlines the guidelines for an audit.

The third motive is scientific. Centrally, the large amount of prospective standardised material provides possibilities for the analysis of the overall panorama of hospitals, diagnoses and modes of treatment. It also provides unique possibilities for studying special rare indications that need the multi-centre approach to collect enough material. Locally, it is possible to use the audit forms as a basis for a study, e.g. comparison between two operation methods, introduction of new types of rehabilitation and so forth, especially when someone can use the audit for his/her thesis work. The hip re-arthroplasty project and also the knee arthroplasty project have benefitted from this incentive.

Performance

In the very long perspective (decades) of follow up for the hip and knee arthroplasties, the ambition of registering details has been changed to a focus on whether or not reoperations are performed. For the hip fracture study much more detailed functional parameters are registered, as this is important in the short-term perspective of these elderly patients. Previous studies[6] have shown that over 80% of the complications needing reoperation occur within two years after the hip fracture. The registered hip fracture patients also have a considerable mortality with time due to high mean age and concomitant diseases.[2,7]

In Sweden all persons have a social security number, e.g. 05 03 15 – 1649. This person was born as child number 164 in Sweden on the 15th of March 1905. The last digit is a control based on the other digits. Due to this social security number, which is unique to the person, it is possible to trace the patient. The number is generally used for all kinds of identification in Sweden. This is a great advantage when checking data with files from different departments and when patients change their address.

Computing

The use of PC programs and handling data on desktop computers, as described for the Swedish multicentre hip fracture study, has shown definite advantages. The knee arthroplasty project has recently also started to use this model. Reports from the participant to the centre have to be made on computer discs due to the large amount of patient data. The possibility for the participating centres continuously to make their own calculations on their data is important. Permits from the Swedish Data

Inspection have been given to all these projects. Access to the central collection of data is limited to the permit holders to protect individual patients.

Centres and communications

The registering centres and project leaders are now:

for the Swedish multicentre hip structure study:

> Professor Karl-Göran Thorngren,
> Department of Orthopaedics,
> Lund University Hospital, S-221 85 Lund, Sweden.

for the Swedish knee arthroplasty project:
> Professor Lars Lidgren,
> address as above in Lund.

for the national hip re-arthroplasty project:
> Professor Peter Herberts,
> Department of Orthopaedics,
> Sahlgren Hospital, S-413 45 Göteborg, Sweden.

Feedback to the participants with regular reports containing their own data as well as collected mean values for the country are necessary. The hip fracture study reports twice a year whereas the arthroplasty projects report once a year. To keep the enthusiasm for the project on a high level, regular discussions are required, e.g. in connection with the Swedish Orthopaedic Societies meetings.

Funding

Great amounts of energy and idealism are necessary to start a large-scale audit project. Furthermore, economic resources are necessary to print forms, to communicate with the other centres and to register data on computer, as well as to do calculations and print reports. The Swedish Medical Research Council has funded all these projects during their initial years. From 1990 the Swedish Government has decided to fund the projects, which are still to be run at the original centres. It has been decided to be advantageous that the profession itself outlines the guidelines for an audit and keeps it running. The goodwill and enthusiasm of the orthopaedic community is the basis for managing the Swedish audit projects.

References

1. Ceder, L., Thorngren, K-G. & Wallden, B. (1980). Prognostic indicators and early home rehabilitation in elderly patients with hip fractures. *Clinical Orthopaedics and Related Research*, **152**, 173–184.
2. Thorngren, M., Nilsson, L. T. & Thorngren, K-G. (1988). Prognosis-determined rehabilitation of hip fractures. *Comprehensive Gerontology*, **2**, 12–17.
3. Dobbs, H. S. (1980). Survivorship of total hip replacement. *Journal of Bone and Joint Surgery*, **62B**, 168–173.
4. Knutson, K., Lindstrand, A. & Lidgren, L. (1986). Survival of knee arthroplasties. A nation wide multicentre investigation of 8000 cases. *Journal of Bone and Joint Surgery*, **68B**, 795–803.
5. Ahnfelt, L., Herberts, P., Malchau, H. & Andersson, E. B. J. (1990). Prognosis of total hip replacement. A Swedish Multicenter Study of 4664 revisions. *Acta Orthopaedica Scandinavica*, **61(Suppl 238)**.
6. Holmberg, S., Kalen R. & Thorngren, K-G. (1987). Treatment and outcome of femoral neck fractures: An analysis of 2,418 patients admitted from their own homes. *Clinical Orthopaedics and Related Research*, **218**, 42–52.
7. Holmberg, S. & Thorngren, K-G. (1985). Rehabilitation after femoral neck fracture. 3053 patients followed for 6 years. *Acta Orthopaedica Scandinavica*, **56**, 305–308.

24
Performance indicators
W. JONATHAN BOYCE

Introduction

Managers in private sector industries can measure their performance in a variety of ways, for example by changes in the volume of sales or by financial ratios such as return on capital employed or net profit margin. Such measures are integral to the accounting systems necessary to run the businesses concerned. In nationalised industries, especially those such as the NHS where income is largely fixed, such measures either do not exist or would not be a fair index of management performance. In such situations alternative measures are required for managers and others to evaluate their performance. The Department of Health's latest *health service indicators* (HSI) represent the current state of play in the attempt to meet this requirement in the NHS.

Even though it may be clear exactly what aspect of performance is to be measured, there may be considerable uncertainty about how to encourage people to use the information. At one extreme is simple publication – a take it or leave it approach. At the other extreme the indicators can be linked to a formal performance review mechanism or used to illuminate decisions in a market place, and in such cases the likelihood of change can be increased by tying them to personal targets and incentives. The issue of how to secure appropriate use of performance indicators is extremely important and often overlooked.

This chapter describes the development of *performance indicators* in the National Health Service, considers some of the problems with them, and finally looks at their relationship with clinical audit.

The term '*performance indicator*' can have many different meanings, ranging from '*any statistical indicator used to assess performance*' to the most specific '*one of the 400 (or so) indicators in the Department of Health's package*'.[1]

376

The Department of Health: performance indicators initiative

Since the inception of the NHS there has been routine collection of many different kinds of data. For example, patient activity data began with the SH3 returns in 1948, to which was added the *hospital in-patient enquiry* (HIPE) in 1952 and then *hospital activity analysis* (HAA) in 1969. It is noticeable that both the extent and the complexity of routine data have increased throughout the history of the NHS but it is only in the last ten to 15 years that the processing of such data and their subsequent use have been given much attention. In 1981 the Public Accounts Committee of the House of Commons examined financial control and accountability in the NHS, and identified a need 'to monitor key indicators of performance'.[2] In 1982 the Secretary of State for Health and Social Security introduced a review system with formal annual reviews of District Health Authority by regions and of regions by the DHSS. Linked to this the DHSS and one region jointly developed pilot indicators for comparing and assessing the performance of health authorities in the efficient use of resources. The first list of indicators was published in 1982 based on routinely available data.[3]

The Department of Health was at this point sceptical of the value of performance indicators, other than as a means of asking pertinent questions. The Permanent Secretary at the time, in evidence to the public accounts committee said:

We are addressing a service the end product of which is whether patients are better or cured and that is the supreme performance indicator. The very real difficulty – it is both conceptually and technically difficult – is to bring into a direct relationship the outputs of the health service in that sense and the inputs in terms of money and manpower. What we are addressing are performance indicators which will be of a very broad nature and will in the early stages enable us to ask questions. With experience it will be possible to ask pertinent and relevant questions. I really would not like the Committee to think that by running together a whole string of data in an equation we are going to produce a cost–benefit analysis of appendicectomies ... We have now got a range of indicators which we think will be a relevant base for enabling regions to ask districts, and for us to ask regions, relevant questions about their performance. But the point that we want to stress is that they will not of themselves take you much beyond the stage of asking questions. They will be pointers rather than definitive judgements of performance.[4]

At the same time as the DHSS was starting, with great caution, to develop performance indicators, the Health Services Management Centre of the University of Birmingham was experimenting with inter-district comparisons on a national scale.[5] They also developed a new way of displaying the information on a percentile bar in relation to other districts – see Figure 24.1 and Table 24.1. In those early days the main use of the

Table 24.1 *1977 trauma and orthopaedic profile*
(for 202 English health districts)

Indicator	Range (%)	Value for East Sampleshire	Position relative to other districts (expressed as a percentile)					
Descriptive			0	20	40	60	80	100
Balance of cross boundary flows	0.0–32.5	82.6		*				
% Residents over 65	9.1–26.2	12.3	*					
Demand								
Waiting list per population	0.0–8.9	5.5						*
% Non-urgent cases waiting over 1 yr	0.0–80.0	58.2					*	
Input								
Beds per population	0.1–1.0	0.35	*					
Out-patient sessions per population	0.9–10.5	2.6		*				
Process								
Length of stay (days)	6.5–24.4	20.3						*
Turnover interval (days)	0.0–13.2	3.1			*			
Day cases as % of all in-patients	0.0–51.5	37.8						*
Total attendances per new out-patient	2.0–15.5	4.6					*	
Total attendances per clinic	13.0–81.0	45.0					*	

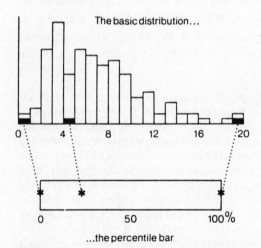

Fig. 24.1. The Health Services Management Centre in Birmingham developed the percentile bar and used it to compare districts on a variety of indicators. Conversion of a distribution to a percentile bar.

comparisons was identification of outliers on a variety of resource and process measures (tail gunning); and it was argued that at the extremes such measures were likely to be good proxy indicators of outcomes.[6] But perhaps the main contribution of the Birmingham initiative was to make the indicators readily accessible to local management both by innovative presentation and by making them available on micro-computers at the moment when interest in information technology began a rapid expansion.

From 1983 to 1987 the *DHSS performance indicator package* and the Birmingham work ran in parallel. Many health authorities possessed both. However, following the introduction of the Körner minimum data set, the two systems have been merged and expanded into a much more extensive set of health service indicators published by the Department of Health.[1]

Health service indicators (HSI)

The current package contains in excess of 400 indicators based on routine data from a variety of sources including Department of Health returns on finance, manpower and activity, the NHS *hospital episode system* (HES), and population data from the *Office of Population, Censuses and Surveys* (OPCS). Each indicator is a ratio of two variables. For example, indicator AM43 is the number of emergency patient journeys in the relevant year in each ambulance authority expressed per thousand resident population of that authority.

The indicators are organised into 42 family groups each of which focuses on a particular type of measure (e.g. hospitalisation rates) or a particular area of health care (e.g. medical physics). Within each of the families indicators are either financial, manpower or activity indicators, or combinations of these. Many indicators are given separately for different medical specialties and some, such as length of stay for finished consultant episodes (LS41), are also given for particular tracer conditions or procedures (LS54). Figures 24.2, 24.3 and 24.4 are examples of output from the HSI package. A certain amount of ingenuity is needed to interpret some of the abbreviations and codes but with a little experience the information is quite accessible.

There has also been a certain amount of pre-processing of data. For example, catchment populations have been pre-calculated from OPCS data on resident populations and HES data on cross-boundary flows, and some indicators are standardised rates where actual values are expressed as a percentage of values expected if average conditions of (say) age distribution were to apply in that district. All of this is somewhat prescriptive, and although it simplifies matters and encourages use for many, has been a source of irritation and frustration to others who would prefer to have access to the basic data.

The number of indicators has increased considerably with the in-

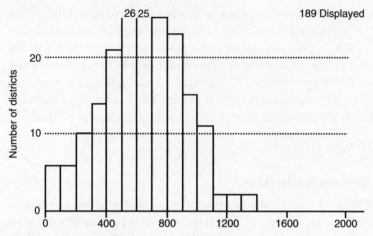

Fig. 24.2. Hospitalisation rate for cataract surgery, 65 +, accessible by condition, 1988.

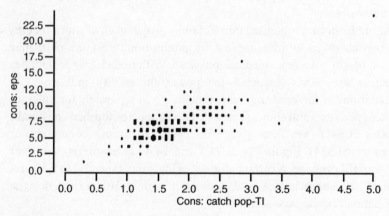

Fig. 24.3. 1988 general surgery scattergram.

Indicator	Oxfordshire value	Nat. min.	middle 80% of national values are between		Nat. max.
% adms no. op.	43.02	0.00	| < * > |		91.92

Fig. 24.4. 1988 general surgery boxplot.

troduction of specialties and tracer conditions and expert systems have been developed that are aimed at guiding busy managers in selecting relevant indicators.

As performance indicators (PIs) have become more refined, and managers have become more familiar with them, the ways in which they are used have diversified. As well as the focusing of attention on extreme values (tail gunning) mentioned earlier, techniques include the setting of targets based on distributions of performance across many organisations; monitoring an indicator for changes over time; and attempts to associate performance on a particular indicator with other variables such as management structure, in order to identify good or bad practice. But as the use of performance indicators has become more widespread, so the problems have become clearer.

Problems with performance indicators

Performance indicators have not had a good press. There is a variety of real problems with their validity, cost and interpretation that lay them open to attack. Those who oppose them or feel threatened by them have not been slow to point out their weaknesses. But one has only to look at their provenance to realise that performance indicators are here to stay, and their weaknesses need to be acknowledged and publicised so that they may be improved in the future and to ensure that those who use them are alert to current limitations. The remainder of this section examines some of the weaknesses.

Validity

All PIs are based on routine data sets, the accuracy and completeness of which are notoriously patchy. Even the simplest investigation of what might be thought to be hard facts in routine data sets can be quite alarming. A recent comparison by the Audit Commission of dates of admission and discharge found in one hospital's patient administration system, with the dates as stated in the medical records, showed that at least one of the dates did not match in 36% of the episodes.

The effect of incompleteness or inaccuracy in a data set may depend on the particular indicator that is going to be derived, or the use to which it is to be put. For example, random incompleteness in a patient administration data set may not significantly alter the derived average length of stay (although it ought then to be expressed with attached confidence intervals) but could have a devastating effect on derived turnover intervals, as there would be a significant underestimate of the occupied bed days.

Equally, the use to which an indicator is to be put is critical. Errors in an indicator that is used to create a distribution may be acceptable, especially if there is reason to believe that the errors are likely to be distributed symmetrically around zero. On the other hand, it would be unwise to assess a single district against a target without attempting to validate the indicator.

Finally, it is worth remembering that a set of data that is valid today may not be valid tomorrow. Practices change and very often the data-collection system can be left behind. For example, the tendency to place patients in beds belonging to another specialty and even to designate different beds on the same ward as belonging to different specialties has reduced the accuracy of data on beds belonging to specialties so much that specialty turnover intervals, once a stable and reliable indicator, are now acknowledged to be unreliable. They will probably be dropped from the HSIs in the future.

Lack of detail

Performance indicators tend to raise more questions than they answer, especially the so-called first line indicators that are often used to screen for extreme values that require explanation. The answers to these further questions require either completely new data sets or else the ability to disaggregate existing data using variables such as age and diagnosis.

Sometimes the more detailed data simply have not been collected for practical reasons or cost considerations. Where they have been collected they are less likely to be accurate than the simpler broad measures. Problems such as local interpretation or loose definitions can have a disproportionate effect in small subsets of data.

Finally, there is a dilemma in presenting detailed indicators between a prescriptive definition of which ratios are available and simple presentation of the basic data. Potential users will have different requirements.

These problems create a dilemma for cross-district comparisons, between on the one hand making crude comparisons that ignore variations in other factors known to be important and on the other hand taking account of such factors but introducing unacceptable inaccuracy.

Interpretation

Accuracy of indicators is by no means the end of the story. Most indicators are measures of one or two variables in a complex interactive system that is in turn subject to outside influences, and so an extreme value or a change in the value of an indicator can have many possible causes. For example, if the provision of general medical beds in a district was higher than average in relation to the catchment population there could be several underlying reasons:

1. There might be more elderly people in the population than usual.
2. The admission rates or lengths of stay within (say) five-year age bands might be higher than average, and either of these might in turn reflect an unusually high incidence of certain types of cases in the community.
3. The long average lengths of stay may be due to a small number of particularly long-stay patients which might in turn reflect a relative paucity of long-stay residential and nursing places.
4. The beds in that hospital might simply be used inefficiently.

The list could be extended, but is sufficient to make the general point.

To explain an extreme value of a first-line indicator requires a good analytical understanding of the system and a further mass of detailed information. These problems lie behind some of the more recent initiatives with the performance indicator package, such as organising the indicators into first-line indicators at the top of a hierarchy of increasing detail, and expert systems that aim to help the user with the analytical framework.

But even when the initial finding has been fully analysed and explained there may be disagreement about the right action to take or the right level for a target.[7] Some people may feel that the length of stay is too short and compromises quality of care. Others may feel that it is not short enough and that the system is inefficient. Targets and thresholds are usually arbitrary and not amenable to resolution by analysis. Having said that, values can sometimes be so extreme that the majority will agree on the need to correct them and on the required direction of movement.

Cost

To be useful, performance indicators need to be detailed, and the more detailed they are the higher the cost of collection and processing. The cost probably ought to be viewed as the opportunity cost of the staff time involved. It can be considerably greater than the simple unit of labour costs if there is a limited supply of the relevant skills; essential tasks elsewhere in the district may be neglected. This may explain why the completeness and accuracy of data collected to central requirements are often so low compared with data that are collected because they are needed locally – the local cost is far higher than is at first imagined.

Lack of outcome indicators

The term performance indicator begs the question of what is meant by performance. The ultimate goal of managers and clinicians alike should be to improve the service to patients (this includes both better clinical outcomes and improved patient satisfaction). A recurring criticism of the indicators developed by the Department of Health is that they almost exclusively measure process and activity rather than outcome. If performance is limited to meaning economy and efficiency then such criticism is unfounded. But something more is then needed in the way of evaluation, or we could end up developing a service that is highly efficient but that has no effect on health.

It is interesting in this respect to note that the *Joint Committee on the Accreditation of Healthcare Organisations* (JCAHO) in the United States has recently embarked on a so–called 'agenda for change', the aim of which is to extend the measurement of performance from simply looking at an organisation's capability to assessing patient care outcomes.[8]

The problems discussed so far tend to be even greater if the indicators are meant to measure change in health status or patient satisfaction with the process. Many of the measurements need careful definition, and carry a higher risk of observer bias. Changes in health status have to be judged against measurements made before the intervention, which necessitates considerable detail. Finally, the cost of collecting good outcomes data is considerably greater than that for processes and activity, not least because the measurements ought to be made at pre-determined times (for example, mobility three months after hip replacement) by which time patients will usually have been dispersed back into the community. The long-term answer to this problem must surely be integration of data from primary and secondary care.

Not surprisingly, outcomes data have only been collected sporadically, usually by doctors with an interest in particular clinical areas, in the centres in which they work. The absence of routine data on outcomes is reflected in the performance indicators, where the only outcomes indicators are based on mortality data or on items recorded statutorily about birth such as birthweight or unintended home delivery.

But if it is clear that we ultimately need reliable outcomes indicators to plan and deliver the best value for our health service money, and if the Department of Health does not try to move in this direction with its health service indicators, then where will the indicators come from? The most obvious place to look is clinical audit.

Performance indicators and clinical audit

While performance indicators have been developed by the DoH and NHS management, professionals in most disciplines have been taking an increasing interest in measuring their own performance. This has recently received formal recognition and encouragement with the attention given to medical audit in the Government's 1989 reform of the health service.[9] Although the broad long-term aims of both movements must surely be the same, they do differ in a number of ways. Fifteen years ago the distinctions were clear. Clinical audit was concerned with patient outcomes, it was the property of professionals, mainly doctors, and almost its sole purpose was educational.[10] Performance indicators, on the other hand, were concerned with structures and processes, were the province of management and were seen as an aid to achieving greater efficiency.

Since then there has been considerable convergence, with professional organisations recognising improved efficiency as a legitimate goal of clinical audit[11] and with managers expressing more and more interest in outcomes and patient satisfaction.

This recognition of an overlap of goals is a necessary first step and is to be welcomed. There is little point in studying the efficiency of different capabilities without regard to their effectiveness. But equally there is little point in measuring outcomes unless one is able to link those outcomes to variation in the structures and processes that produce them so as to understand the causes of good or bad outcome and present remedies. Doctors and managers need to share both types of information but it will be some time before they can be integrated into a single performance indicator system.

Common goals are only a first step. The second step is to have comprehensive, comparable outcomes data and indicators. Most clinical audit to date is local, but there are some examples of 'global audit' that aim to compare clinical outcomes data between centres. For example, the Royal College of Surgeons recently invited consultant general surgeons to submit clinical audit data on their own work for a whole year and received 149 responses (out of a total of just over 1000). This covered 140 000 in-patient admissions and 100 000 operations and has enabled interesting analyses of outcomes and how they vary between centres (D. C. Dunn, pers. commun.). Similar initiatives have been started in other surgical specialties including orthopaedics and ENT. Such initiatives will undoubtedly become more common and we can hope eventually to see a national system of coding and classification underpinning routine data on both health status and patient satisfaction.

The third and final step to the (perhaps unattainable) state of information Nirvana will be the ability to link outcomes to structures and process, and indeed costs. At this point cost-effectiveness studies on a whole range of activities and using routine data become a real possibility, but many will by then doubtless be questioning whether the ends justify the means. We are, however, unlikely to have the luxury of this particular debate for many years yet.

References

1. Department of Health (1989). *Health Service Indicators Guidance – Dictionary*. London: HMSO.
2. Public Accounts Committee (1981). *Financial Control and Accountability in the National Health Service. 17th Report, Session 1980–81*. London: HMSO.
3. DHSS (1982). *Performance Indicators in the NHS*. RA (82)34. London: DHSS.
4. Public Accounts Committee (1982). Paragraphs 1621 and 1634. In *Financial Control and Accountability in the National Health Service. 17th Report, Session 1981–2*. London: HMSO.
5. Yates, J. (1982). *Hospital Beds – A problem for Diagnosis and Management?* London: Heinemann Medical Books Ltd.
6. Yates, J. & Vickerstaff, L. (1982). Inter-hospital comparisons. *Mental Handicap*, **10**, 45–47.
7. Charny, M. (1990). Facing up to demand. *Health Service Journal*, **100**, 52–53.
8. Schyve, P. M. & Roberts, J. S. (1990). Using clinical performance data to stimulate quality improvement. In *Measuring the Outcomes of Medical Care*, ed. A. Hopkins & D. Costain. London: Royal College of Physicians.
9. Department of Health (1989). *Working for Patients*. London: HMSO.
10. Alment, E. A. J. (1976). *With Competence to Practice*. London: Committee of Enquiry.
11. The Royal College of Physicians (1989). *Medical Audit: A First Report. What, Why and how?* London: RCP.

25

Measuring outcome and quality control

DAVID W. YATES AND CHARLES S. B. GALASKO

Introduction

The progression of a disease state can be characterised in terms of input, process and output. Medical audit seeks to compare actual and ideal outcome by examining the management of the patient, taking into account the severity of the disease and the general health of the patient. Was it appropriate to the presenting complaint? Did it make the most effective use of existing resources? Did it offer the best value for money in terms of that particular disease and also in relation to other demands on the health service? These questions cannot be addressed in any scientific manner unless there are objective measurements for the severity of the presenting condition, the type of treatment and the outcome. This chapter examines ways of measuring outcome and the limitations of their use in clinical audit. In an ageing population chronic diseases are becoming more prevalent and cure is unusual. Outcome is often a balance between the activity of the disease process and the effectiveness of treatment. Much of the discussion will therefore overlap into the measurement of disease severity, investigation and treatment.

Gordon[1] has contrasted the significant improvement in weather forecasting over the recent years with our more modest achievements in medicine. Is this true? There has been a massive increase in meteorological information from many sources and it is collated in large computers. In contrast, medical information is sparse, often mixed with anecdote, and rarely is it immediately available in a form that can be directly fed into the computer. Despite this, the achievements in medicine during the past two or three decades have been dramatic and, as medical practitioners, we should not sell ourselves short. There have been major advances in transplantation, joint replacement, minimal invasive surgery, pharmacology and immunology. Yet clinical computation and audit have not featured prominently in these developments.

However, one of the major problems in medicine is the inconsistent application of these new therapies. This is usually due to financial constraints, but occasionally stems from a reluctance to adapt to changing circumstances. Clinical audit addresses this imbalance, usually comparing present performance with 'the ideal', and assesses how we can improve our own services to achieve the outcome available in the best centres using modern equipment and technology. Taking a wider view, this might not be the best for the whole population, but it is a simplistic approach that is commonly used because it is immediately attractive and easy to compute.

Measurement of input

The severity of a disease process is easier to measure when numerical data are available. Hence most progress has been made in scoring severity of illness in intensive care patients and in those who have been injured. Knaus postulated that there were five determinants of outcome in patients admitted to an intensive care unit (Table 25.1).[2]

He emphasised the importance of classifying the underlying disease process first. This assumes an understanding of basic mechanisms. The classification system must be exhaustive, mutually exclusive and must be easy to use by non-specialist assessors. This last point is particularly important as the collection of data upon which a future audit is to be based is usually in the hands of the non-specialist.

The International Classification of Diseases can be used to identify the nature of the disease but, in most cases, it is of little value in measuring severity. This is, of course, essential and should be determined ideally before treatment has started. The criteria used to measure severity must distinguish between cause and effect. For example, it would be inappropriate to choose blood pressure as a measure of severity of major burns – percentage surface area involved would be more appropriate. Criteria are often chosen by 'expert opinion' or by a review of the appropriate literature. They subsequently become refined by experience and anecdote, but more importantly by 'validation studies' against a clearly defined outcome. Examples include staging of colonic cancer, severity of myocardial infarction, extent of ankle fracture and risk of suicide. The most scientific approach is to measure many variables in a large population with varying outcomes and determine those that are the best prognostic indicators.

Table 25.1 *Determinants of outcome after admission to the intensive care unit*

1. Type and severity of disease
2. Physiological reserves (including age and chronic health status)
3. Response to therapy
4. Type of treatment
5. Application of treatment

From Knaus (1987).[2]

Table 25.2 *ASA Classification of physical status*

Class	Physical status
I	A healthy patient with no systemic disease
II	A patient with a mild to moderate systemic disease process…that does not limit the patient's activities (e.g. mild diabetic)
III	A patient with a severe systemic disturbance…that imposes a definite functional limitation (e.g. ischaemic heart disease with limited exercise tolerance)
IV	A patient with severe systemic disease that is a constant threat to life (e.g. advanced chronic liver failure)
V	A moribund patient who is unlikely to survive 24 h with or without surgery
E	Emergency operation on any patient in above classes. Prefix letter E to class

Adapted from American Society of Anesthesiologists (1963).[5]

The use of an ordinal scale is common to most scoring systems. Whilst this is useful in allowing clinicians to rank patients according to severity of a disease process, it has limited statistical value. The scales usually employ variable intervals, i.e. the difference between Grade 1 and Grade 2 state is not necessarily the same as the difference between Grade 2 and Grade 3 state. The validity of the ranking is often determined by comparison with mortality. Whilst this approach has much to commend it, it does not measure the quality of survival and is, of course, only valid as a general retrospective assessment. It has no place in the assessment of individual patients or the determination of prognosis.

Outcome is determined not only by the severity of the disease process and the application of treatment but also by the physiological reserves of the patient. In most adult diseases age does not appear to have a major influence on survival until the sixth decade. From the mid-fifties there is an increasing effect. This is reflected in weighting factors used in the APACHE II system of measuring illness in intensive care patients[3] and in ASCOT, a measure of injury severity.[4] Chronic health evaluation is also represented in the APACHE II system, but perhaps the most widely used measure of chronic disease is that drawn up by the American Society of Anaesthesiologists (Table 25.2).

A further difficulty is the conflict between the use of numerical data such as biochemical findings with a defined normal range and other parameters of health that do not have a definite range of normality. Data from the latter are softer and more difficult to compute and analyse. An example would be psychiatric morbidity, in contrast to the crisper measurement of renal failure.

Management and outcome

Outcome is influenced by the investigations carried out, the type of treatment prescribed and the execution of that treatment. The distinction between the latter two is important as a close inspection of any treatment system will identify discrepancies between what the physician intended and what the patient received. The knowledge of the timing of an intervention is also important. An example of the therapeutic intervention scoring system of Knaus is given in Table 25.3.

The consequences of treatment can also be measured. Examples include the length of stay in hospital and the type of bed occupied, together with the expense of each part of the treatment. However, these measurements are not particularly helpful unless they are judged against the final outcome. Unfortunately, this process can take many years. A good example would be the outcome following a total joint replacement. Several parameters are important. In the short term the incidence of infection and other complications can be used to monitor management. There is no value in reducing the time spent in hospital or reducing other costs, for example using an inferior theatre suite, if these money saving exercises result in a higher rate of infection. In the longer term the rate of loosening and the revision rate can be used to compare the results between one prosthesis and another, between one unit and another and between one hospital and another. However, it may take in excess of 20 years before the eventual outcome can be established and unless very detailed records are kept for this length of time, it may not be possible to assess the standard of overall management.

Table 25.3 *Examples from the therapeutic intervention scoring system*

1 point	ECG Urinary catheter Chest physiotherapy
2 points	CVP monitoring Hourly neurological observation 2 peripheral IV lines
3 points	Cardiac output measurement Arterial blood gas measurements Chest drain
4 point	Cardiac arrest within 48 hours Paralysis and ventilation Haemodialysis

Measurement of outcome

There have been many attempts to assess prognosis accurately, based on presenting features. For example, in 1962 Peel *et al.*[6] proposed a 'coronary prognostic index' to grade the severity of myocardial infarction. It was not widely used, presumably because at that time clinicians were predominantly concerned with individual case management rather than strategic planning. With the advent of increasingly expensive treatment regimes, greater therapeutic possibilities and an apparently ever-tightening budget, it is now generally acknowledged that such indices have a relevance to practising clinicians and there is now more interest in their use in everyday practice.

The development of scales to measure the severity of injury and thereby assess the effectiveness of treatment is a good example of the transformation of audit from anecdote to statistical analysis. The complex and interrelated responses to tissue damage and the activation of homeostatic mechanisms combine to frustrate attempts to characterise in simple terms the physiological responses to, and the severity of, an injury. Clearly an initial measurement of blood pressure and pulse do not reflect the extent of damage. Nevertheless, these and many other measurements are routinely collected and many analyses have been undertaken in order to identify those parameters that are most accurate in determining outcome. In 1980 Champion *et al.*[7] published the results of the assessment of the association between 16 physiological variables and survival. These included systolic blood pressure, pulse rate and strength, capillary refill, respiratory rate and expansion, Glasgow coma scale and pupil size and reaction. By multivariant analysis of these recordings on 1084 patients the authors refined this to best reflect outcome whilst keeping data collection as simple as possible. This 'triage index' was later refined to the trauma score[8] and the revised trauma score.[9]

Measurement of the severity of anatomical disruption after injury has undergone a similar evolution. Early assessments based on the size of the wound were replaced in 1969 by the abbreviated injury scale (AIS) which scores all known injuries on a scale from 1 (minor) to 6 (unsurvivable). This scale has been refined over the years and the 1990 edition of the abbreviated injury scale coding manual now contains over 1200 injuries. Although there is general consensus that it ranks the severity of injury to individual organs and tissue it does not claim to be an interval scale. For example, the difference between AIS 3 and AIS 4 is not necessarily the same as the difference between AIS 1 and AIS 2. The scale was initially used by crash investigators to measure the effectiveness of safety devices but is now used extensively in trauma research and trauma audit. Patients who have sustained multiple injuries are represented by summating the squares of the AIS scores of the three most severely injured body regions. This *injury severity score* (ISS) has been validated against mortality statistics. The fit is not perfect and further refinements are constantly being proposed. For example, it is clear that the ISS does not necessarily reflect the severity of multiple injuries to one body region, as shown in Table 25.4. Neither does it always represent the extent of the ensuing disability.

To resolve such difficulties, modification of existing predictors of outcome may well be desirable but this does create problems for those who are undertaking longitudinal studies. Changes to well-established scoring systems must therefore be introduced with caution and only after widespread consultation.

Combining scoring systems measuring different features of the disease process may improve overall accuracy. For example, the combination of the revised trauma score (RTS) and the ISS together with an adjustment for age is now widely used (as the 'TRISS methodology') to audit trauma care.[11] The probability of survival is calculated by the introduction of weighting factors to the RTS, ISS and age based on the known outcome of patients on a large database. Although this concept is attractive, it is of questionable statistical validity as each component may measure the same variable in different ways (e.g. Glasgow coma score in the RTS, versus level of consciousness in ISS) or measure interrelated features of the same disease process. Expert statistical advice is essential, therefore, before combining scoring systems to assess overall performance.

The TRISS methodology has been used to extend audit from the

Table 25.4 *Examples of the failure of the injury severity score to indicate the severity of injury and ensuing disability*

	AIS	Body region	ISS
Case 1			
Left femoral artery laceration resulting in left high thigh amputation	3	Extremities	9
		Total score	9
Case 2			
Open fracture left tibia and fibula	3	Extremities	9
Fracture left 3rd, 4th and 5th metatarsals	2	Extremities	*
Dislocation left 2nd tarsometatarsal joint	2	Extremities	*
		Total score	9
Case 3			
Transverse displaced fracture right femur	3	Extremities	9
Fracture dislocation left hip	3	Extremities	*
Fracture right ulnar	2	Extremities	*
Fracture left metatarsal	2	Extremities	*
Limb lacerations and abrasions	1	External	1
		Total score	10

* Only the highest score is used in the ISS calculation, thereby ignoring any effect the other injuries may contribute towards the overall threat to life and the ensuing disability. From Galasko *et al.* (1986).[10]

particular to the general. By comparing groups of patients with similar ranges of injury it is possible to compare the performance of different hospitals or indeed different trauma systems. This has now been formally incorporated into the '*major trauma outcome study* (MTOS)' established by Champion in Washington, USA and now being developed in the UK and elsewhere.

Similar systems of analysis and prediction are being applied to other diseases. For example, Poungvarin *et al.*[12] reported a method to distinguish supratentorial intracranial haemorrhage from infarction. They used the same system of expert opinion to identify relevant criteria, applied them in a prospective study, used discriminant analysis to develop a scoring system and then validated it against a new larger data set. This method is commended as a pragmatic and rapid way of establishing a scoring system in many disease states.

Whatever the disease under study, calculation of probability is merely what it says, not a forecast of outcome. For example, if a patient with a probability of survival of 80 % dies the outcome is unexpected in that four out of five patients with a similar disease state and similar pre-existing health and age could be expected to survive. The fifth patient would be expected to die and this could indeed be the patient under study.

Disability

All these calculations are based on the probability of death or survival. No account is taken of the potential disability of survivors. Clearly many more people survive injury and disease than succumb and it is increasingly recognised that our ability to measure the quality of this survival is inadequate. This in turn has hindered our ability to audit care of patients with non-fatal diseases.

The measurement of severity of disability has been the concern, for many years, of those responsible for the chronically ill such as geriatricians and rheumatologists and those who care for victims of stroke, head and spinal injury.[13–16] The currently available methods of assessing 'activities of daily living' have been reviewed by Eakin.[17,18] Although many were designed for specific use with particular diseases they all measure long-term disability and the potential for rehabilitation and yet there is no commonly accepted standard disability scoring system. The *functional independence measure* (FIM) has been designed to overcome this problem by providing a minimum data set for all disciplines (*Uniform Data System for Medical Rehabilitation* 1987).[19] It has a seven level scale assessing activities of daily living, mobility, sphincter control, communication and social awareness.

The qualitative information contained in the International Classification of Diseases index has been extended to cover impairments, disabilities and handicaps (*International Classification of Impairment, Disability and Handicap*, WHO, Geneva 1980, ICIDH).[20] It is essentially a descriptive system and unfortunately cannot be used to measure outcome in any way that would permit statistical analysis. Attempts to introduce ICIDH into routine clinical practice have not been very successful.[21] Scales designed to measure disability after injury and acute illness are in their infancy and much work is required in this area before we are able to measure outcome in terms of morbidity as well as mortality.[22]

Not only do we have difficulty in measuring disability, but there also is some confusion about the terminology. The ICIDH defines impairments, disability and handicap as follows:

An '*impairment*' is defined as 'any loss or abnormality of psychological, physiological, or anatomic structure or function'.

A '*disability*' is defined as 'any restriction or lack (resulting from an impairment) of ability to perform an activity in the manner, or within the range considered normal for a human being'.

A '*handicap*' is defined as 'a disadvantage for a given individual, resulting from an impairment or disability, that limits or prevents the fulfilment of a role that is normal (depending on age, sex and social and cultural factors) for that individual'.

A handicap is concerned with the value attached to an individual's situation or experience when it departs from the norm. It is characterised by a discordance between the individual's performance or status, and the expectations of the individual him/herself, or of the particular group of which he/she is a member. A handicap thus represents socialisation of an impairment or disability, and as such it reflects the consequences for the individual – cultural, social, economic and environmental – that stem from the presence of impairment and disability.

For example, if someone injures a knee and it remains stiff or unstable, that is an impairment. If as a result he/she has problems with walking, climbing, running, etc., the latter are the disabilities. If the individual was a professional footballer and could not return to sport, he would be severely handicapped as a result of the injury. However, if the individual had a sedentary job and neither his occupation, his social activities, nor his hobbies were affected by the stiff knee, then he would not be handicapped by the injury.

Quality of life

Another way of measuring outcome is to measure the quality of life as a function of mortality, morbidity, mobility, and quality of survival and the effect of treatment. Health economists have moved from a simple analysis of health outcome in terms of financial implications for the patient and society, through attempts to assess effectiveness in non-monetary terms, to the concept of '*quality adjusted life years*' or QALYs. Williams[23] was one of the first to use this system to measure the economics of coronary artery by-pass grafting. This approach to measurement of quality of outcome and the implication that the method of treatment should be based on reasons other than medical efficacy, prompt discussion of ethical and moral issues. These aside, it is now generally accepted that with limited financial resources there must be some equity in their distribution.

The QALY approach uses quantitative data on survival, qualitative data on disability and distress, and economic data, for example on drugs,

---

Box 25.1   *Well years of life lost*

Man with life expectancy of 75 years is killed in road crash aged 40

WYLL = 35 (75 - 40 = 35)

Woman with life expectancy of 80 years has subarachnoid haemorrhage aged 60. Quality of life diminished by 0.75 per annum.

WYLL = 15 (80 - 60 = 20; 20 x 0.75 = 15)

Rehabilitation programme improves mobility, bringing benefit of 0.25 per annum

WYLL saving = 5 (20 x (0.75 - 0.25) = 10; 15 - 10 = 5)

---

surgery and other forms of treatment. Various models have been postulated. Torrance[24] introduced the concept of *time trade-off*. He asked people to choose between different options of health status (e.g. remaining in a clearly defined state of ill health that would lead to death at a specified time, compared with a different state of health that would result in death at an earlier or later time). By asking subjects to make judgements on a wide variety of possibilities, narrowing the time intervals until they felt indifferent to the choices offered, he was able to produce a schematic model relating chronic disease status to optimal survival. These results can be combined with information about the influence of treatment on prognosis at various stages of the disease process to improve the model.

There are of course criticisms of this approach. The physical aspects of chronic disease have received most attention and little importance has been attached to the psychosocial variables that can affect the quality of life. Perhaps the most important criticism is the assumption that death is the worst possible outcome. In many of the modern methods of assessing quality of life the concept of release from suffering, through death, has been acknowledged ('If we grumble at sickness God won't grant us death', *War and Peace*). Another approach to measuring the quality of life, based on decision theory, is that of Kaplan and Bush.[25] They introduced the concept of '*well years of life lost*' by integrating mortality and morbidity data. This is explained in Box 25.1.

Rosser and Kind[26] based their QALY evaluations on a cross-tabulation of disability and distress that was developed from interviews with doctors, nurses and patients (see Box 25.2). These definitions have formed the basis

Box 25.2 *Rosser and Kind's classification of disability and distress*

Disability

1. No disability.
2. Slight social disability.
3. Severe social disability and/or impairment of performance at work.
   Able to do all housework except heavy tasks.
4. Choice of work or performance at work severely limited.
   Housewives and old people able to do light housework only, but able to go out shopping.
5. Unable to undertake any paid employment.
   Unable to continue any education.
   Old people confined to home except for escorted outings and short walks and unable to do shopping.
   Housewives only able to perform a few simple tasks.
6. Confined to chair or to wheelchair or able to move around home only with support from an assistant.
7. Confined to bed.
8. Unconscious.

Distress

A. None
B. Mild
C. Moderate
D. Severe

Box 25.3 *Some Concern about QALYs*

- Statistics often based on small samples

- Significant variations between subjects

- Original population used to obtain data set may differ from new population to which it is applied

- Opinions on disability will vary depending on current health status of respondent

- Complex relationship between previous health status and duration of new disability

- Cost–benefit comparisons between different diseases/operations may use QALYs based on different populations with different valuation systems for QALY calculations in the UK. Whilst it is generally accepted that this is an important development there are several major criticisms which are of relevance not only to this study but also to other scoring systems.[27-29] They are summarised in Box 25.3.

The use of QALYs to support the more scientific evaluation of outcome is a laudable aim but it should not be assumed that the replacement of the present informal process (which relies heavily on peer review and value judgements) by statistical analysis, graphs and tables, is necessarily an improvement. There are major problems with the methodology and small variations in the way in which data are collated can produce big differences in accumulated figures and in the subsequent analysis. Furthermore, the original tables of Rosser and Kind are based on the analysis of very small numbers. However, this is not a justification for abandoning such tools, rather a stimulus for their improvement. Many aspects of life which provide 'purpose' and 'fulfilment' can be affected by treatment. Value judgements will remain an important part of outcome measurements and will probably continue to defy attempts to attach numbers to them.

More recently there has been some interest in assessing disability in financial terms. For example, the costs of road improvements could be contrasted with those of injury or the costs of a cervical screening programme with cervical cancer.

The *human capital* method assesses increased risk by earnings foregone through incapacity or premature death. The method is fully actuarial and uses full age-specific accounting to evaluate changes in mortality. It is based on the gross national product (GNP) and includes no indication of the individual's desire to pay. A medical breakthrough that prolonged life from 70 to 80 years would have no particular social justification – it would not raise GNP. In contrast, the *willingness to pay* approach recognises the desire to live longer and is grounded solidly on welfare theory logic. The method is not actuarial, e.g. it has difficulties in discriminating between activities with equal risk but with different age patterns of incidence. A scheme that increases life from 70 to 80 years would be socially justified if those who benefitted were willing (in theory at least) to pay more for the extra years than the cost of the scheme. Both methods share a common deficiency in that they ignore the chain of wider economic transfer set up through society when life is lengthened.

The Department of Transport have reviewed the evaluation of a fatal casualty on a willingness to pay method, and found that using this method the cost of a fatality was double that previously calculated. In other words, for improvements in road safety to be cost effective, fewer lives would need to be saved once the willingness to pay calculation had been added into the overall calculations.

Limitations in clinical practice

There have been major advances in our ability to measure outcome in recent years. Clinicians are now more receptive to the concept of audit and increasingly understand the importance of basing this on accurate information. Problems have been encountered. Scoring systems have been introduced that have no face validity, thereby immediately attracting ridicule. Recently, Thomsen *et al.*[30] analysed two widely used systems for the radiographic classification of ankle fractures and showed that the inter-observer and intra-observer errors for one of these classifications were sufficiently serious to call into question its practical usefulness. Since the outcome of treatment may well depend more upon the severity of the original injury than upon the method of management, it is easy to imagine the potential to mislead. They concluded that 'in future, classification systems should be subject to reliability analysis before they are accepted'.

Audit alone will not indicate the validity of a classification system. Detailed research into its methodology is essential. It is also essential to ensure that the whole clinical team is involved with the introduction of any new scoring system. Whilst some information can usually be collected retrospectively some will be 'new' and only available if the clinician asks the relevant question or carries out the relevant measurement at the appropriate time. In order to obtain co-operation in data collection it is essential that the clinician understands the reason for this additional work. Those inflicting this extra burden must be receptive to new ideas and able quickly to demonstrate the value of their work. It is particularly important that this whole process does not lead the clinician away from patient management. Improved patient care must remain the goal and those introducing new scoring systems and supporting clinical audit must not distance themselves from patients behind mission statements and statistical bureaucracy.

If audit is successful, it will either improve the efficiency and cost effectiveness of care without reducing quality, or it will improve the distribution of good-quality care. It cannot alone result in the development of new methods of treatment, improved methods of diagnosis, or a better understanding of the underlying physiological and pathological processes. The latter are dependent upon research – and audit has a role in helping to identify the most appropriate avenues to pursue.

Audit and research also have a role in education. One of the main criticisms of medical training and medical practice in general is that undergraduates and postgraduates are taught rather than educated. Research is an essential part of every doctor's education in order to develop a critical approach, an enquiring mind and logical thought, and to stir his or her imagination. Audit can help, but it cannot stir the doctor's imagination, nor can it develop an enquiring mind to the extent that research can.

References

1. Gordon, I. J. (1987). Predicting the outcome: a new crystal ball? *Journal of the Royal Society of Medicine*, **80**, 133–134.
2. Knaus, W. A. (1987). Prediction of outcome. *Medicine International*, **160**, 5–8.
3. Knaus, W. A., Draper, E. A., Wagner, D. P. & Zimmerman, J. E. (1986). An evaluation of outcome from intensive care in major medical centres. *Annals of Internal Medicine*, **104**, 410–418.
4. Champion, H. R., Copes, W. S., Sacco, W. J., Lawnick, R. N., Bain, L. W., Gann, D. S., Gennarelli, T., MacKenzie, E. & Schwaitzburg, S. (1990). A new characterisation of injury severity. *Journal of Trauma*, **30**, 539–546.
5. American Society of Anesthesiologists (1963). New classification of physical states. *Anesthesiology*, **24**, 111.
6. Peel, A. A. F., Semple, T., Wang, I., Lancaster, W. M. & Dall, J. L. G. (1962). A coronary prognostic index for grading the severity of infarction. *British Heart Journal*, **24**, 745–760.
7. Champion, H. R., Sacco, W. J., Hannon, D. S., Lepper, R. L., Atzinger, E. S., Copes, W. S. & Prall, R. H. (1980). Assessment of injury severity: the triage index. *Critical Care Medicine*, **8**, 201–208.
8. Champion, H. R., Sacco, W. J., Carnazzo, A. J., Copes, W. & Fouty, W. J. (1981). The Trauma Score. *Critical Care Medicine*, **9**, 672–676.
9. Boyd, C. R., Tolson, M. A. & Copes, W. S. (1987). Evaluating trauma care: the TRISS method. *Journal of Trauma*, **27**, 370–378.
10. Galasko, C. S. B., Murray, P., Hodson, M., Tunbridge, R. J. & Everest, J. T. (1986). Long term disability following road traffic accidents. *Transport and Road Research Laboratory*, *Research Report* 59, Crowthorne, Berkshire, UK.
11. Yates, D. W. (1990). Scoring systems for trauma. *British Medical Journal*, **301**, 1090–1094.
12. Poungvarin, N., Viriyavejakul, A. & Komontric, C. (1991). Siriraj stroke score and validation study to distinguish supratentorial intracerebral haemorrhage from infarction. *British Medical Journal*, **302**, 1565–1567.
13. Coulter, A. (1987). Measuring morbidity. *British Medical Journal*, **294**, 203–204.
14. Katz, S., Ford, A. B., Moskowitz, R. W., Jackson, B. A. & Jaffe, M. W. (1963). Studies of illness in the aged. The index of A. D. I.: a standardised measure of biological and physiological function. *Journal of the American Medical Association*, **185**, 914–919.
15. Editorial (1986). Assessment of disability. *The Lancet* **i**, 591–592.

16. Royal College of Physicians (1987). Physical disability in 1986 and beyond. *Journal of the Royal College of Physicians of London*, **20**, suppl., 3–37.
17. Eakin, P. (1989). Assessments of activities of daily living: a critical review. *British Journal of Occupational Therapy*, **52**, 11–15.
18. Eakin, P. (1989). Problems in the assessments of activities of daily living. *British Journal of Occupational Therapy*, **52**, 50–54.
19. Buffalo General Hospital (1987). *Uniform Data System for Medical Rehabilitation*. New York: Buffalo General Hospital.
20. WHO (1980). *International Classification of Impairments, Disabilities and Handicaps*. Geneva: World Health Organisation.
21. Ford, B. (1984). International classification of impairments, disabilities and handicaps: exercises in its application in a hospital medical record. *International Rehabilitation Medicine*, **6**, 191–193.
22. Yates, D. W., Heath, D. F., Mars, E. & Taylor, R. J. (1991). A system for measuring the severity of temporary and permanent disability after injury. *Accident Analysis and Prevention*, **23**, 323–329.
23. Williams, A. (1985). Economics of coronary artery bypass grafting. *British Medical Journal*, **291**, 326–329.
24. Torrance, G. W. (1986). Measurement of health state utilities to economic appraisal: a review. *Journal of Health Economics*, **5**, 1–30.
25. Kaplan, R. M. & Bush, J. W. (1982). Health related quality of life measurement for evaluation research and policy analysis. *Health Psychology*, **1**, 61–80.
26. Rosser, R. M. & Kind, P. (1978). A scale of valuations of states of illness: is there a social consensus? *International Journal of Epidemiology*, **7**, 347–358.
27. Carr-Hill, R. A. & Morris, J. (1991). Current practice in obtaining the Q in QALYs: a cautionary note. *British Medical Journal*, **303**, 699–700.
28. Fallowfield, L. (1990). The health economist's view of quality of life. In *The Quality of Life*, pp 204–220. Souvenir Press.
29. McTurk, L. (1991). A methodological quibble about QALYs. *British Medical Journal*, **302**, 1601.
30. Thomsen, N. O. B., Overgaard, S., Olsen, L. H., Hansen, H. & Nielson, S. T. (1991). Observer variation in radiographic classification of ankle fractures. *Journal of Bone Joint Surgery*, **73B**, 676–678.

26

Audit: will it work?

CHRISTOPHER BULSTRODE, ANDREW CARR,
PAUL PYNSENT AND MANFRED WILDNER

Introduction

When I use a word it means just what I choose it to mean – neither more nor less.
(Humpty Dumpty in Alice Through the Looking Glass)

Audit is the flavour of the month in clinical medicine. The concept is not new; the attention being paid to it is. Its great attraction appears to be that it is all things to all men. To the seekers after efficiency, it offers the tool by which waste can supposedly be identified and eliminated. To the managers of the health service it is a handle which may be used to bring spending under control. To the heads of clinical departments it provides the data needed to support the firm belief that their particular service is grossly underfunded. To the competitive clinician it is the source of an eternal well-spring of information from which invidious comparisons can be made with the work of colleagues. To the computer addicted individual it provides a use for a machine that until now has proved an engrossing toy but nothing more.

To each of these people the dictionary definition of audit is the same, but the type of information and the way it is gathered to perform audit is completely different. The methods used to analyse information, the conclusions drawn, and the use to which these conclusions are put by these different groups may be so diverse that it is sometimes hard to credit that they are derived from the same clinical material.

It might appear to some that the introduction of audit is inevitable in order to control costs in the health service and to plan logically for the future. This may not be true. Costs can be controlled in other less-formal ways; for instance, there are only a finite number of hours that even the most committed surgeon can operate, and there are only a finite number of scans that an expensive MRI machine can perform in a year. These types

402

of control are simple and self regulating and involve no expenditure on administration. In terms of planning there is no evidence that health care provision in those countries where cost has been strictly audited for some time is any better organised or more logically distributed than in those where it has not.

We feel that much of the thinking about audit has become bogged down in the minutiae of techniques of data collection. Audit leads to informed decisions based on the analysis of reliable data. The quality of the decisions relies on the data and the analysis being correct. The collection of data in itself does not lead to 'good' decisions, it just creates a lot of work. The key to good audit is the identification of useful questions that can be answered by collection of certain clearly defined data. The corollary to this is that audit for one group (management) may be addressing completely different questions to those being asked by another group within the same organisation (clinicians). Because both the questions being asked and the answers sought are completely different an audit system designed to cover both is unlikely to work.

The purpose of this chapter is to question the value of the adoption of audit. It will present some simple principles, which although self-evident are frequently ignored. It will then go on to give some examples of audit in the authors' experience and will demonstrate the limitations on conclusions that can be drawn from these data. It may well be that clinical audit is an over-worked term and that each of the so-called aims of audit in the Royal College guidelines[1] should be correctly titled as 'peer review', quality control, etc., depending on what it does, but for this chapter we will follow Humpty Dumpty and use audit to mean all these things and a few others besides.

General

Types of audit

Audit can be performed in different ways. In its simplest form it can be performed on paper without the use of computers (paper audit). It can also be performed on simple desktop computers. This type of audit initiated directly from the providers of the service itself is described here as 'bottom-up'. The third type is audit initiated by management centrally and is 'top-down' in its organisation.

Table 26.1 *Pros and cons of paper audit*

Advantages	Disadvantages
The system is very cheap to initiate. Running costs can be lost in secretarial budgets.	The equipment and staff are paid for out of your budget.
The system is very flexible.	The system is cumbersome and slow, making analysis difficult.
The data collected are usually owned and controlled by you.	The system is not easy to link to audit systems in other units.

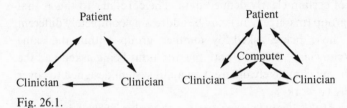

Fig. 26.1.

Paper audit

It is commonly assumed that the data for audit can only be gathered by computer. This is obviously not true. There are powerful reasons for considering simple paper audit. Paper audit is cumbersome, time-consuming and distinctly unfashionable (Table 26.1), but because of its flexibility it should always be considered for use in the early stages while teething problems are being ironed out. Paper audit requires no specialist training to use: it is intuitive and user-friendly. It is fully portable. It provides (with modern photocopiers) infinite numbers of hard-copies. It is not usually in a form suitable for analysis but compared with computer audit it is cheap, reliable and flexible. It is the ideal technique for starting audit when various strategies are being tested and flexibility is vital. Paper audit has one less level of complexity than computer audit in that the data does not have to be 'coded' before it can be entered into the computer (Figure 26.1).

Bottom-up

'If you want something done then do it yourself' applies in the Health Service as everywhere else. For the computer numerate the fashion for audit offers an ideal opportunity to introduce computers into the work environment. Modern desktop computers provide more than adequate

Table 26.2 *'Pros and cons' of peripheral data collection ('bottom–up')*

Advantages	Disadvantages
The system is cheap compared with 'top-down'.	The equipment and staff are paid for out of your budget.
The system is flexible, and user friendly (to you) and does what you want.	Colleagues who are not computer confident will not use the system.
The data collected are primarily owned and controlled by you.	The system may not be compatible with others. Data cannot be compared easily.
It is in your interests to ensure that the data entered are complete and correct.	The responsibility and cost of maintaining the system lies with you.

power. Entering data may seem like a simple and pleasant task to someone who enjoys using computers, but to a colleague who shares neither your enthusiasm for audit nor the fearless passion for computers the prospect may be so unattractive as to be insuperable. Software written by enthusiastic amateurs is never user-friendly except to the author. It is full of bugs and lacks all but the most primitive self-check routines. Furthermore any audit data collected in this way are unlikely to be in a form that can be compared with another unit's data. There is only a limited amount of professional software available for desk-top medical audit. However, bottom-up systems do remain relatively flexible as the programs can be rewritten at least for as long as the author's enthusiasm remains in the face of carping criticism of his programming ability. The systems are cheap, a desktop computer with hard disc and printer need cost no more than £1500. The fundamental advantage of this type of audit is the fact that you own the data, and can use them as you wish. To most readers of this book this single fact will outweigh all other considerations (Table 26.2).

Top-down

Top-down systems are introduced by management to gather information about clinical activity on which rational management decisions can be based. To the paranoic this means that the data may be used by management to force through decisions that may not be supported by clinicians for whatever reason. The data may be taken down and used in evidence against you, a statutory caution if ever there was one. The computers used for this type of audit are impressively large and may cost

Table 26.3 *Pros and cons of central data collection ('top–down')*

Advantages	Disadvantages
The equipment and staff are not paid for out of your budget.	The data collected are primarily owned and controlled centrally.
The system is powerful and may interconnect with many other departments.	The system is cumbersome and inflexible, responding slowly if at all to changing needs.
The responsibility for maintaining the system lies with professionals paid to do it not you.	There is little motivation to ensure that the data entered are either complete or correct.

hundreds of thousands of pounds. They will be staffed by many professionals, none of whose salaries will come directly from your budget. The software is professional and should be bug-free and user-friendly (usually it is neither). The data collected are not directly relevant to clinical practise, being geared to activity levels and costing rather than diagnosis and treatment. Once the information has been passed to the central computer it is exceedingly difficult to get back in any form. Even if management wanted you to have access to the data (which they do not) the lack of flexibility in the system makes it difficult to respond to any analysis that has not been pre-planned. A monolithic audit system, based on large computers or networks imposed centrally lacks flexibility. Firstly, this is because the organisers of the system are remote from the service being audited and are less likely to be sensitive to its needs. Secondly, a large cumbersome system is both expensive and difficult to change; a minor modification in one part having unexpected effects on other parts of the system. The standard cry of software writers is 'just tell us what you want and we will write it'. At the moment most units do not clearly know what they want, so software must be written with built-in flexibility to allow for as much change as possible. Top-down systems are not suitable for this (Table 26.3).

Criteria for audit to be acceptable (Box 26.1)

Flexible

Audit systems must be flexible. At first, information may be recorded in a clumsy way which is inconvenient or wastes time. Categories into which data are placed may be inappropriate, and lead to bad coding. Often data

---

Box 26.1   *Criteria for the successful introduction of audit*

- Flexible
- Cost – minimum
- Work – minimum
- Collection integral to provision

---

are recorded that are not needed. This wastes the time of the collectors and creates resentment. Conversely, data that initially were not thought relevant, or not thought of at all, may have been omitted. Serious omissions can have a knock-on effect by reducing the value of all the other information already being collected. These problems occur initially even in the best-designed audit systems. Time as well as facilities must be available to allow the correction of these problems, and the system must be designed to allow these changes to be introduced, even after the system has started running. Later, further modifications to an audit system will be needed to allow it to evolve as the service being audited evolves. Clinical services are not static but should be continuously adapting to new requirements. The introduction of audit should accelerate this process by strengthening the feedback loop that initiates change. The audit system must be flexible enough itself to respond to these changes if it is to continue to be relevant. This is very difficult to do.

Cost–benefit

In the long term, the improvement in medical care and practice brought about by audit should more than justify the cost of implementing audit. This can be difficult to measure. In the short term the costs may be high (with added training costs and capital outlay). The benefits may be some time in coming and even when they do may be difficult to quantify. In the short term one solution is to take the money for the implementation of audit from a separate budget, provided the use of those funds does not affect the provision of any other service. Otherwise, the cost of introduction must be allocated to an administrative change being introduced at the same time. The computerisation of a clinical unit is often used as this justification but the risks of introducing both together should be borne in mind, as mentioned earlier.

It is to be hoped that audit will also improve quality of care as well as just saving costs. This can be very difficult to measure and before audit is started methods should have been devised to provide and if possible give a financial value to improvements in quality of care. This may be as crude as calculating the extra cost in terms of staff and equipment that would have been required to obtain a similar improvement by conventional means. If a method cannot be devised then audit should not be attempted for that problem. Improvements in care can be introduced and justified without audit. It is just so much nicer if audit can be used to justify the decisions.

Work: the same or less

There is a danger that the introduction of an audit system may create extra administrative work, which may detract from time that could otherwise be devoted to the provision of a clinical service. Every effort should be made to avoid this, as otherwise there will inevitably be resistance to the introduction of audit and inevitably much of its benefit will be lost. A well-designed audit system should greatly reduce the amount of administrative work being done in a unit in the long term. Implementation of an audit system inevitably involves teething problems. This extra work must be budgeted for. If it is not, the staff involved in collecting the data will become antagonistic to audit. The priority for audit will then fall, reflected by the comment 'We are too busy to fill in the forms'. Audit will then be incomplete. This situation, which is depressingly common, is the worst of all worlds. The audit data lack input from the 'busy' units and the work being done to gather data by the other co-operative staff continues to occupy time and resources without providing any benefit. The value of the data gathered is then likely to be far outweighed by the cost of collection. Clinical audit systems that automatically generate a discharge letter from the data-base are an example of a situation where collection of audit data may in fact reduce work-load elsewhere in the system. However, it is virtually the 'only' example that has actually been shown to work. Ideally, those individuals who are involved in the audit process should all perceive a benefit in terms of either less work or improved work quality.

Collection integral to provision

The collection of audit data should be an integral part of the provision of the service itself. If collection of data is tacked onto a service as 'an extra form to fill in' then it will not always be done. There will be no immediate detriment to the service provided but the effect on the value of the audit is serious. If the data are incomplete this weakens the conclusions that can be drawn from those data by an amount quite disproportionate to the small amount of data missing. Even if data points are not missing, but could be without anyone having any way of knowing, great care must be taken with the reliance put on any conclusions that are drawn from the data. Validation of the data at a later stage is time consuming, expensive and rarely performed because the results are only likely to show the poor quality of the data collected. Far better to make data collection an integral part of provision of the service. An example of this is found when comparing the collection of audit data from doctors in the National Health Service (NHS) compared with private practise. Coding of diagnosis and operation is currently proving very difficult to the NHS. Great difficulty is experienced by the clinicians in a hospital we are studying in coding cases at discharge. They currently find themselves unable to code over 50 % of the cases and leave the forms blank despite prodigious efforts to provide appropriate codes. However, these same clinicians are able to code immediately and with apparent 100 % reliability all private cases passing through the same unit. Immediate completion of data on the private patients is integral to the provision of the service – no account, no payment. Nevertheless validation of the completeness and accuracy of data collected remains vital before analysis is attempted. Just like backing-up hard discs it is a vital process and is too rarely performed.

Collection of data

Collection of data onto paper suffers from several weaknesses. The first is that entry onto paper is liable to error. There is no automatic self-validating system. Questions can also be skipped, so data collection can easily be incomplete. The forms are then usually transposed onto computer for analysis. This is a further source of error as well as being a mind-numbingly boring exercise. The advantage of paper is its cheapness and flexibility. This is very helpful in the early stages when ideas about what needs to be collected have not been fully formatted (i.e. not thought out at all).

Collection directly onto computer requires computers to be available wherever data is being collected. For a 'top-down' system this is simply a few extra tens of thousands of pounds for extra terminals. For a cheap 'bottom-up' system this means moving computers around or having expensive and very stealable portables. These are usually very slow to use or have quite illegible screens. Most doctors are unwilling to use a QWERTY keyboard and make as many errors as when entering onto paper. Well-designed programs that require the minimum of data entry and tools such as bar-code readers for patient identification minimise the effort of data entry but require expensive programming. The ability of computers to recognise speech will become commonplace within the next decade and should greatly speed data entry.

The amount of data collected must be kept to an absolute minimum. There is a temptation to collect as much as possible simply because there is a system in place for doing so. This must be resisted. The acid-test for data entry is to ask yourself what possible different outcomes could the collection of this data reveal, and then ask what you would do if each or any of those outcomes did occur. If there would be no action then there is no purpose in collecting the information. The temptation to collect data for the sake of completeness serves no purpose.

The most valuable reason to collect data is in order to identify ways in which outcome can be improved. This might be done by collecting data that identified which step in a clinical process caused the greatest delay, or which gave the most reliable result. In the second case audit has drifted into the field of clinical research. There is no harm in that: the borders are ill-defined. However, the rules of clinical research must then be obeyed. A definable and testable hypothesis must be tested in a statistically rigorous way. This is very difficult to do and requires careful planning before any effort is made to collect the data. If you do not agree with this then try now to design a simple question about the way that your clinical practice is managed that could be answered by the collection of a set of data that are readily available. Exclude those examples where you already know the answer or where whatever the answer there is nothing you can or will do about the situation. Finally, calculate how much time and money would be required to collect those data and then ask yourself whether the answer would justify the costs (especially in terms of your time).

Coding

Diagnostic coding is performed by a clerk in most units. The codes (such as the International Classification of Disease, ICD) remain clumsy and difficult to apply. When validation is attempted errors in coding are large and variable. This situation will prevail until such a time that clinical team leaders finally decide that they alone can code their own patients. In a study carried out in our own unit a tenfold difference was found between the postoperative mortality between two units for a standard operation (total hip replacement). The difference was statistically highly significant and also highly gratifying to one unit, which made the results public immediately. The other unit was not so happy and asked for the data and analysis to be checked. It transpired that one unit was performing the operation for arthritis in otherwise healthy patients. The other unit had a much higher proportion of very elderly patients with a fractured neck of femur for whom they were performing this same operation. In this latter case the postoperative mortality is known to be high (related to the trauma, the age and frailty of the patients). When this confounding factor was removed (which was not separable in the diagnostic coding) the difference in mortality disappeared completely.

Analysis of data

Comparison between units

There has always been considerable interest in the use of data collected for audit to compare the 'success' of individual units. This is particularly important to a subgroup, that of computer numerate clinicians, who combine a highly competitive nature with a touching belief in the truth of numbers. The pitfalls in this type of analysis are so great that it may be well nigh impossible to use audit to make any valid comparisons that can be used to improve clinical practice.

Casemix

Some units concentrate on providing an excellent service for uncompli-cated cases. Those cases in which risk factors are identified are sent elsewhere to units with expertise in those problems. This selection procedure can vary from an absolute unit policy (as may occur in a day surgery unit) to a subconscious bias against performing elective surgery on patients with any identified risk factor. At the receiving end some units have a general casemix while other units have become so specialised that they never treat uncomplicated cases. It is self evident that any comparison without checking for casemix bias is invalid but it is surprising how often such results are reported. Checking for differences in casemix is difficult particularly because such small differences can make such a great difference to outcome. It may be that casemix is always so different that it will swamp all but the most self-evident differences between units. This problem cannot be overcome by increasing the number of patients in the comparison, the difference remains the same.

Measuring outcomes

Hard outcome measures are those that can be recognised by different recorders in different units reliably and consistently. They are such things as death of a patient and on the whole are rare outcomes (certainly in elective orthopaedic surgery). Soft outcome measures are those that depend on the observer's or the patient's subjective interpretation of what has occurred. Wound infection after surgery is an example. Presence of infection may be recorded every time there is reddening of the wound (up to 30% of cases) or it may be recorded as negative unless pus is obtained that grows organisms (less than 1% of cases). Even if the condition is graded, differences in interpretation of the borders between grades makes comparison difficult or impossible. Care must also be taken not to assume the validity of outcome measures without first checking the literature. Many measures are in general use simply because they bear the name of an eminent surgeon. A recent study demonstrated that two experienced orthopaedic surgeons did not agree, amongst other things, about what back pain meant[2]. A second study revealed that a group of chest physicians showed poor agreement about some of the most basic signs elicited from using a stethoscope.[3]

Comparing outcomes

If studies are confined to hard outcomes then there are statistical problems in the comparison of rare events. The occurrence of rare events fits a Poisson distribution. In this case the confidence limits can be looked up in a statistical text book. If the incidence of such events in two units is to be compared a calculation of the likelihood of difference of the observed magnitude occurring by chance can be made from a binomial distribution in the following way. The total number of patients from which the complication arose (e.g. the number of patients receiving a given operation each year) is known for each unit. The probability of a single complication occurring by chance in unit A and not in unit B can be calculated simply by saying that if for example there are equal number of patients passing through each unit the chance is 50:50. If the numbers are different the chance of this random event alters according to the ratio but can still be calculated exactly. The chances of the second complication occurring again in unit A is $\frac{1}{2}$ times $\frac{1}{2}$ or $\frac{1}{4}$. The same goes on until the number of complications in unit A is reached assuming there are none in unit B. For there to be a difference that could only have occurred by chance less than one time in twenty ($p < 0.05$) there would have to be five complications in

Table 26.4 *Significant difference ($p < 0.05$) in rare outcome calculated from Binomial distribution applicable when n > 50*

Number of cases in each unit which are
significantly different at the level $p < 0.05$

A	B
0	5
1	7
2	9
3	10
4	12

unit A and none in unit B. Surprisingly, this figure is independent of the total number of patients being studied provided that it is more than approximately 50. If Unit B also has some complications then the number that must occur in A for there to be a significant difference can be calculated in the same way (Table 26.4). It would not require an audit system or complication statistics to ring alarm bells in unit A if this difference occurred in real life. Analysis of the statistics only serves to demonstrate that in the past the differences in postoperative deaths between practices and hospital that have resulted in urgent reviews of clinical practice may in fact have simply been a result of chance.

Analysis bias

If the analysis of the data is performed by the clinician who has gathered the data and whose clinical standing depends on the outcome there is a danger that he or she may affect the results subconsciously or even consciously. Every clinician has been tempted to remove from his/her results the patient who subsequently turned out to have good reasons for the operation to fail. This error is especially important if the data set is already incomplete. Technically, if data are missing such cases should be entered as a result on the side of supporting the null hypothesis whatever that is (usually that there is no difference). When this is done with more than one or two missing data points it is very unusual to achieve statistical significance. A further error commonly occurs in the use of computers in the analysis of the data. The availability of a multitude of statistical tests at the press of a button may tempt the committed clinician to regroup his/her data or even change his/her statistical test until the result produces the difference he/she has worked so hard to find. This form of trawling invalidates the use of statistics in the analysis of data unless a major correction factor is applied. This factor removes the statistical significance of all but the most gross differences.

Application of audit

He who pays the piper calls the tune.

In the first instance the way in which data are collected and analysed will determine who has the first opportunity to make use of the data. If the audit system has been created by individual clinicians who have collected and analysed the data on their own desktop computers then that information 'belongs' to the clinicians and can be used by them to further their own ends. In fact 'bottom-up' audit can be positively threatening to central management. It gives those clinicians whom they are trying to manage access to information that the clinicians can use in their negotiations with central management. Worse still, because they own the data they can suppress conclusions drawn from that data if those conclusions do not support their own ends. Small wonder then that management has been less than eager to provide the relatively small amounts of money needed for clinically based 'bottom-up' audit.

A centrally organised audit system has the advantage that powerful computers and staff skilled in using them are used and that these are paid for from budgets remote from provision of the clinical service. However, in the first instance the data gathered are likely to be relevant to management problems not clinical ones. Secondly, the data collected belongs to management and can be used or suppressed by them when pursuing their ends. A situation can then arise where a clinician may be using his/her 'valuable' time to gather data that then become the property of management. The managers may then use conclusions drawn from this data to curtail the activities of the clinician in question. Even if this were never to happen, the perception by a clinician that it could, would make it very difficult to persuade him/her to co-operate in the collection of data. The weakness of this system is therefore in the collection of data. Management must rely on the goodwill or gullibility of clinicians, neither of which they are likely to have in great measure for any length of time.

Conclusion

In conclusion there are no simple answers to audit. It does provide one way in which controls may be applied to health care provision and increased efficiency obtained, where efficiency may be in terms of costs, service provision or both depending on your interpretation of audit. Some clinicians may prefer to pay the penalty of decreased efficiency in return for clinical freedom. In this case audit may be seen as costly, time consuming and counter-productive. Furthermore, even if you are committed to audit there may be others in your unit who are not. If they refuse to co-operate in the collection of data your audit will be greatly weakened by its incompleteness to an extent that it may not be worth your time collecting the data however much you wish to. Audit used to compare outcome from different units is so unreliable that we doubt that real changes will ever be demonstrated statistically before they become obvious clinically. Audit imposed from the top down is very dangerous indeed. The data gathered are unreliable, the analysis and interpretation is by managers who may have no knowledge of the confounding factors involved and who are collecting information primarily for the purpose of bringing the health service under their control. Devoting valuable clinical time to gathering data to provide controls for the management may not be the optimum use of a clinician's time. The introduction of audit is not inevitable: it depends totally on the will of clinicians who must decide whether to collect their own data to protect their position or to collect data for the management to help them manage 'better'. Furthermore, it depends on all clinicians wishing to act in the same way for its true strength to be realised. This is such an improbable scenario that the future of audit must be questionable.

References

1. The Royal College of Surgeons of England (1989). *Guidelines to Clinical Audit in Surgical Practice*. London: RCS.
2. McCombe, P. F., Fairbank, J. C. T., Cockersole, B. C. & Pynsent, P. B. (1989). Reproducibility of physical signs in low-back pain. *Spine*, **14**, 906–918
3. Spitteri, M. A., Clark, S. W. & Cook, D. G. (1978). Reliability of eliciting physical signs in examinations of the chest. *The Lancet*, **1**, 873–875.

27

What has been achieved so far?

SIMON P. FROSTICK

Introduction

Why should clinicians be involved in clinical audit? Amongst some clinicians there is open hostility to the concept of formal audit of medical practice. Further, with the introduction of the National Health Service (NHS) reforms and the devolvement of financial control to the level of consultant clinicians the resistance to particularly the resource aspects of audit is even more apparent.

The managers want waiting lists reduced, waiting times in clinics to be at a minimum and a cost-effective service provided, but they also expect the clinicians to be directly involved in the management structure and to provide much of the managerial information. The 'big brother' concept plays a significant role in the fears of the imposition of formal audit. Cries of loss of *clinical freedom* abound as clinicians are asked to justify their actions to the purse holders.

Before the answer posed in the title of this chapter can be approached it is necessary to define what has been the role of audit to date. The *Working for Patients*[1] White Paper and Royal College[2,3] directives on clinical audit have changed the perception of clinical audit and along with this change in perception the fears have grown. Audit of all aspects of medical practice has been around and undertaken for many years. The medical journals have reported the review of clinical practice from the time of their initial publication and groups of clinicians have met and discussed clinical problems and their management for centuries. The main change now is in accountability. Clinicians are expected to account for all decisions appertaining to each clinical case and give reasons if problems arise. This, of course, has both medical and resource implications so that clinical colleagues and hospital management expect to audit these decisions. The

416

justification for this is that resources are limited and so must be used most efficiently.

Therefore, the role of audit has not changed but has become polarised into two linked areas:

1. Review of clinical decision making and management.
2. Making the most efficient use of resources for the patients.

The various authors in this book have attempted to describe the philosophy of medical audit and to illustrate the particular needs of individual specialties. If we ask the question 'What are the aims of medical audit?' three broad but inseparable areas can be addressed:

1. The aims as determined by Central Government.
2. The aims as determined by the Royal Colleges and specialty professional bodies.
3. The aims as determined by individual clinicians.

Hopefully, all three factions agree that the ultimate aim of audit is to improve the quality of care for the patients provided by the health care system. The emphasis by each group will differ. Central Government is concerned, and always will be concerned, with the potentially escalating costs of health care in the Western nations of the world. Demand will always outstrip supply especially in a state-run system because of the restrictions of resources. Though unpalatable a state-run system cannot have a bottomless purse. Government and clinicians must, therefore, determine priorities in health care that are of benefit to the maximum number of patients. The inefficiency and cost of the other extreme, the privately based health care system, is exemplified by the USA. The iniquity of such a system is demonstrated by the fact that 37 million people in the USA are not covered by any form of health care insurance and cannot reap the benefits of modern day medicine. However, even in the USA moves are being made to start to reverse the trends.

The colleges and specialty bodies are primarily concerned with education and the maintenance of high standards of medical care. Audit is fundamental to education and it is correct that nationally recognised bodies should lay down general guidelines for such activities.

Individual clinicians are directly concerned with providing a quality and efficient service to patients. Many clinicians, especially in the surgical specialties, have long waiting lists for treatment. The patients, Central Government and local management are all demanding an improvement in waiting times for out-patient appointments and subsequent in-patient care. Government and management are demanding improvements in cost effectiveness. Audit for the clinicians is, therefore, a means of reducing complications and eliminating inappropriate or inefficient means of treatment. It is also a means of estimating the usefulness of a particular form of treatment and the long-term benefits to the patient. If appropriate comparisons are available, consultants can also compare aspects of their work with their peers. In this fashion they would be able to estimate whether their practice is broadly similar to others or if not these comparisons should stimulate them to consider the reasons for any major variation.

Can the aims of audit be achieved?

In simple terms the answer is yes. All aspects of health care must be oriented towards an improvement in the quality of care provided for the population. The need for audit implies that:

1. quality of care is less than perfect and constant review helps to reduce the imperfections;
2. there are changing *needs* in health care;
3. there are changing ways of delivering the health care requirements.

The reasons why there is a less than perfect delivery of health care are partly related to human nature and partly due to the changing nature of health care. The need to make value judgements as to the cost effectiveness of particular treatments also contributes to a less than ideal quality of care.

In reality it may be much more difficult to achieve the aims of audit. The reasons for this are multiple:

1. Resistance by members of the medical staff to expose their shortcomings and to accept criticism.
2. A lack of resources to perform audit activity in such a fashion that it is worthwhile and results in a change in delivery of health care.
3. A tendency for management to look for cost effectiveness at all costs without considering the overall effect on health care.

If the clinicians could review their clinical activities in isolation then it would be a fairly simple procedure for consultants to achieve an adequate audit of their activities and to effect appropriate changes, thus completing the audit cycle. However, increasingly clinical activity cannot be separated from resource management, which inevitably introduces a large number of factors outside the control of the individual consultants. Therefore, in order to achieve the aims of audit a considerable amount of time and resources must be devoted to the audit activity. Clinicians will need to accept that this will mean time away from directly treating patients. Management will have to accept that there will be a reduced commitment to the service as a result of the audit activity and in the short term a possible increase in waiting lists.

Levels of audit activity

We must consider how extensive our audit activity must be. At what level should we perceive the benefit of audit?

1. to the individual patient;
2. to all patients under a consultant's care;
3. to the hospital and local community;
4. to the nation.

Many clinicians would probably argue that *we* can only be concerned with the provision of treatment for *our* patients and that the other aspects must be left to others. The view of the author would be that although we must resist all attempts to use economic factors solely to dictate how we treat patients we must bear in mind the overall effects on the health and wealth of the nation as a whole.

It is self evident that under defined criteria we must consider all the levels of audit suggested above. Each patient is entitled to feel that they are receiving the best possible care; we must be certain that a particular treatment regimen is appropriate and effective for a group of patients; the local community must derive the maximum and most cost-effective service from its local hospitals, and the nation as a whole is entitled to know that the delivery of health care is resulting in a positive effect on the GNP and that the ill, the disabled and the handicapped are appropriately cared for.

How has audit changed?

For the enthusiasts very little has changed in their perception, under-standing or indeed practice of audit. These individuals have been reviewing their clinical activity and effecting change for much of their working lives. The most important change for these individuals has been in the formalisation of the audit activity and the need to persuade the whole of the medical community to be involved. This has been aided by some of the reforms of the NHS. Managerial responsibility is gradually being devolved to the unit level and it is the responsibility of the Clinical Director to ensure that resources are used most effectively; adequate and effective audit of the unit's activities is fundamental to this. Recommendations and directives from the Royal Colleges concerning training of juniors have also had an effect on the promotion of audit.

For the unenthusiastic clinician probably little has also changed. Some consultants have never undertaken any review of their activity and may even deny that they ever have any complications after treatment. It will be very difficult to persuade these individuals that audit is necessary. Others have been examining their clinical practice consistently but not in a formalised way and not calling the activity audit. The change in this group is one of definition – when is review audit and when is review clinical research? A considerable amount of confusion has ensued which has been exacerbated by so-called experts on audit failing to distinguish audit and clinical research. A rapid review of the journals confirms this confusion. Certainly, in the main orthopaedic journals many of the papers purporting to be clinical research are in reality poor quality audit papers – retrospective reviews of groups of patients. The value of these as audit papers is limited as often the numbers of individuals reviewed are but a small percentage of the total in each original group so that general conclusions can be drawn but specific recommendations resulting in change cannot be made.

Therefore, the only real changes in audit have been the formalisation of the activity and an increased awareness amongst the medical population that clinicians need to review their clinical activity. The main value of this will eventually be:

1. better data;
2. validation of collected data;
3. a better understanding that even clinicians are fallible but are willing to admit the fallibility and most importantly are willing to improve.

Major achievements of audit

Throughout the book examples of the benefit of audit have been described. It is evident from these surveys that the value of audit data is in the fact that the studies are trying to obtain the maximum amount of data available about the topic under discussion; further, that these data are validated. It is very easy to argue the benefit of a particular activity if only the real enthusiasts or experts are reviewed. The true value is only apparent once data from all sources are looked at including that obtained from individuals who undertake a particular treatment regimen very occasionally. At an individual level, it is only once all the data about a particular subject are reviewed that the clinician will be able to make any decisions about the activity; bias will be introduced if samples are selected inappropriately either consciously or unconsciously.

Over the years observations have been made that have resulted in major improvements in the health of the nation. In the nineteenth century the incidence of cholera in London was very high, but the observation that the sewage outlets were up-stream from the places where the water companies were taking their water from the Thames resulted in a change in the collection of water and a very rapid fall in the disease. During the early part of this century it was noted that the mortality rate following acute appendicitis decreased well before the introduction of antibiotics had occurred. This decrease in mortality was due to an overall improvement in nutrition and general health of the population.

The survival of soldiers in the First World War following injury at the front improved dramatically with the introduction of field stations. Observations during that war and subsequently in both the Second World War and the Korean War led eventually to the modern concepts of trauma care, including immediate resuscitation and early surgical intervention. The system of notifiable diseases has also helped in understanding diseases and has at the very least recorded the reduction of many major pathologies and the contribution made by public health measures as well as specific treatment regimes.

These are all examples of observing outcome and completing the audit loop to effect change. The surveys have required large amounts of resources to achieve the necessary result but similar principles can be applied by an individual clinician to an individual patient.

The maternal mortality surveys started in Scotland in the 1930s have served to highlight the need to improve obstetric care. They have demonstrated risk factors and have lead to an improvement in public awareness and an improvement in the way in which all doctors care for pregnant women. Over the years these surveys have been one factor in the reduction of maternal mortality.

The perinatal mortality survey has, in some ways, paralleled that of the maternal mortality survey, and similar to the latter has demonstrated a marked fall in the perinatal mortality. Some hospitals still have a

significantly higher perinatal mortality than the expected national median
level. An individual unit will know where in the league it falls but this
information will only be known by that unit. This form of peer pressure
should encourage the outliers to improve. Further, some hospitals will
hold case conferences if a neonate is stillborn or dies in the postnatal period
in order to discuss the causes, and effect changes in process.

The National Confidential Enquiry into Perioperative Deaths[4] is a very
important and totally confidential survey. It has highlighted many
problems associated with the provision of surgical services. The continuation of the survey and the willingness by the majority of surgeons to
participate will hopefully influence surgeons to consider closely the services
they provide.

A number of reports during the 1980s have been fundamental in the
alteration of orthopaedic services. The Duthie Report[5] discussed the
overall problems of provision of an adequate orthopaedic service in the
UK and suggested ways in which improvements could be made. This
report came at a time when orthopaedics itself was starting to undergo
major changes with rapid increases in surgery for total joint replacement
and other important developments.

The Royal College of Physicians[6] report on the treatment of elderly
patients with fractures of the neck of the femur highlighted the delays in
performing appropriate surgery and recommended that all patients with
this injury should be operated upon within 24 hours. Most orthopaedic
surgeons would support this principle but often the 'structure' is not
available to achieve the acceptable standard.

How can audit be improved?

Adequate data collection and data validation are required to ensure that
the value of audit improves. Further, the establishment of national
standards of activity and achievement are required. The maternal and
perinatal mortality studies are good examples of where national standards
have been established by the profession and centres that vary from the
national 'norm' are encouraged to find out why by peer pressure and not
by threat of punitive action as only they themselves can identify their
position in the league.

A major initiative has been established by the Royal College of Surgeons
of England – the *confidential comparative audit*[7] meetings. These meetings
have been held to allow surgeons to compare their activity with that of
others across England and Wales. At present the numbers of surgeons

willing to take part is quite small (the enthusiasts?) so that national standards cannot be recommended from the analysis of the data. The main reason why only 10–20% of surgeons are involved is partly that many surgeons still lack adequate data and partly due to a fear of exposing one's shortcomings. The absolute confidentiality of the survey hopefully will persuade more individuals to be involved. Further, as computer technology becomes more readily available the standard of the data should improve.

At an individual or unit level the major improvements in use of audit will become apparent once individuals accept the need to improve the quality of care and any unnecessary victimisation is eliminated. Many individual clinicians already review their activity and try to determine reasons for failing to achieve a high quality of care. Systematic review of activity may reduce complications, for example, and lead to an overall improvement in the quality of care.

Most specialties are developing acceptable outcome measures. Defining outcome measures has been a very difficult process. It is obvious that objectivity is frequently impossible especially if we wish to measure patient satisfaction as part of the overall quality assurance. Clinicians are being asked by the managers to develop outcome measures for contract purposes. However, if we consider complications of surgical procedures, in many instances the ability to diagnose an adverse event accurately may be poor so that trying to estimate an 'acceptable' level is impossible. Referring to the medical literature may not be particularly helpful as suitable ways of comparing like with like are not available. In order to enable different groups of clinicians within the same specialty to compare data it is necessary for them to develop a common minimum data set. Problems of detail still exist even when using an accepted minimum data set but this would be a first step towards being able to perform comparative audit.

Extrapolating a finding in one specialist area to another is fraught with problems as there may need to be validation for each specialty. For example, using the ASEPSIS[8] scoring system for wound infection, developed in cardiothoracic surgery, in the assessment of infection in orthopaedic patients requires validation of the system to demonstrate that it is appropriate and meaningful.

Small specialties have a particular problem in developing audit methods and holding appropriate meetings. There is a critical mass of clinicians required for audit meetings to be meaningful. Small specialties will probably need to organise regionally based audit or will need to hold meetings in conjunction with allied specialties. Further, even the major specialties should hold joint audit meetings on a regular basis: surgeons

and anaesthetists; orthopaedists and geriatricians; oncologists and surgeons, etc. These meetings will focus on particular areas of activity and can
also serve as 'update' tutorials for all concerned.

Should we continue with audit?

At present the real benefits of clinical audit are not apparent to many
clinicians. Shaw[9] defined four phases in the introduction of audit:

1. Philosophical – should doctors be involved in audit?
2. Organisational – are resources available?
3. Practical – how and what to audit.
4. Invasive – publication of results.

Individual clinicians and units are in different phases. The real
enthusiasts are in phase 4; they already have decided that audit is
worthwhile, have found appropriate resources, have decided approaches
to audit and indeed have published useful data. The enthusiasts, however,
see that there are no hard and fast rules and that audit is continually
evolving. For the unenthusiastic clinician the decision in phase 1, to some
extent, has been pre-empted by the Government and Royal Colleges and to
some extent by their own personal requirements for review of their own
practice. However, these clinicians cannot be persuaded to enter the other
phases as there is little tangible evidence that true benefit will accrue in
terms of an improvement of patient care. Further, sheer pressure of work
often prevents many clinicians from being able even to consider the
possible benefits of audit.

The reasons for continuing audit can be summarised as follows:

1. self examination;
2. clinical review;
3. education;
4. management demands;
5. reassurance of the general public and purchasers of health care.

Audit for the purpose of self examination has been emphasised
throughout this book. It is the most fundamental form of audit that must
be undertaken. Clinicians must be honest with themselves as to their
abilities and have the insight that they have shortcomings; they must also
have the courage to admit that there is always room for improvement.
Clinicians must allow themselves to be part of the peer review process and
take note of recommendations for change.

In most specialties advances in health care have resulted from an individual observing the effects of a treatment regime and then organising a formal clinical research project. Audit for the purpose of clinical review of the effects of treatment will continue to stimulate advances in medical science.

The Royal Colleges have emphasised the role of audit in the educational process. It is fundamental for seniors and juniors alike to learn from their clinical activities.

The reorganisation of the NHS has resulted in a greater emphasis on audit. As far as the managers are concerned audit is necessary in order to develop strategic plans for hospital activity and for the formulation of contracts. Clinicians often perceive the demands for information by managers as threatening. However, managers must plan the activities of the hospital to meet the health care requirements of the local population and with a major restriction of the resources available; clinicians must demonstrate that they can undertake to fulfil the health care needs of the public and provide a quality service. In order for this to work, adequate and often common information is required by both managers and clinicians. Therefore, communication in a non-adversarial way must be set up between the two groups and data appropriately shared without eliminating patient confidentiality.

The general public are becoming increasingly aware of the shortcomings of doctors; they can be at least partially reassured if doctors are seen to review their activity and are willing to admit mistakes. Similarly, purchasers of health care are seeking to be assured that the quality of care is sufficiently high with the minimum of adverse events.

In continuing with audit a mechanism of audit must be chosen that removes any threat from the activity. Some units are introducing *occurrence screening*[10] as the major audit method. In the USA this type of audit is widespread. Although monitoring failure is relatively easy it is the most threatening form of audit and ignores many positive features such as the successful provision of treatment in the majority of cases. Moreover, responses from patients when asked about quality are subject to normative bias, i.e. the patients like to please. Occurrence screening will be useful as one element in the audit spectrum. Its introduction may be indicated if particular problems have become apparent from other sources, such as morbidity and mortality meetings, but it should only be used on a short-term basis once the problems have been highlighted and appropriate action taken. Alternatively, occurrence screening could be used on a random basis.

It is important to ensure that audit and audit meetings are interesting and in turn are seen to have a positive effect on process. Therefore, audit methods need to be constantly reviewed and audited to ensure they are continuing to benefit the medical community.

Conclusions

Audit has achieved a great deal but further effort is required to ensure that audit continues to contribute to the improvement in quality of care for patients. Methodologies, outcome measures, minimum data sets, etc. are gradually being developed and will continue to evolve for some time. Hopefully, increasing numbers of clinicians will become interested in audit and will see that benefits do accrue both to themselves and to their patients.

References

1. Department of Health (1989). *Working for Patients*. London: HMSO.
2. The Royal College of Physicians (1989). *Medical Audit – a First Report: What, Why and How?* London: RCP.
3. The Royal College of Surgeons of England (1989). *Guidelines to Clinical Audit in Surgical Practice*. London: RCS.
4. Buck, N., Devlin, H. B. & Lunn, J. N. (1987). *The Report of a Confidential Enquiry into Perioperative Deaths*. London: Nuffield Provincial Hospitals Trust.
5. *Orthopaedic Services: Waiting Time for Out-patient Appointments and In-patient Treatment* (1981). Report for Working Party to the Secretary of State for Social Services (Chairman Professor R. B. Duthie). London: HMSO.
6. Royal College of Physicians (1989). *Fracture Neck of Femur: Prevention and Management*. London: RCP.
7. Emberton, M., Rivett, R. & Ellis, B. W. (1991). Comparative audit: a new method of delivering audit. *Annals of the Royal College of Surgeons of England (Suppl)*, **73(6)**, 117–120.
8. Wilson, A. P. R., Treasure, T., Sturridge, M. F. & Gruneberg, R. N. (1986). A scoring method (ASEPSIS) for postoperative wound infections for use in clinical trials of antibiotic prophylaxis. *The Lancet*, **i**, 311–313.
9. Shaw, C. D. (1990). Criterion based audit. *British Medical Journal*, **300**, 649–650.
10. Bennett, J. & Walshe, K. (1990). Occurrence screening as a method of audit. *British Medical Journal*, **300**, 1248–1251.

28

A practical guide to audit

SIMON P. FROSTICK

This chapter will provide various lists that may aid the development of audit in clinical departments. It is not designed to be comprehensive or dogmatic but contains items for consideration. Figure 28.1 is an algorithm that might be employed when introducing audit. Table 28.1 compares audit methods.

Hardware – computers

Hospital based mini computers with peripheral terminals
Advantages

1. Centrally based systems organised and run by the hospital information technology department.
2. Maintenance costs will be covered.
3. Direct links with PAS and other networked programs.
4. Cost to directorate may be low as system might be installed as part of resource management initiative.
5. Training of staff may be undertaken using central resources.

Disadvantages

1. Individual departments will not have control over data.
2. Individual departments may not have control over type and form of data acquired and stored.
3. Processing of data may be limited.
4. May not fulfil the complete computing requirements of a department.

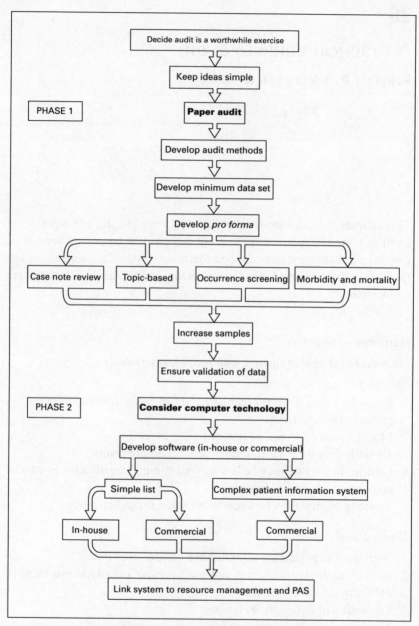

Fig. 28.1. An algorithm for introducing audit into clinical departments.

Table 28.1 *Audit methods*

Method	Advantages	Disadvantages
Case record review	1. Simple 2. Educational 3. Easily see changes 4. Should result in a marked improvement of case record keeping	1. Can be boring 2. Potentially threatening to individuals 3. ?Medicolegal consequences if major defects are found
Topic-based audit	1. Variety 2. Educational 3. Plenty of scope for completing audit loop 4. ?Small publications for juniors	1. Needs to be prospective to be most effective 2. Difficulty getting missing data from case records
Occurrence screening	1. Short bursts of prospectively acquired data 2. Shows up adverse events 3. Useful for assessing nursing/theatre/hotel process as well as other events 4. ?Helpful for contract purposes	1. Very threatening 2. May identify rogue data which can be regarded as typical by the unwary
Morbidity and mortality	1. Traditional 2. Educational 3. Can identify particular problems	1. Threatening 2. Simple counting is not sufficient 3. Care must be taken with rogue data 4. ?Medicolegal if patients identified

Networked personal computers
Advantages

1. Department will exert control over the extent and type of system that is installed.
2. Department can control the software, including the items for data entry, processing, etc.
3. Department can control access to data.
4. All computing needs of the department can be fulfilled.

Disadvantages

1. The system will be expensive to set-up and maintain.
2. Expert advice is needed to ensure that the hardware is suitable and will fulfil long-term aims of the department.
3. There may not be a link to PAS, etc.
4. An in-house systems manager will need to spend a considerable amount of time ensuring that the system is functioning properly.
5. The hospital information technology department may be very reticent to provide any help or advice.
6. Maintenance contracts will have to be funded from directorate sources.

Software

In-house database
Advantages

1. Simple.
2. Cheap.
3. Department has complete control.
4. Obligatory entry fields can be included.
5. Very good as a simple list to fulfil basic audit functions.

Disadvantages

1. Probably not possible to achieve objectives without a lot of time and several revisions.
2. Requires an enthusiastic and good-quality programmer familiar with relational databases.
3. May not be secretary friendly.
4. May not generate reports such as discharge summaries.
5. Usually will not be possible to link to other programs.

NB:

1. Define what is required from the data, then,
2. Define data entry fields.

Commercially produced software
Advantages

1. Amount of data being stored will be far greater than for an in-house system.
2. Program will probably come integrated with one or more of the recognised coding systems.
3. Links with PAS, etc. may be available allowing the downloading of demographic data and uploading of data for contracts, etc.
4. May be secretary friendly allowing secretaries to automatically produce reports, discharge summaries and letters. Managers can have access to regular reports generated automatically by the software.
5. May be possible to develop links to wordprocessors, spreadsheets, statistics, graphics, etc.
6. A patient information system would take over all functions of traditional case records.
7. Obligatory fields of data entry, including the Department of Health minimum data set.
8. Data that are common to clinicians and managers will be readily available.

Disadvantages

1. The software will be expensive.
2. Updates and revisions may only be available at times defined by the software house. These will also incur a cost. Most software houses include a maintenance cost in the contract based upon a percentage of the original cost. Resources will have to be available to cover these recurrent costs.
3. It may not be easy to perform *ad hoc* audit interrogations of the software without a knowledge of some form of programming.
4. Software houses may not be financially stable businesses and may cease trading before software is complete.
5. There may be a tendency to make the program too complicated and so fail to achieve the aim of recoding data accurately.

NB:

1. All audit data will be subject to the Access to Patients Records Act
   (1991) and to the Data Protection Act (1984). Therefore, if patients can
   be identified they have the right to gain access to both paper based and
   computer based audit data.
2. Computer data must be validated.

It is the author's view that the best system to install is one based on a
local area network, PC based but linked to the hospital mainframe for
appropriate electronic transfer of data. Further, it is the author's opinion
that hospital based audit programs do not fulfil the needs of an individual
department, they will be very inflexible and it will not be possible to obtain
regular updates to improve the situation. It is the author's opinion and
experience that a relationship can be developed with a software house to
write a comprehensive patient management system that is specialty based.
This requires (i) a co-operative and farsighted software house and (ii) a
clinician who is interested in spending the time directly involved in the
development.

Minimum data set

1. Develop a data set appropriate to the specialty. This should be
   developed by the national specialty bodies so that all departments are
   attempting to acquire and store similar data items. If possible obtain
   basic demographic data from the central hospital computers.
2. Develop a minimum data set that will be completed on all patients. It
   may not be possible to find missing items at a later stage. Therefore, do
   not make it excessively complex.
3. Validate the data entry. This can be performed at the end of the weekly
   consultant ward round.

Complications

1. Record all complications as they occur.
2. Record data about the general health status of the patients (including
   all co-morbidity).
3. Record data about the physiological status of the patients.
4. Record data about the severity of the complications themselves.
5. Record patient risk factors.
6. Record method of diagnosis of the complication.
7. Develop a simple pro forma upon which to record the complications.

Outcome measures and quality measures

A nationally based system of outcome measures is required for each specialty and often between specialties. Hard outcome measures are rare. Some quality measures such as waiting times for out-patients, being introduced as a result of the '*Patients*' *Charter*' may not be achievable. Discussion between clinicians and managers must be undertaken to determine an acceptable list of quality measures which may be included in contracts.

Final word

Audit is a waste of time, money and effort if the audit loop is not closed and a change in structure/process does not occur.

Index